HANDBOOK OF PRESCHOOL MENTAL HEALTH

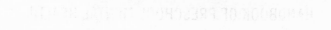

HANDBOOK OF PRESCHOOL MENTAL HEALTH
Development, Disorders, and Treatment

Edited by
JOAN L. LUBY

THE GUILFORD PRESS
New York   London

© 2006 The Guilford Press
A Division of Guilford Publications, Inc.
72 Spring Street, New York, NY 10012
www.guilford.com

Paperback edition 2009

Printed in the United States of America

This book is printed on acid-free paper.

Last digit is print number: 9 8 7 6 5 4 3

Library of Congress Cataloging-in-Publication Data

Handbook of preschool mental health : development, disorders, and treatment /
  edited by Joan L. Luby.
     p. ; cm.
Includes bibliographical references and index.
ISBN 978-1-59385-313-6 (hardcover : alk. paper)
ISBN 978-1-60623-350-4 (paperback : alk. paper)
1. Child psychiatry—Handbooks, manuals, etc. 2. Preschool children—
Mental health—Handbooks, manuals, etc.
 [DNLM: 1. Mental Disorders—physiopathology. 2. Child Development.
3. Child Psychology. 4. Child, Preschool. 5. Mental Disorders—therapy.
WS 350 H23597 2006] I. Luby, Joan L.
  RJ499.H36 2006
  618.92′89—dc22

                                                                      2006000352

"For Warmth" reprinted from *Call Me by My True Name* (1999) by Thich Nhat Hanh
with permission of Parallax Press, Berkeley, California, www.parallax.org.

To my parents, Elliot and Ideane Luby,
who, with tremendous love and generosity,
helped me to realize my intellectual dreams

About the Editor

Joan L. Luby, MD, is an infant/preschool psychiatrist and Associate Professor of Child Psychiatry at the Washington University School of Medicine in St. Louis, where she is the founder and director of the Early Emotional Development Program. This clinical and research program focusing on mood disorders in preschool children was the first of its kind nationally. Dr. Luby has been awarded grants from the National Institute of Mental Heath and the National Alliance for Schizophrenia and Depression, which have supported her research on the phenomenology of early-onset mood disorders. She currently chairs the Infancy Committee of the American Academy of Child and Adolescent Psychiatry and serves on several scientific advisory groups focused on the development of age-appropriate diagnostic criteria for preschool disorders.

Contributors

Thomas F. Anders, MD, Department of Psychiatry and Behavioral Sciences, University of California, Davis, M.I.N.D. Institute, Sacramento, California

Adrian Angold, MRCPsych, Center for Developmental Epidemiology, Department of Psychiatry and Behavioral Sciences, Duke University Medical Center, Durham, North Carolina

Andy C. Belden, PhD, Department of Child Psychiatry, Washington University School of Medicine, St. Louis, Missouri

Anne Leland Benham, PhD, Department of Psychiatry and Behavioral Sciences, Stanford University School of Medicine, Palo Alto, California

Somer L. Bishop, MA, Department of Psychology, University of Michigan, Ann Arbor, Michigan

Melissa M. Burnham, PhD, Department of Human Development and Family Studies, University of Nevada, Reno, Reno, Nevada

Irene Chatoor, MD, Department of Psychiatry and Pediatrics, George Washington University, and Children's National Medical Center, Washington, DC

Brent R. Collett, PhD, Department of Psychiatry and Behavioral Sciences, University of Washington School of Medicine, and Children's Hospital and Regional Medical Center, Seattle, Washington

Geraldine Dawson, PhD, Department of Psychology and University of Washington Autism Center, University of Washington, Seattle, Washington

Susanne A. Denham, PhD, Department of Psychology, George Mason University, Fairfax, Virginia

Helen Link Egger, MD, Center for Developmental Epidemiology and Department of Psychiatry and Behavioral Sciences, Duke University Medical Center, Durham, North Carolina

Susan Faja, MS, Center on Human Development and Disabilities, University of Washington, Seattle, Washington

Erika E. Gaylor, PhD, Center for Education and Human Services, Policy Division, SRI International, Menlo Park, California

Rebecca Goodvin, MA, Department of Psychology, University of Nebraska, Lincoln, Nebraska

Amy K. Heffelfinger, PhD, Departments of Neurology and Neurosurgery, Medical College of Wisconsin, Milwaukee, Wisconsin

Audrey Kapilinsky, LCSW, Child Development Center, University of California, Irvine, Irvine, California

Deepa Khushlani, MD, Department of Psychiatry and Behavioral Medicine, Children's National Medical Center, Washington, DC

Ron Kotkin, PhD, Department of Pediatrics and Child Development Center, University of California, Irvine, Irvine, California

Marc Lerner, MD, Department of Pediatrics, University of California, Irvine, Irvine, California

Alicia F. Lieberman, PhD, Department of Psychiatry, University of California, San Francisco, San Francisco, California

Catherine Lord, PhD, Department of Psychology and Psychiatry, University of Michigan Autism and Communication Disorders Center, Ann Arbor, Michigan

Joan L. Luby, MD, Department of Psychiatry, Washington University School of Medicine, St. Louis, Missouri

Jon M. McClellan, MD, Department of Psychiatry and Behavioral Sciences, University of Washington School of Medicine, and Children's Hospital and Regional Medical Center, Seattle, Washington

Sara Meyer, MA, Department of Psychology, University of California, Davis, Davis, California

Christine Mrakotsky, PhD, Department of Psychiatry, Harvard Medical School, and Children's Hospital Boston, Boston, Massachusetts

Carol M. Rockhill, MD, PhD, Department of Psychiatry and Behavioral Sciences, University of Washington School of Medicine, Seattle, Washington

Michael S. Scheeringa, MD, MPH, Institute of Infant and Early Childhood Mental Health and Department of Psychiatry and Neurology, Tulane University School of Medicine, New Orleans, Louisiana

Carol Fisher Slotnick, MSW, PhD, Department of Psychiatry and Behavioral Sciences, Stanford University School of Medicine, Palo Alto, California

Matthew L. Speltz, PhD, Department of Psychiatry and Behavioral Sciences, University of Washington School of Medicine, and Children's Hospital and Regional Medical Center, Seattle, Washington

Brian S. Stafford, MD, MPH, Department of Pediatrics and Child Psychology, Denver Children's Hospital, and The Kempe Center, Denver, Colorado

Robin Steinberg-Epstein, MD, Department of Pediatrics, University of California, Irvine, Irvine, California

Kenneth W. Steinhoff, MD, UCI Child Development Center, University of California, Irvine, Irvine, California

James M. Swanson, PhD, UCI Child Development Center, University of California, Irvine, Irvine, California

Ross A. Thompson, PhD, Department of Psychology, University of California, Davis, Davis, California

Patricia Van Horn, PhD, Department of Psychiatry, University of California, San Francisco, San Francisco, California

Sharon Wigal, PhD, Department of Pediatrics, University of California, Irvine, Irvine, California

Tim Wigal, PhD, Department of Pediatrics, University of California, Irvine, Irvine, California

Charles H. Zeanah, MD, Department of Psychiatry and Pediatrics, Tulane University, New Orleans, Louisiana

Preface

For *Warmth*
I hold my face between my hands
   no I am not crying
I hold my face between my hands
   to keep my loneliness warm
      two hands protecting
      two hands nourishing
      two hands to prevent
my soul from leaving me
   in anger.
            —THICH NHAT HANH

In so few words, this poem beautifully captures what is so vital about early emotional development and its importance in the human condition. It is the willingness and ability to embrace fully and experience the broad spectrum of emotional states, including those that are painful and distressing, that may be key to mental health and adaptive personal development. As psychoanalytic theory has suggested for decades, by achieving this emotional developmental capacity, one gains the ability to have a clear view of oneself and others, and to engage fully and honestly in the human experience and all of its vicissitudes. Guiding young children's development in this area early in life could be as empowering as learning to walk or talk. However, because of its intangible quality and our own limited mastery of this as adults, this goal has eluded us thus far.

This volume aims to discuss early-onset mental disorders in preschool-age children from a fundamentally developmental perspective. To achieve this goal, the first section of the book is devoted to a review of the available empirical developmental literature pertaining to those areas that have a direct relevance to mental disorders. This includes a review of new data on the development of self-concept (Chapter 1), emotions and socialization (Chapter 2), and cognition (Chapter 3). There are surprising gaps in the developmental literature on many basic elements of the development of emotions, although key elements of the available literature in this area are reviewed in Chapter 10 on mood disorders as they pertain to our understanding of normative and aberrant affect early in life.

Although child mental health providers would agree in principle that a fundamental knowledge of normative development is essential to practice, this is often given short shrift in training and in clinical application. When developmental principles are applied, they tend to be anecdotal, informal, and therefore inexact. As we attempt to identify mental disorders in younger and younger populations, a more detailed knowledge of these elements becomes essential as we aim to differentiate clinically significant problems from the normative and transient emotional and behavioral extremes and difficulties of early development.

Over the last decade, significant progress has been made in the understanding of mental disorders in preschoolers, who range in age from 3 to 6 years, while much has been known about children older than 6 for some time. Part II provides a comprehensive review of the available empirical findings for each diagnostic category in which a substantial body of data was found. Chapters 6 and 9 on eating and sleeping disorders, respectively, give an up-to-date and clinically pragmatic account of how these problems that cross the clinical threshold present in the preschool period. Chapters 7 and 10 on anxiety and mood disorders, respectively, as well as Chapter 8 on posttraumatic stress disorder (PTSD), review the empirical database. Work on mood disorders and PTSD has achieved considerable momentum in the area of validation and clarification of age-adjusted symptoms.

There is a substantial body of work on the identification of autism spectrum disorders in the preschool period, which is the latest developmental period that one should aim to capture these disorders. New empirical findings have emerged on preschool attention-deficit/hyperactivity disorder from a multisite treatment study (see Chapter 4). These findings are useful to inform both diagnosis and treatment. These chapters are designed to be of use to clinicians of all disciplines as a source of information on how to diagnose properly and begin to formulate treatment strategies for very-early-onset disorders.

Although the area of specific treatments for preschool disorders remains a largely empirically unexplored area, the chapters contained in Part III review the state of our knowledge of treatment modalities specifically designed for preschoolers. Areas covered range from dyadic play therapies (Chapters 15 and 16) to psychopharmacology (Chapter 14). Chapters focus on the theoretical (e.g., play therapy) to highly empirical (e.g., treatment of autism spectrum disorders; Chapter 17), varying with the available data base specific to each diagnostic area.

Chapter 14 on psychopharmacology broadly reviews the scant available empirical studies as they apply to the range of conditions identified and treated in young children. Given the substantial gaps in the literature, the chapter outlines recommendations for future research. Basic guidelines and principles for the prescribing physician are also offered to help inform clinical decision making in this area in which there is substantial social pressure on the physician to prescribe in the absence of empirical data to guide these treatment decisions. Part III also includes Chapter 13 on neuropsychological assessment of preschool-age children. This is a developing area, with new, age-specific assessment methods that may serve as a useful adjunct to a diagnostic assessment.

Whereas the chapters presented in this volume are of obvious use to clinicians and researchers who focus on young children, the principles outlined may also be useful and applicable for practitioners who assess and treat mental disorders across the lifespan. In particular, the developmental perspective can be used to formulate more informed hypotheses about etiologies and may also be surprisingly useful to assess adaptive functioning in individuals across the age range. In this way, they may also be applicable to prevention and personal growth models.

The Buddhist spiritual leader and author Thich Nhat Hanh, and others like him, serve as a model for individuals seeking greater emotional sentience, as well as for those seeking relief from emotional suffering. I am grateful and humbled by my own experiences of suffering, which I continue to try "to keep warm." As his gracefully crafted words convey, the practice of fully experiencing and simultaneously regulating a broad array of appropriate emotions is important, because it enhances one's ability to experience joy in all its intensity, as joy emerges from anguish (as one example), and in this way to participate fully in and enjoy human relationships. These principles have also helped me to have a clearer view of emotions, their range and repertoire, and to apply this view to my own area of interest, early-onset mood disorders. I believe it is important to keep our loneliness "warm"—as Thich Nhat Hanh suggests, to stay in touch with but not become overwhelmed by loneliness and emotions like it—for balance and understanding to help us identify, tolerate, experience, and modulate these emotions in our children and ourselves.

I hope that this book will be useful to clinicians, developmentalists, and researchers interested in young children. The field of preschool mental health has made substantial progress as advances in our understanding of early development have emerged. The greater awareness of the emotional and cognitive capacities of the young child has opened the door for clinicians and researchers to design age-appropriate approaches to tap internal emotional states in preverbal children. Subsequent findings reviewed in this volume, demonstrating an even earlier onset of many mental disorders than previously recognized, hold promise for investigations of early and potentially more effective intervention. Whereas such advances are welcome news for preschool children, and alone would likely gratify those of us committed to that population, they may also hold promise for impacting the trajectory of mental disorders across the lifespan. It is tremendously exciting and gratifying that the field of preschool mental health has made sufficient progress to fill an edited volume of this size.

Contents

Part I

Normative Development in the Preschool Period

1

Social Development

Psychological Understanding, Self-Understanding, and Relationships

ROSS A. THOMPSON, REBECCA GOODVIN, and SARA MEYER

All preschoolers are developing individuals. Whether or not they are challenged by autism, anxiety, mood disorders, or other problems of mental health, they are acquiring new forms of self-awareness and social understanding, are striving to understand and manage their emotions, and their psychological development is profoundly influenced by their close relationships with caregivers. The view that typical and atypical children alike face comparable developmental challenges and opportunities is central to the developmental psychopathology perspective that is incorporated into this volume, and has guided theory and research concerning early childhood mental health for the past quarter-century (see Cicchetti & Cohen, 2005). Such a view integrates the special concerns of early mental health problems with the broader challenges of typical development during the preschool years. This integrated view is especially important in light of the pioneering new advances in the conceptualization, prevention, and treatment of early mental health problems in infants and young children. Understanding the developmental processes and influences that shape early social, emotional, and personality development contributes to improved knowledge of the sources of vulnerability and support that can inform the study of preschool mental health.

This chapter, and Chapter 2 by Denham, provides a survey of normative processes of emotional, social, and personality development (see Thompson, 2006, for a more extended discussion of these topics). Here we focus on three facets of early psychological growth that are especially prominent in the preschool years. First, young children dramatically advance in their comprehen-

3

sion of other people and the intentions, desires, emotions, and beliefs that cause people to act as they do, and we summarize these accomplishments in psychological understanding. These achievements are important to mental health because individual differences in social and emotional understanding are associated with social competence, and lack of social competence is a key feature of some psychological disorders. Second, early childhood is a time of equally dramatic advances in self-understanding as young children begin to represent themselves and their characteristics in psychologically relevant ways, and we describe these accomplishments in the next section. Finally, because young children's experiences in close relationships are central to these and other facets of psychological growth, we consider the nature of these relationships and their developmental importance in the third section. Throughout this chapter we consider the mental health implications of these developmental processes and the influences on them.

DEVELOPMENT OF PSYCHOLOGICAL UNDERSTANDING

The traditional view is that young children are egocentric, limited in their comprehension of others' feelings, desires, and thoughts by their cognitive preoccupation with their own viewpoint. Contemporary developmental scientists are, by contrast, amazed by how early and successfully the young child begins to grasp the mental states of other people, even when those emotions, beliefs, and desires are different from the child's own. Young children may sometimes seem egocentric because of their limited social knowledge, such as when they are judging what would be a desirable snack or gift for an adult. But closer examination (using more incisive research methods) has shown that even infants begin to comprehend that subjective mental states are the key to understanding people's behavior, and during the preschool years children acquire a surprisingly sophisticated understanding of the nature of those mental states. The hallmark of psychological understanding during the preschool years is children's developing "theory of mind," which consists of (1) the realization that mental states underlie actions, (2) the diverse sources of those mental states, (3) the realization that mental states are associated with other mental states, and (4) that mental representations of the world may not always be consistent with the reality they represent. These conceptual accomplishments are important, because the capacity to understand the feelings, desires, and thoughts that govern behavior contributes to other essential skills, such as social competence, emotion sensitivity, and a dawning psychological understanding of self.

Infancy: Social Catalysts to Dawning Psychological Understanding

The earliest origins of developing theory of mind begin in infancy, as babies first become intrigued by the social partners surrounding them and seek to discern predictable regularities in their behavior. During episodes of face-to-face play in the early months after birth, for example, infants and their caregivers engage each other in close proximity while interacting with facial expressions, vocalizations, touching, behavioral gestures, and in other ways (Malatesta, Culver, Tesman, & Shepard, 1989; Tronick, 1989). These brief but ubiquitous episodes of focused social interaction have no agenda other than mutual entertainment, but they also provide an early forum for the development of social skills and the growth of the baby's social expectations for the adult. From these exchanges, infants gradually learn that people respond to their initiatives in ways that create excitement; that social interaction is dynamic and changing; and that facial, vocal, and behavioral expressions of emotion go together. Furthermore, because episodes of face-to-face play shift frequently between periods of well-synchronized behavioral coordination and periods of dyssynchrony, infants also learn how their actions and feelings can influence the continuing course of social interaction with a partner (Thompson, 2006).

The importance of this learning can be seen in studies of the "still face" effect in young infants, in which mothers alternate episodes of face-to-face interaction with an episode in which they look at the baby but are impassive and unresponsive. During these intervening perturbation episodes, infants reliably respond with diminished positive affect, withdrawal, self-directed behavior, and sometimes with social elicitations (e.g., brief smiles, momentarily increased vocalizing and reaching) alternating with negative affect. These responses seem to reflect their expectation that the adult should continue to interact animatedly with them. When mothers subsequently respond normally, infants become more sociable but also remain subdued (see Adamson & Frick, 2003, for a review of this literature). Studies have revealed that depressed mothers are less responsive and emotionally more subdued and negative in face-to-face play than are nondepressed mothers, and the offspring of depressed mothers are themselves less responsive and emotionally animated than are typical infants as early as 2–3 months of age (e.g., Cohn, Campbell, Matias, & Hopkins, 1990; Field et al., 1988). Moreover, if maternal depression persists, by the end of the first year, infants exhibit atypical patterns of frontal brain activity related to emotion that are also evident in interaction with other, nondepressed partners (Dawson et al., 1999). Differences in early social responsiveness therefore seem to be important for the development of social expectations and social skills, which may be particularly important for mental health if these capacities develop atypically owing to difficult early relational experiences.

Later in the first year, infants become capable of moving about on their own, and this locomotor accomplishment is accompanied by greater goal directedness and intentionality as babies become capable of approaching objects and people that interest them. This achievement is also accompanied by greater parental monitoring and intervention and, perhaps inevitably, conflicts of will between the infant and protective parents when the infant approaches dangerous or forbidden objects. These conflicts may be conceptually important, however, because they expose infants to social encounters that underscore how others' intentions differ from those of the self (Campos et al., 1999). Perhaps because of experiences like these, elegant experimental studies by Woodward and others have shown that by 9–12 months infants begin to perceive other people as intentional, goal-oriented actors (see Woodward, Sommerville, & Guajardo, 2001). It appears, in other words, that when watching other people reaching, pointing, or acting in an object-oriented way, infants begin to perceive those actions as goal-directed. They are assisted in this realization by sensitive caregivers who are themselves attuned to the intentional orientation of behavior, and who often punctuate their verbal responses to their own goal-oriented activity, or to the infant's goal-directed efforts, with affirmative utterances whenever the goal has been accomplished.

By the end of the first year, therefore, infants have begun to perceive other people as subjective, intentional agents whose goals may or may not be the same as the infant's own. They show this awareness in many ways, such as in the creation of joint attentional states with adults, and in social referencing behavior. Infants create joint attention with adults when they look in the direction of the adult's gaze or look from an object to the adult's face and back to the object again. Such initiatives reflect a rudimentary awareness of the association between attentional direction and subjective focus, and sometimes also seem intended to alter the adult's subjective orientation to elicit a desired response (e.g., getting access to the object, such as a toy, by redirecting the adult's attention to it; see Tomasello & Rakoczy, 2003). "Social referencing" occurs when a person uses another's emotional cues to interpret an uncertain event, and can be observed when 1-year-olds scan the mother's face in an unfamiliar situation (Baldwin & Moses, 1996). Such events show that by the end of the first year, infants are good consumers of emotional cues, and they are acquiring an understanding that others' emotions can be evoked by specific objects or events that the infant also sees, and infants can use this understanding to guide their own interpretation of that event. Taken together, research on joint attention and social referencing portrays the 1-year-old as having a surprisingly nonegocentric regard for people as intentional agents with subjective viewpoints that can, at times, be monitored and altered.

Understanding People's Desires and Emotions

Toddlers expand their developing theory of mind as they comprehend how people's actions are guided by their desires and emotions. These psychological states are actually quite challenging for young children to comprehend, because they are invisible, multidetermined motivators of behavior. But as early as 18 months, children already exhibit a rudimentary comprehension of the importance of differences in desire. In one study, Repacholi and Gopnik (1997) presented 14- and 18-month-olds with two snacks: goldfish crackers (the children's favorite) and broccoli (which the children disliked). Then the adult tasted each snack, smiling and exhibiting pleasure ("Mmmm!") with one, and frowning and saying "Ewwww!" with the other. In the "match" condition, the adult's preferences were the same as the child's; in the "mismatch" condition, the adult preferred the broccoli and disliked the crackers. Then the adult extended her hand and said, "I want some more; can you give me more?" The 18-month-olds reliably gave the adult the food she desired in both the match and mismatch conditions. By contrast, the 14-month-olds overwhelmingly gave the adult more goldfish crackers in each condition. The sensitivity to differences in desire among 18-month-olds (especially when the adult's desire contrasted with the child's own preferences) is consistent with evidence that spontaneous verbal references to desire emerge by 18 months, and that somewhat later children begin to offer constrastive statements about desire, such as comparing what one person wants with what another desires (Bartsch & Wellman, 1995).

By age 2, toddlers also begin spontaneously to talk about emotions, the causes of emotions, and even emotional regulatory efforts (e.g., Bartsch & Wellman, 1995; Wellman, Harris, Banerjee, & Sinclair, 1995). Careful analyses of the content of these utterances show that children of this age regard emotions as subjective, psychological conditions that can vary between people, with young children often contrasting another's emotions with their own. Later in the third year, toddlers comprehend the connections between desires and emotions (e.g., people are happy when they get what they want, and unhappy when they do not) (Wellman & Woolley, 1990). By age 3, children have begun to understand how emotions are associated with beliefs and expectations about events, such as the surprise a visitor feels after seeing giraffes on a farm (Wellman & Banerjee, 1991). Young children's comprehension of the connection between emotion and thought is also revealed in their appreciation of how feelings can be evoked by mental reminders of past emotionally evocative experiences. By age 5, for example, children understand that someone can feel sad when seeing a cat that reminds her of a pet who ran away (Lagattuta & Wellman, 2001). These insights not only help young children comprehend the origins and consequences of others' feelings but also contribute to children's understanding of their own emotions and how to manage them (Thompson, 1994).

Comprehending Beliefs—and False Beliefs

Consider the following situation: An experimenter shows a child a candy box and asks the child what she thinks is inside. The child replies, naturally, "Candy!" The box is opened, and the child discovers that inside are stones, not candy. The box is closed again, and the experimenter now asks what another child, who has not looked inside the box, will think is inside. A child age 5 or older would probably reply that a naive child would think that the box contains candy. However, a much younger child is surprisingly likely to claim that the naive child would expect to find stones and, in fact, this child will deny that she *ever* expected to find anything else in the box! The difference can be understood in terms of developing theory of mind. Younger children do not understand how mental representations can be inconsistent with reality; for them, your beliefs about the world *must* be consistent with how things are. By contrast, 4- and 5-year-olds comprehend that reality can be represented in multiple ways and that people act on these mental representations, even though they may be incorrect (Wellman, 2002). Young children's dawning understanding of false belief is significant not only because it reveals an awareness of the independence of mental events from objective reality, but also because it is a gateway to the comprehension of other psychological realities, such as the privacy of personal mental experience, the creation of mistaken beliefs in others, and the mind's interpretive activity independent of experience. In short, young children begin to understand that how you feel or think need not be revealed, that others can be fooled, and that the mind operates independently of experience.

Understanding false belief, and other early achievements in developing theory of mind, emerges because young children are careful observers of other people and think insightfully about what they observe. As they watch people in goal-directed activity and see them express pleasure in their accomplishments and other emotions in different situations, and begin to overhear language incorporating mental state references (e.g., "I *thought* you were leaving . . . "), young children gradually construct an understanding of the mind. In addition, other social experiences are important catalysts for developing psychological understanding. In particular, young children's exposure to, and participation in, simple conversations with adults, siblings, and peers are a rich source of insight into mental events. In these conversations, children can learn about mental events through language that helps to make feelings and thoughts more explicit, they can compare their beliefs and expectations with those of others, and they can benefit from the insight provided by another into the psychological origins of the behavior of others whom they observe (Thompson, Laible, & Ontai, 2003). Thus, when parents discuss mental states (including emotions) more frequently and with greater elaborative detail, especially the causes of mental states in the child and others, preschoolers acquire a better understanding of people's thoughts, feelings, and intentions (Astington & Baird, 2005; Thompson et al., 2003). Indeed, some of the conceptual catalysts in social interaction to the development of theory of mind may arise surprisingly early, such as in the sensitivity of mothers to the psychological experiences of their infants (Meins et al., 2002).

More broadly, everyday conversations may also be important to children's acquisition of values, self-referent beliefs, causal assumptions, moral attributions, and other complex psychological inferences. Studies have shown, for example, that mothers' conversations about feelings contribute to early conscience development, and that disciplinary procedures requiring the child to reflect on the victim's feelings contribute to preschoolers' psychological understanding (Ruffman, Perner, & Parkin, 1999; Thompson et al., 2003). This may help to explain why individual differences in children's theory of mind understanding, particularly their comprehension of false belief and emotion understanding, are associated with children's social competence in friendship with peers (Denham et al., 2003; Dunn, Cutting, & Demetriou, 2000).

These remarkable advances in psychological understanding in early childhood set the stage for greater insight into people and the self. By ages 5 and 6, for example, young children begin to perceive others in terms of psychological motives and traits, and create expectations for others based on the traits they infer in them (Heyman & Gelman, 2000). They are also beginning to consider fairness in their peer relationships, particularly in relation to gender exclusion, although they have much to learn about social groups (Killen, Pisacane, Lee-Kim, & Ardile-Rey, 2001). Preschoolers are, in short, becoming more insightful in their psychological understanding of others, and these insights also extend to themselves.

There are important implications of these discoveries about developing psychological understanding for preschool mental health. Infants and young children clearly respond not only to people's behavior but also to the emotions, intentions, desires, and beliefs that they infer in others' actions and from what they learn about the psychological world from conversations with family members. Understanding the intergenerational influences that contribute to risk for internalizing and externalizing disorders in troubled families (e.g., inherited vulnerability, emotional climate of the home, coercive family interactions) must include the early sensitivity of young children to the intentions and emotions underlying their interactions with family members, and how attributional biases, moral judgments, and motivational evaluations are conveyed intergenerationally through parent–child conversation. Moreover, early peer relationships are also affected by developing psychological understanding; thus, the emotional vulnerability derived from interaction in a troubled family is likely to be manifested in young children's greater difficulty in peer sociability. Finally, although it is apparent that preschoolers are not sophisticated at misleading others concerning their thoughts and feelings, a rudimentary comprehension of the privacy of personal psychological experience is established in early achievements in theory of mind. This provides a foundation for psychological dissembling in the years that follow, together with a dawning awareness of how the mind itself constructs its own reality that can become enlisted for therapeutic purposes.

DEVELOPMENT OF SELF-UNDERSTANDING

Developing self-understanding in early childhood is important to mental health, because the self organizes experience and guides behavior. How young children represent themselves establishes continuity between an awareness of how one has been in the past and expectations for how one will be in the future. Developing autobiographical memory during the preschool years embeds self-understanding in representations of past events (Nelson & Fivush, 2004), and as children develop an awareness of their personal characteristics, it provides a guide to future action (Froming, Nasby, & McManus, 1998). For example, a young child's belief that she is shy may, when activated, discourage the child from interacting with a new child at school. Moreover, self-related beliefs can cause children to structure their experiences and environments in particular ways that influences the range of partners, challenges, and opportunities that children are likely to permit for themselves. Strong, coherent, and positive self-representations may offer a psychological buffer even in negative circumstances, whereas negative self-representations may be a risk factor for early clinical problems (Cicchetti & Rogosch, 1997; Harter, 1999). Both the development of a coherent, autonomous self and the specific characteristics of the developing self-concept have significant consequences for psychological development and risk of mental disorders.

Developmentally Emergent Features of the Self

Although the growth of an autonomous sense of self has traditionally been viewed as an accomplishment of childhood, many of the foundations of self-understanding emerge in infancy (Thompson, 2006). Early in the first year, for example, infants develop a prerepresentational form of self-awareness that derives from the perceptual experiences arising from their sensorimotor activity, affect, and experiences of agency in interaction with the world (Neisser, 1993). Young infants are highly attuned to the contingency between their own actions and the perceptual experiences that derive from them, and from this a nascent sense of "self" becomes constructed (Gergely & Watson, 1999). Later in the first year, the contingency of social interaction contributes to a dawning form of interpersonal or intersubjective self-awareness as infants strive to coordinate their own intentional, subjective states with those of others (e.g., in joint attention), and in their awareness that they can be the object of another's attention and affect. By age 18 months, another aspect of self-awareness emerges as toddlers become capable of featural self-recognition when identifying themselves in a mirror (Lewis & Brooks-Gunn, 1979), which heralds, to some researchers, the birth of the cognitive self-concept (Howe & Courage, 1997). These are each significant foundations to the gradual development of self-awareness and highlight that the emergence of the "self" is not a unitary process, but involves different facets of self-representation emerging at different periods in the early years.

It is not until around the second birthday that children's self-understanding begins to resemble the qualities of self that we recognize in older children. At this time, young children begin verbally self-referencing (e.g., "Me, too!"), as well as asserting their competence (e.g., by refusing assistance) and describing their experiences using internal state words, such as references to feelings and desires (Bretherton & Beeghly, 1982; Stipek, Gralinski, & Kopp, 1990). Young children are also sensitive to how others evaluate them, partly because they are beginning to conceptualize and apply standards of conduct to their own behavior; thus, others' evaluations of them are important and influential (Stipek, Recchia, & McClintic, 1992; Thompson, Meyer, & McGinley, 2006). This contributes to the earliest experiences of self-referential emotions, such as pride, shame, guilt, or embarrassment, that expand emotional experience and link the development of emotion and self (Lewis, 2000; Stipek et al., 1992).

By the third year, therefore, self-representations have become globally affective and evaluative in nature. Moreover, in contrast with the traditional view that young children perceive themselves exclusively in terms of physical appearance and behavior (e.g., brown hair, runs fast), there is growing evidence that even young children develop a coherent, psychologically oriented self-concept by 3½ to 4 years of age. This becomes apparent when researchers, rather than asking children to describe themselves using open-ended questions (which tend to elicit concrete self-descriptors), instead invite children to describe their characteristics by choosing from contrasting pairs of descriptive attributes (e.g., "I like to be with other people" vs. "I like to be by myself") (e.g., Brown, Mangelsdorf, Agathen, & Ho, 2004; Eder, 1990; Marsh, Ellis, & Craven, 2002; Measelle, Ablow, Cowan, & Cowan, 1998). Studies using such measures show that young children are capable of representing their psychological and emotional qualities in conceptually coherent ways, describing individual differences in their physical skills, academic capabilities, relationships with parents and peers, social competence, and even self-characterizations of feelings relevant to depression, anxiety, and aggression or hostility. Moreover, young children's self-descriptions show stability over time and are consistent with mothers' and teachers' reports of children's personality characteristics (Brown et al., 2004; Eder & Mangelsdorf, 1997; Measelle et al., 1998).

In summary, although further research is needed to elucidate the meaning inherent in young children's use of trait labels (which probably lack the rich meaning inherent in how older people use these concepts), and there is considerable growth yet to occur in their self-awareness, it seems apparent that children are thinking of themselves in psychologically relevant ways from late in the preschool years. This raises at least two important considerations for preschool mental health. First, it suggests that a psychological self-concept emerges surprisingly early and is thus likely to be significantly affected by the family emotional climate in early childhood, as discussed below. Second, because psychological self-awareness is slowly emerging in the early years, child clinicians must be cautious in their inferences from preschoolers' statements about themselves by remembering that young children often have different underlying conceptions in their use of trait labels than do adults (see Luby & Belden, Chapter 10, this volume, on mood disorders). A young child who proclaims that she can accomplish impossible feats or does not like to be with other people may not be reflecting the same self-attributions that would be true if these statements were from an older child or adult.

By the end of the preschool years, therefore, young children's self-understanding provides a foundation for how they will see themselves in the years to come, although there remains significant growth in the depth, complexity, and nuance of self-understanding to come. Even so, by age 5, children perceive themselves in psychologically complex ways, evaluate their characteristics and accomplishments (with contributions from others' evaluations of them), and experience a range of self-referential emotions. Moreover, children of this age can also regard themselves within a broad temporal framework—relating their past experiences to future expectations—that constitutes a conceptual foundation for autobiographical memory (Nelson & Fivush, 2004; Povinelli, 2001). These accomplishments also contribute to the significant advances in self-regulation that occur during the preschool years, with children becoming more capable of managing their behavior, attention, thinking, and emotions than was true in infancy, although important advances are yet to come (Fox & Calkins, 2003; Kopp, 1982). The preschooler has become a psychologically complex individual in his or her own eyes, as well as in the eyes of others.

One implication is that early childhood influences have important consequences for developing psychological self-understanding, and that self-concept might receive clinical attention in evaluation of young children at psychological risk for mood disorders and other difficulties. There is evidence, for example, that aversive early caregiving experiences can profoundly affect many features of developing self-representation in early childhood. Maltreated toddlers and young children exhibit more negative or neutral affect in visual self-recognition, for example, and less frequently use verbal self-reference and internal state words (particularly negative emotion words) compared with nonmaltreated children (Beeghly & Cicchetti, 1994; Schneider-Rosen & Cicchetti, 1991). Moreover, consistent with their sensitivity to others' evaluations of themselves, young children are not only prone to negative self-evaluations when caregivers likewise appraise their performance, but these negative self-assessments may also, in some circumstances, contribute to risk for later depressive disorders (Kistner, Ziegert, Castro, & Robertson, 2001). The findings of studies such as these underscore the associations between caregiving relationships, the development of self-understanding, risk for psychopathology, and manifestations of clinical disorders arising in early childhood.

Influences on Developing Self-Representations

Early relational experience is important to developing self-understanding in several ways. As earlier noted, caregivers and others who matter to the child contribute a valuational dimension to self-understanding, arising from how they regard the child and how it is expressed, from the affect with which they view the child's mirror image to how they evaluate the child's accomplishments, misbehavior, and characteristics. In light of the importance of these relationships to young children, it is unsurprising to find these external assessments of the self incorporated—or internalized—into young children's developing self-regard. In this respect, influences on self-concept arise in many daily and seemingly mundane interactive contexts, from how parents respond to a toddler's insistence on "do it myself" to the manner in which disobedience is managed, and including expressed and implied evaluations of the child's initiatives, performance, and attributes. Although research in our laboratory indicates that early self-concept is more than just the "looking glass self" described by Mead (1934), because young children independently appraise themselves as well, it is apparent that the evaluations of others are important and formative.

Another significant influence is young children's dialogues with parents or other caregivers who structure children's understanding of personal experiences, thus contributing to autobiographical self-representation (Nelson & Fivush, 2004). Like language about emotion and beliefs, language about the self from a mature partner provides young children with unique explicitness and clarity about personal psychological processes that are otherwise complex, invisible, and difficult to comprehend. Even before they can directly participate in conversations about events involving themselves, young children are often present for stories being told about them between their caregivers and others. Children attend to these conversations and are aware of when the self is a central actor, and children appropriate messages about their characteristics that are embedded in these stories (Miller, Potts, Fung, Hoogstra, & Mintz, 1990). Somewhat later, parents talk with their young offspring about shared experiences that include both explicit labels and implicit messages about children's feelings ("You were sad when your puppy ran away") and behaviors ("You're being very shy today"), and provide children with assessments of those emotions and behaviors ("You shouldn't be scared," or "You're a good listener"), sometimes in relation to standards of conduct. Children from different cultures and sociodemographic groups begin to think about themselves differently based on how their characteristics are differently regarded and valued by parents and other caregivers (Mullen & Yi, 1995; Wiley, Rose, Burger, & Miller, 1998). Furthermore, the quality of the adult's conversational discourse is important. Studies have shown that when mothers speak about children's experiences in an elaborative manner, incorporating rich detail and background information, their young children develop more coherent and detailed personal, autobiographical narratives than do the children of mothers with a less elaborative conversational style (e.g., Haden, Haine, & Fivush, 1997).

These relational influences on developing self-understanding occur within a broader relational environment. Infants and young children develop strong emotional attachments to their parents, and these have an important influence on psychological development, especially as these attachments influence emergent early representations of others, relationships, and the self. Attachment theorists suggest that a child's secure attachment to a parent should foster a more positive affective sense of self because of a history of sensitive, positive, and warm interactions. The rejecting or inconsistent responsiveness of the parent associated with an insecure attachment, however, may engender a more affectively negative global self-concept. Research on attachment security and the self in young children provides support for these formulations, with the additional finding that securely attached young children are also capable of a balanced understanding of the self as having both positive and negative qualities (Cassidy, 1988; Clark & Symons, 2000; Goodvin, Meyer, Thompson, & Hayes, 2006; Verschueren, Marcoen, & Schoefs, 1996). These findings indicate that the broader emotional quality of the parent–child relationship is also an important influence on developing self-understanding.

RELATIONSHIPS AS ENVIRONMENTS OF PSYCHOLOGICAL DEVELOPMENT

The most important environment of early development is the environment of relationships that shapes psychological growth. This is because young children's experiences with caregivers who know them well, and who provide individualized, emotion-laden interactions that are ubiquitous in the early years, are profound influences on social and emotional development. Furthermore, the emotional attachments that infants and young children develop with their caregivers heighten the influence of relational partners on developing self-awareness, psychological understanding, emotional growth, and sociability in early childhood. The importance of early relational influences is a double-edged sword with respect to risk for developmental psychopathology, however. Although positive relationships can provide a secure foundation for healthy psychological growth and a buffer against stress and difficulty, it is also true that troubled, violent, or dysfunctional early relationships constitute a significant risk for the development of psychopathology (Thompson, Flood, & Goodvin, 2006).

Relational Processes and Psychological Health

Recent studies have highlighted the early vulnerability of young children to clinically significant problems and the importance of relationships to their vulnerability. The development of conduct problems in preschoolers, for example, derives from an interaction of the child's temperamental vulnerability with maternal rejection and depression, parental conflict, and other kinds of family difficulty (Owens & Shaw, 2003; Shaw, Gilliom, Ingoldsby, & Nagin, 2003). A depressed caregiver's sadness, irritability, helplessness, and guilt-inducing behavior contributes to a young child's enmeshment in the emotional problems of the adult and his or her own vulnerability to internalizing problems (Goodman & Gotlib, 1999). Young children in homes characterized by marital conflict and domestic violence show heightened sensitivity to parental distress and anger, tend to become overinvolved in their parents' emotional conflicts, have difficulty regulating the strong emotions that conflict arouses in them (in a manner resembling "emotional flooding"), and exhibit other indications of internalizing problems (Cummings & Davies, 1994; Grych & Fincham, 1990). The difficulties of children with anxiety disorders are often exacerbated rather than alleviated by parents who themselves become anxious as a result of the child's distress and thus accede to the child's wishes to avoid fear-provoking events, even though they are also critical of the child's difficulties (Thompson, 2001; Vasey & Ollendick, 2000). More generally, parental "expressed emotion," manifested in criticism, distress, and/or emotional overinvolvement in the child's problems, has been implicated in a wide variety of clinical problems in childhood and adolescence (see review by Thompson et al., 2006).

These studies suggest that there are diverse ways that relational experience affects early psychological growth and risk for psychopathology in young children. The warmth and sensitivity of parent–child interaction is a central contributor to the development of secure parent–child relationships, and the importance of secure attachments to healthy psychological development is discussed further below. The broader emotional climate of the home, which is shaped by the marital relationship and external demands on family life, is also important in young children's developing emotional security (Cummings & Davies, 1994; Davies & Cummings, 1994). How parents and offspring mutually cope with conflict, which includes the parents' disciplinary style, the quality of communication between them, opportunities for negotiation and bargaining, and the child's construal of the parents' behavior is an important relational influence on social and emotional well-being, especially as it contributes to the young child's developing behavioral self-control and acquisition of internalized standards of conduct (Grusec & Goodnow, 1994). Shared conversations between parents and young children are also important catalysts for conceptual understanding of others and the self and, because they provide an avenue for conveying values, attributions, judgments, and assumptions, these conversations also contribute to the intergenerational transmission of psychological belief systems and culture. Parents also scaffold the development of emotional competence in young children by carefully managing daily routines and other experiences to remain within the child's capacities for emotional self-control, and also by proactively anticipating new experiences with children (e.g., a visit to the doctor) and coaching them in how to adaptively cope. Beyond these, parents are influential as models of emotional functioning, and as providers of (intended and inadvertent) rewards and incentives for the socioemotional capabilities of their offspring (see Laible & Thompson, in press, for a review).

The value of a developmental psychopathology perspective to preschool social development and mental health is that it highlights how these relational experiences offer support or vulnerability to psychological health depending on whether families are well-functioning or troubled. Furthermore, when this perspective is considered for young children, it becomes clear that when a preschooler exhibits conduct problems (see Rockhill, Collett, McClellan, & Speltz, Chapter 5, this volume), depressive symptomatology (see Luby & Belden, Chapter 10, this volume), heightened anxiety (see Egger & Angold, Chapter 7, this volume), or other problems of clinical significance, it is likely to reflect relational as well as individual pathology. As a consequence, addressing the child's problems often requires addressing the broader family emotional environment in which these difficulties arise. To be sure, parent–child (and especially mother–child) relationships are not the only important relational influences in the early years. Young children's relationships with extended family members, child care providers and preschool teachers, siblings, and peers each constitute significant influences on developing psychological understanding and provide important sources of support (as well as risk). Early parent–child relationships are uniquely important, however, because of their breadth of influence, the sophistication and ubiquity of the adult's influences, and the emotional attachment they share.

Security of Attachment

One of the central features of young children's relationships with caregivers is the security children derive from them, and attachment theory provides a valuable approach to understanding the origins and consequences of the security of attachment in early childhood (for recent reviews, see Cassidy & Shaver, 1999; Thompson, 2006). Sensitive maternal care contributes reliably to a secure attachment, with insensitivity associated with attachment insecurity in infants as young as 1 year of age. Moreover, variations in the quality of maternal insensitivity seem to be associated with differences in the types of insecurity that infants exhibit. In particular, fairly consistent maternal unresponsiveness is associated with insecure–avoidant behavior, whereas mothers who are inconsistently responsive are more likely to have insecure–resistant offspring. A third insecure classification, "insecure–disoriented or disorganized," appears to be associated with maternal behavior that is not only insensitive but also, at times, frightened, or frightening to the infant. Perhaps unsurprisingly, the latter form of insecurity is found more commonly in families characterized by sociodemographic risk, especially involving child maltreatment (Lyons-Ruth & Jacobvitz, 1999). In typically developing nonrisk samples, the majority of infants and young children are securely attached, but the proportion of insecure attachments is higher in clinical or at-risk samples of families (see Stafford & Zeanah, Chapter 11).

Are early differences in the security or insecurity of attachment modifiable? Are they predictive of later behavior? Research indicates that the security of attachment predicts later social and emotional functioning, especially when the sensitivity (or insensitivity) of maternal care remains relatively consistent over time. In other words, infants maintain their security when it is warranted by the continuing sensitivity of caregivers. However, the security of attachment can and often does change over time, usually in response to changes or stresses in the family that can alter familiar patterns of mother–child interaction (Thompson, 2006). Although this indicates that early security is no certain guarantee that a child will remain secure in the future, this conclusion is also optimistic with respect to intervention efforts. Young children who develop insecure attachments owing to insensitive parental care need not remain that way, especially if mothers can be enabled to respond more warmly and sensitively to their offspring.

If the sensitivity of maternal care remains consistent, a secure attachment foreshadows a more positive parent–child relationship as the child matures, and securely attached children also are more successful in other close relationships, such as with friends and teachers (Thompson, 1999, 2006). Securely attached children also score higher on later assessments of emotional health, self-esteem, positive affect, and other emergent personality dimensions. Developmental researchers have also been interested in how a secure or insecure attachment is associated with developing psychological understanding, consistent with the view from attachment theory that early relational experience influences young children's emergent understanding of others, relationships, and self. Securely attached preschoolers are stronger in emotion understanding, conscience development, friendship conceptions, and other features of early social understanding, although much more research on this topic is needed (Thompson, 2006).

Is the security of attachment relevant to risk for later psychopathology? Because of its desirable psychosocial correlates, a secure attachment may contribute to positive mental health and constitute a buffer for the effects of stress and difficulty on emotional well-being. By contrast, insecure attachment may be a risk factor, and the greatest concern has been focused on the disorganized–disoriented form of insecurity. Indeed, researchers have found an association between infant disorganized attachment and risk for later internalizing and externalizing disorders in childhood, although it should be remembered that the same family stresses that initially contributed to the development of disorganized attachment may also contribute to its later outcomes (see Thompson, 2006, for a review). Even so, it is apparent that early relational insecurity heightens the possibility for developmental difficulties in young children whose relational experiences within the family may be troubled or difficult. In more extreme conditions, especially in families characterized by parental psychopathology and/or child maltreatment, these relational problems can be the catalyst for disorders of attachment (see Stafford & Zeanah, Chapter 11, this volume, for further discussion of these issues).

Taken together, research on the security of attachment and on the broader network of relational influences within the family confirms the importance of relational experience to the development of psychological vulnerability or well-being for young children. Although this is not surprising, what is more impressive is the diversity of the relational influences that are important, as noted earlier, and how this reconceptualizes problems of early mental health. Contrary to the long-standing clinical tradition of perceiving psychological health or pathology as existing within the person, a developmental psychopathology perspective to early mental health requires also perceiving health or pathology *in the relationship* between the child and the caregiver(s) who are most influential. Likewise, efforts to provide treatment to a young child must often involve the child's caregiver(s), if such efforts are to succeed, because of how early relationships provide a continuing context for psychological development (see Van Horn & Lieberman, Chapter 16, this volume, on dyadic play therapy).

CONCLUSION

Why is it important for clinicians and scholars concerned with early childhood mental health to be interested in normative aspects of social development? One reason is that contemporary research is revealing young children to be interpersonally and intrapsychically more perceptive and sophisticated than was earlier believed to be true. As traditional notions of early childhood egocentrism and children's concrete, physicalistic self-descriptions are being superceded by an awareness of their psychologically oriented understanding of self and other, it is apparent that young children are more insightfully aware of the mental and emotional processes that exist within the minds of other people, and of their own psychological characteristics. This raises new questions about how children who are challenged by clinical symptomatology, or are growing up in homes characterized by family stress or parental psychopathology, are conceptualizing themselves within their intrapsychic and interpersonal world. Current research in developmental psychopathology reveals that the effects of early clinical problems on emotion understanding, self-awareness, emotion regulation, social competence, and other emerging competencies are profound and are beginning to be understood through the juxtaposition of the research findings in the developmental sciences and the work of clinical researchers.

A second reason why normative aspects of social development are important to understanding early childhood mental health is how they contextualize the child. We have emphasized the importance of the family relational context to psychological development, because research on attachment and other family processes underscores its significance to risk and vulnerability. Viewing the child in the context of close relationships is essential to conceptualize accurately the origins of childhood pathology, and relevant preventive and treatment possibilities. Although it is beyond the scope of this chapter (but it is discussed in other chapters in this volume), early childhood mental health should also be contextualized within the broader social systems of the child and the family. Children at psychological risk are also often children at sociodemographic risk, whose families are beset by poverty, dangerous neighborhoods, and other challenges with direct and indirect consequences for healthy psychological development.

As developmental scientists whose work has regularly included at-risk samples of children, we also recognize the value of a developmental psychopathology perspective for understanding early childhood development for typical children. Because the constellation of risks and supports for children facing difficulty is so much broader than what is usually observed for more typically developing children, it is possible to understand more acutely how development of emotion understanding, self-awareness, and comprehension of the psychological world is affected by relational experiences that sometimes challenge children's understanding. In the end, it is through the thoughtful interchange of ideas from developmental science and clinically relevant research that we construct an understanding of all children as developing individuals.

REFERENCES

Adamson, L., & Frick, J. (2003). The still face: A history of a shared experimental paradigm. *Infancy, 4,* 451–473.

Astington, J., & Baird, J. (Eds.). (2005). *Why language matters for theory of mind.* New York: Oxford University Press.

Baldwin, D., & Moses, L. (1996). The ontogeny of social information-processing. *Child Development, 67,* 1915–1939.

Bartsch, K., & Wellman, H. (1995). *Children talk about the mind.* London: Oxford University Press.

Beeghly, M., & Cicchetti, D. (1994). Child maltreatment, attachment, and the self system: Emergence of an internal state lexicon in toddlers at high social risk. *Development and Psychopathology, 3,* 397–411.

Bretherton, I., & Beeghly, M. (1982). Talking about internal states: The acquisition of an explicit theory of mind. *Developmental Psychology, 18,* 906–921.

Brown, G. L., Mangelsdorf, S. C., Agathen, J. M., & Ho, M. (2004). *Young children's psychological selves: Convergence with maternal reports of child personality.* Manuscript submitted for publication.

Campos, J., Anderson, D., Barbu-Roth, M., Hubbard, E., Hertenstein, M., & Witherington, D. (1999). Travel broadens the mind. *Infancy, 1,* 149–219.

Cassidy, J. (1988). Child–mother attachment and the self in six-year-olds. *Child Development, 59,* 121–134.

Cassidy, J., & Shaver, P. R. (Eds.). (1999). *Handbook of attachment: Theory, research, and clinical applications.* New York: Guilford Press.

Cicchetti, D., & Cohen, D. (Eds.). (2005). *Developmental psychopathology* (2nd ed.). New York: Wiley.

Cicchetti, D., & Rogosch, F. A. (1997). The role of self-organization in the promotion of resilience in maltreated children. *Development and Psychopathology, 9,* 797–815.

Clark, S. E., & Symons, D. K. (2000). A longitudinal study of Q-sort attachment security and self-processes at age 5. *Infant and Child Development, 9,* 91–104.

Cohn, J., Campbell, S., Matias, R., & Hopkins, J. (1990). Face-to-face interactions of postpartum depressed and nondepressed mother–infant pairs at 2 months. *Developmental Psychology, 26,* 15–23.

Cummings, E. M., & Davies, P. (1994). *Children and marital conflict: The impact of family dispute and resolution.* New York: Guilford Press.

Davies, P. T., & Cummings, E. M. (1994). Marital conflict and child adjustment: An emotional security hypothesis. *Psychological Bulletin, 116,* 387–411.

Dawson, G., Frey, K., Panagiotides, H., Yamada, E., Hessl, D., & Osterling, J. (1999). Infants of depressed mothers exhibit atypical frontal electrical brain activity during interactions with mother and with a familiar, nondepressed adult. *Child Development, 70,* 1058–1066.

Denham, S., Blair, K., DeMulder, E., Levitas, J., Sawyer, K., Auerbach-Major, S., et al. (2003). Preschool emotional competence: Pathway to social competence. *Child Development, 74,* 238–256.

Dunn, J., Cutting, A., & Demetriou, H. (2000). Moral sensibility, understanding others, and children's friendship interactions in the preschool period. *British Journal of Developmental Psychology, 18,* 159–177.

Eder, R. A. (1990). Uncovering young children's psychological selves: Individual and developmental differences. *Child Development, 61,* 849–863.

Eder, R. A., & Mangelsdorf, S. C. (1997). The emotional basis of early personality development: Implications for the emergent self-concept. In R. Hogan, J. Johnson, & S. Briggs (Eds.), *Handbook of personality psychology* (pp. 209–240). Orlando, FL: Academic Press.

Field, T., Healy, B., Goldstein, S., Perry, S., Bendell, D., Schanberg, S., et al. (1988). Infants of depressed mothers show "depressed" behavior even with nondepressed adults. *Child Development, 59,* 1569–1579.

Fox, N., & Calkins, S. (2003). The development of self-control of emotion: Intrinsic and extrinsic influences. *Motivation and Emotion, 27,* 7–26.

Froming, W. J., Nasby, W., & McManus, J. (1998). Prosocial self-schemas, self-awareness, and children's prosocial behavior. *Journal of Personality and Social Psychology, 75,* 766–777.

Gergely, G., & Watson, J. (1999). Early socio-emotional development: Contingency perception and the social-biofeedback model. In P. Rochat (Ed.), *Early social cognition* (pp. 101–136). Mahwah, NJ: Erlbaum.

Goodman, S. H., & Gotlib, I. H. (1999). Risk for psychopathology in the children of depressed mothers: A developmental model for understanding mechanisms of transmission. *Psychological Review, 106,* 458–490.

Goodvin, R., Meyer, S., Thompson, R. A., & Hayes, R. (2006). *Self-understanding in early childhood: Associations with attachment security, maternal perceptions, and the family emotional climate.* Manuscript in preparation, University of Nebraska–Lincoln.

Grusec, J., & Goodnow, J. (1994). Impact of parental discipline methods on the child's internalization of values: A reconceptualization of current points of view. *Developmental Psychology, 30,* 4–19.

Grych, J. H., & Fincham, F. D. (1990). Marital conflict and children's adjustment: A cognitive-contextual framework. *Psychological Bulletin, 107,* 267–290.

Haden, C. A., Haine, R. A., & Fivush, R. (1997). Developing narrative structure in parent-child reminiscing across the preschool years. *Developmental Psychology, 33,* 295–307.

Harter, S. (1999). *The construction of the self: A developmental perspective.* New York: Guilford Press.

Heyman, G., & Gelman, S. (2000). Preschool children's use of trait labels to make inductive inferences. *Journal of Experimental Child Psychology, 77,* 1–19.

Howe, M., & Courage, M. (1997). The emergence and early development of autobiographical memory. *Psychological Review, 104,* 499–523.

Killen, M., Pisacane, K., Lee-Kim, J., & Ardila-Rey, A. (2001). Fairness or stereotypes?: Young children's priorities when evaluating group exclusion or inclusion. *Developmental Psychology, 37,* 587–596.

Kistner, J. A., Ziegert, D. I., Castro, R., & Robertson, B. (2001). Helplessness in early childhood: Prediction of symptoms associated with depression and negative self-worth. *Merrill–Palmer Quarterly, 47*, 336–354.

Kopp, C. (1982). Antecedents of self-regulation: A developmental view. *Developmental Psychology, 18*, 199–214.

Lagattuta, K., & Wellman, H. (2001). Thinking about the past: Young children's knowledge about links between past events, thinking, and emotion. *Child Development, 72*, 82–102.

Laible, D., & Thompson, R. A. (in press). Foundations of socialization. In J. Grusec & P. Hastings (Eds.), *Handbook of socialization*. New York: Guilford Press.

Lewis, M. (2000). Self-conscious emotions: Embarrassment, pride, shame, and guilt. In M. Lewis & J. M. Haviland-Jones (Eds.), *Handbook of emotions* (2nd ed., pp. 563–573). New York: Guilford Press.

Lewis, M., & Brooks-Gunn, J. (1979). *Social cognition and the acquisition of self*. New York: Plenum Press.

Lyons-Ruth, K., & Jacobvitz, D. (1999). Attachment disorganization: Unresolved loss, relational violence, and lapses in behavioral and attentional strategies. In J. Cassidy & P. Shaver (Eds.), *Handbook of attachment* (pp. 520–554). Chicago: University of Chicago Press.

Malatesta, C., Culver, C., Tesman, J., & Shepard, B. (1989). The development of emotion expression during the first two years of life. *Monographs of the Society for Research in Child Development, 54*(1–2, Serial No. 219).

Marsh, H. W., Ellis, L. A., & Craven, R. G. (2002). How do preschool children feel about themselves?: Unraveling measurement and multidimensional self-concept structure. *Developmental Psychology, 38*, 376–393.

Mead, G. H. (1934). *Mind, self, and society*. Chicago: University of Chicago Press.

Measelle, J. R., Ablow, J. C., Cowan, P. A., & Cowan, C. P. (1998). Assessing young children's views of their academic, social, and emotional lives: An evaluation of the self-perception scales of the Berkeley Puppet Interview. *Child Development, 69*, 1556–1576.

Meins, E., Fernyhough, C., Wainwright, R., Gupta, M., Fradley, E., & Tuckey, M. (2002). Maternal mind–mindedness and attachment security as predictors of theory of mind understanding. *Child Development, 73*, 1715–1726.

Miller, P. J., Potts, R., Fung, H., Hoogstra, L., & Mintz, J. (1990). Narrative practices and the social construction of self in childhood. *American Ethnologist, 17*, 292–311.

Mullen, M. K., & Yi, S. (1995). The cultural context of talk about the past: Implications for the development of autobiographical memory. *Cognitive Development, 10*, 407–419.

Neisser, U. (1993). The self perceived. In U. Neisser (Ed.), *The perceived self: Ecological and interpersonal sources of self-knowledge* (pp. 3–21). New York: Cambridge University Press.

Nelson, K., & Fivush, R. (2004). The emergence of autobiographical memory: A social–cultural developmental theory. *Psychological Review, 111*, 486–511.

Owens, E. B., & Shaw, D. S. (2003). Predicting growth curves of externalizing behavior across the preschool years. *Journal of Abnormal Child Psychology, 31*, 575–590.

Povinelli, D. (2001). The self: Elevated in consciousness and extended in time. In C. Moore & K. Lemmon (Eds.), *The self in time* (pp. 75–95). Mahwah, NJ: Erlbaum.

Repacholi, B., & Gopnik, A. (1997). Early reasoning about desires: Evidence from 14- and 18-month-olds. *Developmental Psychology, 33*, 12–21.

Ruffman, T., Perner, J., & Parkin, L. (1999). How parenting style affects false belief understanding. *Social Development, 8*, 395–411.

Schneider-Rosen, K., & Cicchetti, D. (1991). Early self-knowledge and emotional development: Visual self-recognition and affective reactions to mirror self-images in maltreated and non-maltreated toddlers. *Developmental Psychology, 27*, 471–478.

Shaw, D. S., Gilliom, G., Ingoldsby, E. M., & Nagin, D. S. (2003). Trajectories leading to school-age conduct problems. *Developmental Psychology, 39*, 189–200.

Stipek, D., Recchia, S., & McClintic, S. (1992). Self-evaluation in young children. *Monographs of the Society for Research in Child Development, 57*(1, Serial No. 226).

Stipek, D. J., Gralinski, J. H., & Kopp, C. B. (1990). Self-concept development in the toddler years. *Developmental Psychology, 26,* 972–977.

Thompson, R. A. (1994). Emotion regulation: A theme in search of definition. In N. Fox (Ed.), The development of emotion regulation and dysregulation: Biological and behavioral aspects. *Monographs of the Society for Research in Child Development, 59*(2–3, Serial No. 240), 25–52.

Thompson, R. A. (1999). Early attachment and later development. In J. Cassidy & P. Shaver (Eds.), *Handbook of attachment* (pp. 265–286). New York: Guilford Press.

Thompson, R. A. (2001). Childhood anxiety disorders from the perspective of emotion regulation and attachment. In M. W. Vasey & M. R. Dadds (Eds.), *The developmental psychopathology of anxiety* (pp. 160–182). London: Oxford University Press.

Thompson, R. A. (2006). The development of the person: Social understanding, relationships, self, conscience. In W. Damon & R. M. Lerner (Series Eds.), N. Eisenberg (Vol. Ed.), *Handbook of child psychology* (6th ed.): *Vol. 3. Social, emotional, and personality development* (pp. 24–98). New York: Wiley.

Thompson, R. A., Flood, M. F., & Goodvin, R. (2006). Social support and developmental psychopathology. In D. Cicchetti & D. Cohen (Eds.), *Developmental psychopathology* (2nd ed.): *Vol. III. Risk, disorder, and adaptation.* New York: Wiley.

Thompson, R. A., Laible, D., & Ontai, L. (2003). Early understanding of emotion, morality, and the self: Developing a working model. In R. Kail (Ed.), *Advances in child development and behavior* (Vol. 31, pp. 137–171). San Diego: Academic Press.

Thompson, R. A., Meyer, S., & McGinley, M. (2006). Understanding values in relationship: The development of conscience. In M. Killen & J. Smetana (Eds.), *Handbook of moral development* (pp. 267–297). Mahwah, NJ: Erlbaum.

Tomasello, M., & Rakoczy, H. (2003). What makes human cognition unique?: From individual to shared to collective intentionality. *Mind and Language, 18,* 121–147.

Tronick, E. (1989). Emotions and emotional communication in infants. *American Psychologist, 44,* 11–19.

Vasey, M. W., & Ollendick, T. H. (2000). Anxiety. In M. Lewis & A. Sameroff (Eds.), *Handbook of developmental psychopathology* (2nd ed., pp. 511–529). New York: Plenum Press.

Verschueren, K., Marcoen, A., & Schoefs, V. (1996). The internal working model of the self, attachment, and competence in five-year-olds. *Child Development, 67,* 2493–2511.

Wellman, H. (2002). Understanding the psychological world: Developing a theory of mind. In U. Goswami (Ed.), *Handbook of childhood cognitive development* (pp. 167–187). Oxford, UK: Blackwell.

Wellman, H., & Banerjee, M. (1991). Mind and emotion: Children's understanding of the emotional consequences of beliefs and desires. *British Journal of Developmental Psychology, 9,* 191–214.

Wellman, H., Harris, P., Banerjee, M., & Sinclair, A. (1995). Early understanding of emotion: Evidence from natural language. *Cognition and Emotion, 9,* 117–149.

Wellman, H., & Woolley, J. (1990). From simple desires to ordinary beliefs: The early development of everyday psychology. *Cognition, 35,* 245–275.

Wiley, A., Rose, A., Burger, L., & Miller, P. (1998). Constructing autonomous selves through narrative practices: A comparative study of working-class and middle-class families. *Child Development, 69,* 833–847.

Woodward, A. L., Sommerville, J. A., & Guajardo, J. J. (2001). How infants make sense of intentional action. In B. F. Malle, L. J. Moses, & D. A. Baldwin (Eds.), *Intentions and intentionality* (pp. 149–169). Cambridge, MA: MIT Press.

2

Emotional Competence

Implications for Social Functioning

SUSANNE A. DENHAM

Four-year-olds Robbie and Jamila are pretending to be firefighters. They have firefighters' hats and boots, and even a fire engine on which to ride. They have a plush Dalmatian dog and cots to lie on until someone rings the big bell. They are having fun! Robbie moves the fire engine to the spot that Jamila points to—they are ready to rescue the people from that fire! But then things get complicated, changing fast, as interaction often does. Jamila suddenly decides that she should be the fire engine driver, and she tries to pull Robbie off its seat. At the same time, Tyrone, hovering nearby, runs over and whines to join in. But Robbie, almost falling off the fire engine, does not want Tyrone to join—he is "too much of a baby." At the same time, Jamila trips over a cot, falls down, and starts to cry. And just then, Tomas, the class bully, approaches, laughing at 4-year-olds making believe and crying.

Much more than simple playtime was going on here. Imagine the skills of social–emotional learning (SEL) that are needed to negotiate these interactions successfully. For example, Robbie has to know how to resolve the conflict over the fire engine, react to Tyrone without hurting his feelings too much, and "handle" Tomas safely. More generally, Robbie needs to learn how to communicate well with others (especially to express his emotions in socially appropriate ways), handle provocation, engage with others positively, and build relationships. Taken together, these abilities are vital for how Robbie gets along with others, understands himself, and feels good in his world, both within himself and with other people.

Thus, important aspects of SEL are required as preschoolers attend to important developmental tasks—in this case, learning to interact with age-mates. If successful in engaging Jamila, Tyrone, and Tomas in play and interacting with them, then Robbie shows many indicators of such developmentally appropriate SEL. He is beginning to demonstrate (1) self-awareness (especially experiencing and understanding his own emotions); (2) self-management (especially emotion regulation); (3) social awareness (especially understanding others' emotions and perspectives); (4) responsible decision making; and (5) relationship management (Collaborative for Academic Social and Emotional Learning, 2003; Payton et al., 2000).

These important components of SEL obviously include many specific emotion-related competencies. Many young boys and girls Robbie and Jamila's age are learning to cope with their own emotions and with the emotional hurdles that arise when interacting with other people. More specifically, emotionally competent young children begin to do the following:

- Purposefully express, and fully experience, a broad variety of emotions, without incapacitating intensity or duration.
- Understand their own and others' emotions.
- Regulate and cope with their emotions—whenever emotional experience is "too much" or "too little" for themselves, or when its expression is "too much" or "too little" to fit with others' expectations.

The goals of this chapter are to consider the SEL repertoire of normally developing preschool-age children, but with a keen appreciation of how lack of SEL can contribute to developmental and mental health difficulties, both during and after preschool. We first define our developmental perspective, which centers on SEL components' relation to aspects of both the child's environment and the child's own cognitive and temperamental makeup. Then we describe the developmentally appropriate manifestations of SEL during the preschool period, along with their implications for social and academic functioning; that is, we review the theoretical precepts and empirical findings on SEL and its importance during preschool, with special attention to the components of emotional competence—experiencing, expressing, understanding, and regulating emotions—that map so directly onto aspects of SEL. We also discuss responsible decision making and relationship management during this age period. Finally, we conclude by considering the meaning of preschool SEL for mental health, along with the need for future research.

DEVELOPMENTAL PERSPECTIVE ON SOCIAL AND EMOTIONAL LEARNING

All strategies for caring adults' promotion of children's SEL, as well as for preschool mental health programming, whether for prevention or intervention, can be derived from normative theories of child development (Shonkoff

& Phillips, 2000). Given this bedrock, I view development through an organizational, bioecological lens, in which different developmental tasks are central to each age level (Weissberg & Greenberg, 1998). Transitions from one developmental period to another are not only marked by reorganization around new tasks but are also based on the accomplishments of the earlier period. Successful mastery of developmental tasks is supported by not only within-child abilities, processes, and biological predispositions, but also the immediate environment of the child (e.g., interactions of the child with his or her parents or teacher), transactions between elements of the child's immediate environment (e.g., parent–teacher communication about the child); elements outside the child's immediate environment that nevertheless impact him or her (e.g., demands on the parents' time and energy, even depression and other forms of parent psychopathology); and the broader social-political context of the child's world (e.g., welfare policy). Thus, complete understanding of young children's SEL must take into account these levels of influence.

These developmental milestones do not unfold automatically; on the contrary, they are heavily influenced, even at the neuronal level, by environmental inputs throughout early childhood (Greenberg, Domitrovich, & Bumbarger, 2001; Greenberg & Snell, 1997); that is, there are environmental conditions that nurture and reward the application of these SEL skills. In fact, much of the individual variation in the components of children's emotional competence derives from experiences within the family and preschool classroom (Denham, 1998; Hyson, 1994).

Socialization of emotions is ubiquitous in preschoolers' everyday contact with parents, teachers, caregivers, and peers. I conceive of socialization of emotion as including three somewhat overlapping dimensions. First, all people with whom children interact exhibit a variety of emotions, which the children observe. Second, children's emotions, which can be both intense and frequent, often require some kind of reaction from their adult social partners. Third, intentionally teaching about the world of emotions is considered by some adults to be an important area of teaching (Dix, 1991; Eisenberg & Fabes, 1994; Eisenberg, Fabes, & Murphy, 1996; Eisenberg, Fabes, Nyman, Bernzweig, & Pinuelas, 1994; Eisenberg et al., 1999; Gottman, Katz, & Hooven, 1997). Each of these three mechanisms of socialization of emotion—modeling emotional expressiveness, reactions to children's emotions, and teaching about emotion—can influence all the components of children's SEL (Denham, 1998; Denham, Bassett, & Wyatt, in press; Denham, Grant, & Hamada, 2002; Eisenberg, Cumberland, & Spinrad, 1998; Halberstadt, 1991).

Of course, intrapersonal contributors are no doubt also important; abilities and attributes of the children themselves can either promote or hinder SEL. For example, some children are blessed with cognitive and language skills that allow them to better understand their social world, including the emotions within it, as well as to better communicate their own feelings, wishes, desires, and goals for social interactions and relationships (Cutting &

Dunn, 1999). A preschooler who can reason more flexibly can probably take another person's unique emotional perspective into account (e.g., "Some people really are fearful of swimming pools, even though they delight *me*"). In a similar manner, children with greater verbal abilities can ask more pointed questions about their own and others' emotions (e.g., "Why is he crying?") and understand the answers to these questions, which gives them a special advantage in understanding and regulating emotions. For example, a preschooler with more advanced expressive language also can describe his or her own emotions more pointedly (e.g., "I don't *want* to go to bed! I am *mad*!"), which not only allows the child to get his or her emotional point across, but also allows others to communicate with him or her and perhaps offer possibilities for solving the problem.

Similarly, children with different emotional dispositions (i.e., different temperaments) are particularly well- or ill-equipped to demonstrate emotional competence. An especially emotionally negative child, for example, will probably find that she has a greater need for emotion regulation, even though it is at the same time harder for her to achieve. Such a double-bind taxes her abilities to "unhook" from an intense emotional experience (see, e.g., Eisenberg et al., 1993, 1994, 1997). Conversely, a child whose temperament predisposes him flexibly to focus attention on a comforting action, object, or thought, and shift attention from a distressing situation, is better able to regulate emotions, even intense ones. Given this developmental foundation from which to view SEL and its promotion, it is time to examine in more detail exactly what does develop.

DEVELOPMENTALLY APPROPRIATE MANIFESTATION OF SOCIAL AND EMOTIONAL LEARNING DURING PRESCHOOL

Setting the Stage: The Developmental Task

In the case of preschoolers, SEL skills are organized around the developmental tasks of positive engagement and managing emotional arousal within social interaction, while successfully moving into the world of peers (Howes, 1987; Parker & Gottman, 1989). Although these tasks are not easy for children just entering the peer arena, successful interaction with age-mates is a crucial predictor of later mental health and well-being, even school adjustment, learning, and academic success—beginning during preschool and continuing thereafter (Birch, Ladd, & Blecher-Sass, 1997; Denham & Holt, 1993; Ladd, Birch, & Buhs, 1999; Ladd, Kochenderfer, & Coleman, 1996; Robins & Rutter, 1990; Smith, 2001). In particular, when developmental milestones of SEL are not negotiated successfully, preschoolers are at risk for psychopathology, both at the time and later in life (Cytryn, McKnew, Zahn-Waxler, & Gershon, 1986; Denham, Zahn-Waxler, Cummings, & Iannotti, 1991; Roff, 1990). I now describe these crucial preschool SEL skills in greater detail.

Skills of Social and Emotional Learning:
Self-Awareness and Emotional Expressiveness

Self-awareness and emotional expressiveness, especially recognizing and sending affective messages, are central to SEL. Emotions must be expressed in keeping with one's goals, in accordance with the social context; the goals of the self and those of others must be coordinated; that is, the self-awareness component of SEL includes experiencing and expressing emotions.

What specifically does the expression of emotions "do for" a child and his or her social group? Most importantly, the experience and expression of emotion signals whether the child or other people need to modify or to continue their goal-directed behavior (see Campos, Mumme, Kermoian, & Campos, 1994). Hence, such information can shape the child's own behaviors. An example is happiness: If one boy experiences happiness while playing in the "block corner" with another, then he may seek out the other child during another activity, and even ask his mother whether the other child can come to his house to play. The experience of joy gives him important information that affects his subsequent behavior. Additionally, emotions are important because they provide social information to other people and affect others' behaviors. Peers benefit from witnessing other children's expressions of emotion. When a girl's friends witness the social signal of her anger, for example, they know from experience whether their most adaptive response would be to fight back or to retreat.

Thus, preschoolers are learning to use emotional communication to express nonverbal messages about a social situation or relationship—for example, giving a hug. They also develop empathic involvement in others' emotions—for example, kissing a baby sister when she falls down and bangs her knee. Furthermore, they display complex social and self-conscious emotions such as guilt, pride, shame, and contempt in appropriate contexts (Alessandri & Lewis, 1993; Garner, 2003; Lewis, Alessandri, & Sullivan, 1992; Strayer & Roberts, 1997, 2004a, 2004b; Walter, 2002).

All of these emotions must be expressed in keeping with one's goals, in accordance with the social context (Halberstadt, Denham, & Dunsmore, 2001). This is no small task, because the goals of the self and those of others must be coordinated; that is, even young children are involved in interactions in which their goals conflict with those of their playmates. Based on their emerging understanding of such conflict, preschoolers can modulate emotional expressiveness to help interactions proceed as smoothly as possible. Thus, emotional competence includes expressing emotions in a way that is advantageous to moment-to-moment interaction and relationships over time. For example, Robbie is generally well liked by the other children in his kindergarten class, in part, because of his generally pleasant, happy demeanor.

Specifically, emotionally competent individuals are aware that an affective message needs to be sent. But for successful interaction, what affective message should be sent? First, children slowly learn which expressions of which emotions facilitate specific goals. Tyrone learns that his whiny voice, downcast face, and slightly averted body posture are not associated with successful entry into play. Second, children learn that the appropriate affective message is the one that "works" in the setting, or with a specific playmate. Tyrone may learn that a smile and otherwise calm demeanor is the better key to unlock the door to shared play with Robbie and Jessica; on the other hand, if he needs to defend himself, an angry scowl might get Tomas to back off, at least temporarily. Children also find out that the method, intensity, and timing of an affective message are crucial to its meaning and eventual success or failure. Robbie has learned that showing slight annoyance for a short while over his disagreement with Jessica is very different than remaining very angry with her for days. The likelihood of Robbie and Jessica enjoying their time together, and continuing to be playmates and friends, is higher when Robbie shows brief annoyance, followed by both children's behavioral adjustments that lead to mutually satisfying play. High-intensity, long-lasting anger has more detrimental effects, arousing and isolating both parties, and making either short- or long-term interaction more difficult.

Finally, children's emotional expressiveness can become even more complex during preschool. Young children are beginning to realize that a person may feel a certain way "on the inside" but show a different outward demeanor (Denham, 1998). In particular, they are learning that the overt expression of socially disapproved feelings may be controlled or suppressed, while more socially appropriate emotions are expressed. For example, disappointment and even rage at being reprimanded by a parent or teacher may be relevant—that is, the adult has indeed blocked the child's goal, such as when Robbie's teacher says it is time to clean up and stop playing firefighters—but expressing such anger with adults is usually imprudent. Some emotional expressions are relevant to the situation but not the context, and some irrelevant ones need to be masked. Anxiety when playing a new game is probably irrelevant to the goal of having fun and needs to be suppressed. Because of their relation to voluntary control and contextual appropriateness, these emerging aspects of preschoolers' expressive repertoire—their ability to use the display rules of their culture—are more clearly related to emotion regulation and are discussed in more detail when that aspect of emotional competence is reviewed.

Implications of Emotional Expressiveness for Succeeding Socially

Accumulating evidence suggests that this SEL component contributes to overall success in interacting with one's peers. At a simple level, emotional expressiveness can refer to the individual child's profile of frequency, intensity, and/ or duration of basic and complex emotions—happiness, sadness, anger, fear, guilt, and empathy, for example. Preschoolers' expression of specific emotions, especially their enduring patterns of expressiveness, relates to their overall success in interacting with peers (i.e., peer status) and to their teachers' evaluation of their social functioning, including their friendliness and aggression. *Positive* affect is important in the initiation and regulation of social exchanges; sharing positive affect may facilitate the formation of friendships and render one more likable (Denham, McKinley, Couchoud, & Holt, 1990; Lemerise, 2000; Park, Lay, & Ramsay, 1993; Sroufe, Schork, Motti, Lawroski, & La Freniere, 1984). Conversely, *negative* affect, especially anger, can be quite problematic within social interaction and may serve as an impediment to successful formation of friendships (Denham et al., 1990; Lemerise & Dodge, 2000; Rubin & Clark, 1983; Rubin & Daniels-Beirness, 1983).

Children who show relatively more joyful than angry emotions (1) are rated higher by teachers on friendliness and assertiveness, and lower on aggressiveness and sadness; (2) respond more prosocially to peers' emotions; and (3) are seen as more likable by their peers (Denham, 1986; Denham et al., 1990; Denham, Renwick, & Holt, 1991; Eisenberg et al., 1997; Rydell, Berlin, & Bohlin, 2003; Sroufe et al., 1984; Strayer, 1980). Sadness or fear, whether observed in the classroom or in interaction with one's mother, is related to teacher ratings of withdrawal and internalizing difficulties (see, e.g., Denham, Renwick, et al., 1991; Rydell et al., 2003).

Finally, there is evidence (Denham et al., 2001) that preschoolers in play groups characterized by negative temperament, anger expressed in the preschool classroom, and negative emotional responsiveness toward others were evaluated by both teachers and peers as lacking in social competence up to 1 year later (Denham, 1986; Denham et al., 1990; Denham, Renwick, et al., 1991; Eisenberg et al., 1997; Rydell et al., 2003; Sroufe et al., 1984; Strayer, 1980); that is, emotionally negative 3-year-old preschoolers engage with equally negative playmates and continue to play in such groups during the next preschool year, perhaps due to their declining sociometric status. These effects held true more often for boys. If such patterns of relationship are forming already in preschool, it is likely that other children would continue to avoid these resentful, disagreeable, threatening peers in later years.

Moreover, some forms of this emotional negativity are quite context-specific. Gleeful taunting, such as laughing while one causes another emotional or physical pain, may look like positive expressiveness on the surface, but it is really a form of emotional aggression. Such gleeful taunting expressed during conflict predicts negative peer status and teacher ratings of social functioning more strongly than does anger within conflicts (Miller & Olson, 2000); after all, most preschoolers openly show anger during conflicts, to the point that such expression is normative. Gleeful taunting, which is not normative behavior, predicts social difficulty.

In summary, it is easy to envision why children's patterns of emotional expressiveness provide such potent intrapersonal support for, or roadblocks to, interactions with age-mates (Campos & Barrett, 1984). A sad or angry child who sits unhappily on the sidelines of a group, with nothing pleasing her, is less able to see, let alone tend to, the emotional needs of others. And it is no wonder that her peers flatly assert, as did a 3-year-old research participant, "She hits. She bites. She kicked me this morning. I *don't like* her." Conversely, a happier preschooler is better able to respond to others. Overall, young children's own expressed emotions often are related to evaluations of their social competence by important persons in their widening world (e.g., teachers, peers, parents).

Implications of Emotional Expressiveness for Succeeding Academically

Children who express more positive and moderately intense emotions overall also are perceived by their teachers as easier to teach and as better performers in school (Keogh, 1992; Martin, Drew, Gaddis, & Moseley, 1988; Palinsin, 1986); in fact, those children who observers rated as less negative during interactions with their mothers on the first day of kindergarten showed better academic performance through eighth grade (Morrison, Rimm-Kauffman, & Pianta, 2003).

Along with expressiveness that is visible to others, the individual's experience of emotion is important as well. Because emotion assists in organizing and directing cognition (Blair, 2002), it is important for children to modulate both their experience and expression of emotion to interact and to learn. Thus, emotion regulation is an important component of emotional competence.

Skills of Social and Emotional Learning: Self-Management/Emotion Regulation

When intensity, duration, or other parameters of the experience and expression of emotion are "too much" or "too little" to meet goals and expectations of the child and/or social partners, emotion regulation is needed (Cole, Martin, & Dennis, 2004; Denham, 1998; Saarni, 1999; Thompson, 1994). Candidates for regulation include emotions that are aversive, those that are positive but possibly overwhelming, and emotions that need to be amplified for either intra- or interpersonally strategic reasons.

Beginning to attend preschool or a child care center is a particularly important transition that taxes young children's emotion regulatory skills. Preschoolers' attention is focused on success with their friends in this context. Unlike adults, however, these newly important peers are neither skilled at negotiation nor able to offer assistance in emotion regulation. At the same time, the social cost of emotional dysregulation is high with both teachers and peers; initiating, maintaining, and negotiating play, and earning acceptance all require preschoolers to "keep the lid on" (Raver, Blackburn, & Bancroft, 1999). Thus, because of the increasing complexity of young children's emotionality and the demands of their social world, with "so much going on" emotionally, some organized emotional gatekeeper must be cultivated.

Children learn to retain or enhance those emotions that are relevant and helpful, to attenuate those that are relevant but not helpful, and to dampen those that are irrelevant; these skills help them to experience more well-being and maintain satisfying relationships with others. For example, Robbie may know that showing too much anger will hurt Tyrone's feelings, but showing too *little* angry bravado with Tomas could make Robbie more of a target. Managing "false" signals is also crucial (e.g., a boy entering other children's game of "chase" had a sudden "tummy rumble" as he neared them, but he did not consider it pertinent—he was *not* afraid!).

Early in the preschool period, much of this self-management is bio-behavioral (e.g., thumbsucking), and/or obtained externally from adults; for example, although very upset when a playmate grabs all the toys, a young child can go to the caregiver for assistance instead of immediately resorting to aggression. Parents and teachers help children gain the cognitive coping strategies they will eventually use (e.g., purposely redeploying attention). Adults also use emotion language to help children regulate emotion by identifying and interpreting their feelings (e.g., "This will only hurt a little"), and helping children process causal associations between events and emotions. They also demonstrate behavioral coping strategies when they problem-solve around emotional situations or structure their child's environment to facilitate regulation (e.g., a mother avoids situations that she knows will frighten her daughter).

Because of increased cognitive ability and control of both their attention and their emotionality (Lewis, Stanger, & Sullivan, 1989), children do develop greater capacities for independent emotion regulation during the preschool period. They become increasingly aware of the need for emotion regulation and more able to use various emotion regulation strategies. Over time, they also notice whether their emotion regulation efforts are successful.

Finally, as they become more flexible in choosing optimal ways of coping in specific contexts, children gradually begin to use specific coping strategies for self-regulation—problem solving, support seeking, distancing, internalizing, externalizing, distraction, reframing or redefining the problem, cognitive "blunting," and denial. Many such strategies are indeed quite useful for emotion regulation; they are sequentially associated with decreased anger (e.g., Gilliom, Shaw, Beck, Schonberg, & Lukon, 2002). Hence, preschoolers who are more able to regulate emotions display more socially appropriate emotions, according to display rules of their culture (Kieras, Tobin, & Graziano, 2003).

Implications of Emotion Regulation for Succeeding Socially

It is clear that emotion regulation is a crucial ability in managing the demands inherent in interpersonal situations (Parker & Gottman, 1989). When the young child begins to regulate his or her own emotions, he or she gets along more successfully with peers and adults alike. For example, Eisenberg et al. (1993, 1994, 1997, 2001, 2003) have found that preschoolers' and primary school children's optimal emotion regulation is related to their socially appro-

priate behavior. Even more specifically, reliance on attention-shifting strategies may correspond with low externalizing problems and high cooperation,
whereas reliance on a more problem-focused regulatory strategy, such as
gathering information to help solve the problem, may be more closely related
to assertiveness (Gilliom et al., 2002). In contrast, lack of emotional and behavioral regulation at age 2 years predicts externalizing problems at 4 years,
even with aggressiveness at age 2 controlled; lack of regulation of exuberant
positive emotions and fear is related to externalizing and internalizing difficulties, respectively (Rydell et al., 2003). In summary, children who are able
to regulate their emotions are more well-liked and are seen by adults and
peers as functioning well socially across a range of ages, from preschool to the
end of grade school. Inability to regulate emotions figures prominently in the
trajectory toward behavior difficulties at school entry.

As already implied (Kieras et al., 2003), emotion regulation and expressiveness often operate in concert. Specifically, young children who are most
emotionally intense and regulate this intense emotion poorly show difficulties
in maintaining positive social behavior and have more troubled relationships
with peers, as evidenced by lower peer status (Eisenberg, Fabes, Guthrie, et
al., 1996; Eisenberg et al., 1995, 1997; Murphy, Shepard, Eisenberg, Fabes,
& Guthrie, 1999). In other research (Denham et al., 2003; Denham, Blair,
Schmidt, & DeMulder, 2002), kindergarten teachers observed that children
who showed much anger but were unable or unwilling to regulate it construc-
tively during preschool had problems with oppositionality 2 years later. In
contrast, even highly negative children are buffered from peer status problems
by the good emotion regulation skills that caring adults can teach them.

It also seems clear that the need to regulate emotional experience and
expression can compete with higher-order cognitive processing demands. In
particular, when the child regulates emotion in reactive ways, through withdrawal, hypervigilance, or venting rather than through effortful processes involving higher cognitive abilities (e.g., problem solving, distraction, reframing
the problem), these higher-order cognitive abilities are underused and consequently underdeveloped (Blair, 2002). For example, 3-year-old Karen's attention and energy for her entire morning in preschool is consumed with fussing
about getting her way, her terrible cold, and who gets to play with certain
toys, then she probably will not have the cognitive capacity left over to attend
to and process the information about stories, rhymes, and songs introduced
by her teachers. In short, emotion regulation is central to young children's social and cognitive functioning, and deserves applied practitioners' full attention.

The conscious appraisal of emotions is considered by some to be beyond
the capabilities of preschoolers (Blair, 2002). This assertion may be true of
young children's awareness of emotions while experiencing them, although it
could be argued that some emotional experiences require conscious reflection,
even during this age period (Denham, 1998). Whichever contention is closer
to the truth, it is probably indisputable that children learn to understand

much about emotions during early childhood. This knowledge, which may be most available to them during "cool," nonemotional moments, forms an important foundation for the development of conscious emotion appraisal of both self and others.

Skills of Social and Emotional Learning: Self- and Other Awareness/ Emotion Knowledge

Emotion knowledge is inextricably related to the capacity for accurate social awareness. As active participants in the social world, preschoolers continually make interpretations and attributions about their own and others' behaviors and emotions (Dodge, Pettit, McClaskey, & Brown, 1986; Miller & Aloise, 1989). In fact, emotions of self and other are central experiences in the lives of young children—immediate, salient, and important in their social transactions. In spontaneous conversations, preschool children talk about and reflect upon their own and others' feelings, and discuss causes and consequences of their own and others' emotional experiences and expressiveness (Dunn, 1994; Fabes, Eisenberg, McCormick, & Wilson, 1988).

Once perceived, affective messages must be interpreted accurately; errors can lead to both intrapersonal and social difficulties. If Robbie misattributes Tomas's scowl as happiness, Tomas may actually punch him. More specifically, emotion knowledge yields information about emotional expressions and experience in self and others, as well as events in the environment. By preschool, most children can infer basic emotions from expressions or situations (Denham, 1986). They have a better understanding of happy expressions and situations than of negative ones (Fabes, Eisenberg, Nyman, & Michealieu, 1991).

Understanding More Complex and Subtle Aspects of Emotion

Throughout the rest of the preschool period, children come to understand many more subtle aspects of the expressions and situations that elicit basic emotions:

- Differentiating among the emotions of self and other—for example, realizing that one feels more sad than angry when receiving a "time out" from the preschool teacher.
- Going even further than recognizing the expressions and situations that elicit discrete emotions to make more complex attributions about the causes of a *particular person's* emotions (e.g., self, peer, parents; Dunn & Hughes, 1998). Through their increased social sensitivity and experience, older preschoolers develop strategies for appraising others' emotions when available cues are less salient and consensual, focusing on personal dispositions as opposed to goal states ("She had a bad day" instead of "She didn't want Billy to play with her").

- Grasping the consequences of emotions for both self and others (Denham, 1997). Clearly, knowing why an emotion is expressed (its cause) and its likely aftermath (its consequences in the behavior of self or others) aids a child in regulating behavior and emotions, as well as reacting to others' emotions.

Furthermore, young children begin to identify other peoples' emotions even when they may differ from their own—for example, knowing that Mother's smile as she comes into the house means her workday was satisfactory, and she probably won't yell tonight. To interpret emotional information even more accurately, information specific to a particular person in a particular situation may be needed. Important emotional information includes (1) whether or not the situation is equivocal (i.e., can elicit more than one emotion), (2) the person's expressive patterns and the situational conflict, and (3) the degree to which the situational conflict is person-specific. Only toward the end of the age range do preschoolers even begin to attain these skills. Although this aspect of emotion knowledge is very important, preschoolers are just beginning to acquire and use it (Gnepp, 1989; Gnepp & Chilamkurti, 1988; Gnepp & Gould, 1985; Gnepp, McKee, & Domanic, 1987).

Toward the end of this developmental period, preschoolers also begin to comprehend complex dimensions of emotional experiences, such as display rules. They also begin to understand these rules as they use them in emotion-eliciting circumstances (Banerjee, 1997; Josephs, 1994; Rozek, 1987), perhaps beginning with emotions that are most subject to socialization pressure, such as anger (Feito, 1997). How skilled older preschoolers are at this complex aspect of emotional understanding is partly dependent on how this knowledge is measured; investigators using developmentally appropriate methodological simplifications generally find that although older preschoolers and kindergartners have much to learn, they have a solid foundation for understanding display rules.

Finally, it is not uncommon for older children and adults to experience and understand "mixed emotions," such as when an older sister is somewhat amused at her younger brother's antics, but is mostly annoyed when he tries to leap over her backpack but lands on it, breaking the earphones inside (Harter & Whitesell, 1989). However, because young children's expressiveness is becoming more intricate as they leave the preschool period and head toward kindergarten, they too may begin to experience and understand simultaneous emotions and ambivalence. Again, researchers who ask questions via an age-appropriate methodology have revealed that preschoolers know more about mixed emotions than was previously assumed (Donaldson & Westerman, 1986; Kestenbaum & Gelman, 1995; Peng, Johnson, Pollock, Glasspool, & Harris, 1992).

Because young children and their peers are beginning to express complex emotions, we might expect them to have some understanding of them; however, such understanding is quite limited, and it develops quite slowly. Even older preschoolers are unable to report feeling pride, guilt, or shame appropriately; instead, they report simpler emotions (Arsenio & Lover, 1995; Berti, Garattoni, & Venturini, 2000; Harter & Whitesell, 1989; Nunner-Winkler & Sodian, 1988).

In summary, preschoolers acquire much emotion knowledge to assist them in social interactions with family and peers. However, it is equally clear that many of the finer nuances of emotion knowledge are either just emerging or not yet within their repertoires at all.

Implications of Emotion Knowledge for Succeeding Socially

Although there are developmental progressions in the various aspects of emotion knowledge, with knowledge of expressions and situations preceding other sorts of understanding, there also are marked individual differences in these developments (Dunn, 1994). Because personal experiences and social interactions or relationships are guided, even defined, by emotional transactions (Denham, 1998; Halberstadt et al., 2001; Saarni, 1999), it follows that one's level of emotion knowledge figures prominently in personal and social success.

Emotion knowledge allows a preschooler to react appropriately to others, thus bolstering social relationships. Interactions with an emotionally knowledgeable age-mate would likely be viewed as satisfying, and render one more likable. For example, the youngster who understands emotions of others may be more helpful when a friend is angry or sad, and the preschooler who can talk about his or her own emotions also is better able to negotiate disputes with friends. Similarly, teachers are likely to be attuned to the behavioral evidence of emotion knowledge—the use of emotion language, the sympathetic reaction—and to evaluate it positively. Thus, children who understand emotions are more prosocially responsive to their peers and are rated as more socially skilled by teachers, and more likable by their peers (Denham, 1986; Denham & Couchoud, 1991; Denham et al., 1990; Roberts & Strayer, 1996; Smith, 2001; Strayer, 1980).

More specifically, emotion situation knowledge and emotion language usage during conversations with friends are involved in conflict resolution; cooperative, shared pretend play; and successful communication (Dunn & Cutting, 1999; Dunn & Herrera, 1997). Furthermore, young children's understanding of emotion situations is *negatively* related to nonconstructive anger reactions during peer interaction (Garner & Estep, 2001). Moreover, preschoolers' understanding of emotion expressions and situations is related to their use of reasoned argument with, and caregiving of siblings (Dunn, Slomkowski, Donelan, & Herrera, 1995; Garner, Jones, & Miner, 1994).

In contrast, preschoolers with identified aggression and oppositionality or peer problems show specific deficits in understanding emotion expressions and situations, both in preschool and at later developmental points (Denham et al., 2003; Denham, Blair, et al., 2002; Denham, Caverly, et al., 2002;

Hughes, Dunn, & White, 1998). Furthermore, first graders' difficulties in understanding emotional expressions were related to their problems with peers and social withdrawal, even when researchers accounted for preschool verbal ability and self-control measures (Izard et al., 2001; Schultz, Izard, Ackerman, & Youngstrom, 2001; Smith, 2001).

Other research has examined in more detail the implications of young children's specific errors in emotion understanding. For example, Barth and Bastiani (1997) discovered a subtle relation that may underlie aggressive children's social difficulties: Preschoolers' overattributions of peers' expressions as angry—a recognition bias similar to older children's hostile attribution bias—was associated with negative social behavior (Dodge & Somberg, 1987). Such overattribution of anger in emotion understanding is also related to preschool boys' aggression and to both boys' and girls' peer rejection (Schultz, Izard, & Ackerman, 2000); see also Denham and colleagues (1990), who found that confusing happiness with any negative emotion, or confusing negative emotions, was negatively related to sociometric likeability.

In summary, these patterns of results suggest that deficits in early childhood emotion knowledge are related to children's social and behavior problems preceding, and extending into, kindergarten. Boosting such emotion knowledge, and doing so before school entry, thus increases in importance. In the future, for example, ascertaining these early social-cognitive difficulties could make it easier to intervene with children, before their difficulties with aggression become entrenched.

Responsible Decision Making

Because cognition (e.g., thinking, attention) and emotion work together, it is important to address each child's skills in *thinking* about interpersonal interactions, going beyond his or her emotional experience, knowledge, regulation, and expression. Responsible decision making assumes importance as the everyday social interactions of preschoolers increase in frequency and complexity. Young children must learn to analyze social situations, set social goals, and determine effective ways to resolve differences that arise between them and their peers. Even preschoolers can begin to learn these important thinking skills that support their increasingly complex social interaction, such as the ability to play positively, to cooperate, and to demonstrate other social skills (Mize & Cox, 1990; Pettit, Dodge, & Brown, 1988).

Social information-processing theory, which forms a foundation for training in responsible decision making (Crick & Dodge, 1994), involves the social information-processing steps of encoding information about the problem from the social surround, interpreting it, forming goals, and selecting and enacting the most favorable response. The theory has been expanded to include emotional information and content at every step (Lemerise & Arsenio, 2000). Each of these steps, with a new focus on emotions, is important in its own right.

In the *encoding and interpreting* steps, the child takes in important information about others' behavior, emotions, intentions, and the likely effect of others' behavior, as well as his or her own arousal level, the intensity of the emotions felt, and his or her relationship with others. Robbie sees, accurately, that Jamila is annoyed about who is currently in charge of the fire engine, that Tyrone is a little scared about asking to play, and that Tomas is looking for a chance to act angry and mean—on purpose.

In the next step, *clarification of goals,* the child formulates goals, which are focused arousal states that function to motivate him or her to produce outcomes. When a child cannot regulate emotion, he or she may focus on external goals, such as revenge, or may retreat into passivity, neither of which promotes successful interaction. A child who more successfully regulates emotions is more able to focus on relationship-enhancing goals. The child's perception of the other's emotions may also affect the goals chosen; for example, a child who showed intense glee at a playmate's distress could render the playmate's need for revenge or withdrawal more likely. If Tomas acts mean if Robbie chooses to stick up for himself, Robbie may switch goals and decide that he wants to act really mean back, even to fight.

The last steps all involve the child's final behavioral response: *response generation, evaluation*, and *decision*. Access to and choice of actual behavioral responses differ depending on the child's goal-related emotions; that is, feeling sad that one's drawing was destroyed by a peer might elicit very different response than anger at the peer for doing such a mean thing.

Furthermore, it is clear that responsible decision making and other aspects of SEL must work together for the child's optimal functioning. For example, a preschooler who can emotionally regulate him- or herself after being pushed, feels better but still might not be able to choose how to act. Without responsible decision-making skills, even a well-regulated child cannot perform the effortful cognitive processing needed to choose the most optimal behavioral response. Conversely, a preschooler who usually has good problem-solving ideas may be able to access these ideas when he or she is extremely emotionally aroused by being pushed.

If Robbie, who seems rather aware of his own emotional processes, can remain calm enough, perhaps via the emotion regulatory strategies listed earlier, such as problem-focused regulation or support seeking, he may choose a response that can enhance his relationships. Even though he is scared of Tomas, he may say something to defuse the bully's nastiness (and to help regulate his own emotions by "fixing" the problem), such as "Quit laughing, Tomas. Do you want to play or not?" Alternatively, he may seek out his teacher to assist in sorting out the difficulties.

Relationship Management

Other relationship skills represent the final component of SEL, including, for example, making positive overtures to play with others, initiating and maintaining conversations, active listening, cooperating, sharing, taking turns, negotiating, and saying "no" or seeking help when necessary (Doyle & Connolly, 1989; Honig, 1999; Honig & Wittmer, 1996). Given the situation on the opening case, Robbie may use many such specific skills in the service of getting along with his playmates. He might figure out a way to cooperate with Jamila, try to negotiate some sort of mutually satisfactory solution with Tyrone, and seek help in dealing with Tomas. These important, distinct abilities enhance the more general strategies of self- and other-awareness, self-management, and responsible decision making.

SUMMARY AND FUTURE DIRECTIONS

The goals of this chapter were to introduce and outline the development of SEL during the preschool period and its importance to mental health and social–emotional functioning. Although these abilities are exceedingly important, I have only scratched the surface of their manifestations and implications, as well as their promotion by adults. Much basic research work needs to be done in this area, particularly in examining how the components of SEL work together rather than viewing them as separable entities. Furthermore, work proceeding from the framework presented here needs to situate SEL abilities within the "whole child," viewing how SEL interacts with cognition, language, and other aspects of development, both concurrently and predictively.

It seems that our state of knowledge is ripe for the exploration of more applied topics. When the developmental tasks that are important for preschoolers' social and preacademic functioning are appreciated, psychology professionals are in a better position to assist parents and teachers in promoting optimal development (Denham & Burton, 2003). More research is particularly needed to discern possible indirect contributors to SEL, such as parental psychopathology, divorce, poverty, child care quality, and their interactions.

Working together, clinicians, parents, and preschool teachers/day care providers can make sure that preschoolers like Robbie continue their early excellent progress in emotional and social competence to successfully meet the challenges of literacy, problem solving, and sustaining more complex, fulfilling relationships with others. We can help children like Tyrone, Tomas, and even Jamila to find better ways to interact, so that their well-regulated behaviors support social, emotional, and academic pursuits throughout their lives.

REFERENCES

Alessandri, S. M., & Lewis, M. (1993). Parental evaluation and its relation to shame and pride in young children. *Sex Roles, 29*(5–6), 335–343.
Arsenio, W., & Lover, A. (1995). Children's conceptions of sociomoral affect: Happy victim-

izers, mixed emotions and other expectancies. In M. Killen & D. Hart (Eds.), *Morality in everyday life: Developmental perspectives* (pp. 87–128). Cambridge, UK: Cambridge University Press.

Banerjee, M. (1997). Hidden emotions: Preschoolers' knowledge of appearance–reality and emotion display rules. *Social Development, 15,* 107–132.

Barth, J. M., & Bastiani, A. (1997). A longitudinal study of emotional recognition and preschool children's social behavior. *Merrill–Palmer Quarterly, 43,* 107–128.

Berti, A. E., Garattoni, C., & Venturini, B. A. (2000). The understanding of sadness, guilt, and shame in 5–, 7–, and 9–year-old children. *Genetic, Social, and General Psychology Monographs, 126,* 293–318.

Birch, S. H., Ladd, G. W., & Blecher-Sass, H. (1997). The teacher–child relationship and children's early school adjustment: Good-byes can build trust. *Journal of School Psychology, 35,* 61–79.

Blair, C. (2002). School readiness: Integrating cognition and emotion in a neurobiological conceptualization of children's functioning at school entry. *American Psychologist, 57,* 111–127.

Campos, J. J., & Barrett, K. C. (1984). Toward a new understanding of emotions and their development. In C. E. Izard, J. Kagan, & R. B. Zajonc (Eds.), *Emotions, cognition, and behavior* (pp. 229–263). New York: Cambridge University Press.

Campos, J. J., Mumme, D. L., Kermoian, R., & Campos, R. G. (1994). A functionalist perspective on the nature of emotion. *Monographs of the Society for Research in Child Development, 59*(2–3), 284–303.

Cole, P. M., Martin, S. E., & Dennis, T. A. (2004). Emotion regulation as a scientific construct: Methodological challenges and directions for child development research. *Child Development, 75,* 317–333.

Collaborative for Academic, Social, and Emotional Learning. (2003). *Safe and sound: An educational leader's guide to evidence-based social and emotional learning (SEL) programs.* Chicago, IL: Author.

Dunn, J. (1994). Understanding others and the social world: Current issues in developmental research and their relation to preschool experiences and practice. *Journal of Applied Developmental Psychology, 15,* 571–583.

Crick, N., & Dodge, K. A. (1994). A review and reformulation of social information-processing mechanisms in children's social adjustment. *Psychological Bulletin, 115,* 74–101.

Cutting, A. L., & Dunn, J. (1999). Theory of mind, emotion understanding, language, and family background: Individual differences and interrelations. *Child Development, 70,* 853–865.

Cytryn, L., McKnew, D. H., Zahn-Waxler, C., & Gershon, E. S. (1986). Developmental issues in risk research: The offspring of affectively ill parents. In M. Rutter, C. E. Izard, & P. B. Read (Eds.), *Depression in young people: Developmental and clinical perspectives* (pp. 163–188). New York: Guilford Press.

Denham, S. A. (1986). Social cognition, social behavior, and emotion in preschoolers: Contextual validation. *Child Development, 57,* 194–201.

Denham, S. A. (1997). "When I have a bad dream, Mommy holds me": Preschoolers' consequential thinking about emotions and social competence. *International Journal of Behavioral Development, 20,* 301–319.

Denham, S. A. (1998). *Emotional development in young children.* New York: Guilford Press.

Denham, S. A., Bassett, H. H., & Wyatt, T. (in press). The socialization of emotional competence. In J. Grusec & P. Hastings (Eds.), *Handbook of socialization.* New York: Guilford Press.

Denham, S. A., Blair, K. A., DeMulder, E., Levitas, J., Sawyer, K. S., Auerbach-Major, S. T., et al. (2003). Preschoolers' emotional competence: Pathway to mental health? *Child Development, 74,* 238–256.

Denham, S. A., Blair, K. A., Schmidt, M. S., & DeMulder, E. (2002). Compromised emotional competence: Seeds of violence sown early? *American Journal of Orthopsychiatry, 72,* 70–82.

Denham, S. A., & Burton, R. (2003). *Social and emotional prevention and intervention programming for preschoolers.* New York: Kluwer Academic/Plenum Press.

Denham, S. A., Caverly, S., Schmidt, M., Blair, K., DeMulder, E., Caal, S., et al. (2002). Preschool understanding of emotions: Contributions to classroom anger and aggression. *Journal of Child Psychology and Psychiatry, 43,* 901–916.

Denham, S. A., & Couchoud, E. A. (1991). Social–emotional predictors of preschoolers' responses to an adult's negative emotions. *Journal of Child Psychology and Psychiatry, 32,* 595–608.

Denham, S. A., Grant, S., & Hamada, H. A. (2002). *"I have two 1st teachers": Mother and teacher socialization of preschoolers' emotional and social competence.* Paper presented at the Symposium submitted to the 7th Head Start Research Conference, Washington, DC.

Denham, S. A., & Holt, R. W. (1993). Preschoolers' likability as cause or consequence of their social behavior. *Developmental Psychology, 29,* 271–275.

Denham, S. A., Mason, T., Caverly, S., Schmidt, M., Hackney, R., Caswell, C., et al. (2001). Preschoolers at play: Co-socializers of emotional and social competence. *International Journal of Behavioral Development, 25,* 290–301.

Denham, S. A., McKinley, M., Couchoud, E. A., & Holt, R. (1990). Emotional and behavioral predictors of peer status in young preschoolers. *Child Development, 61,* 1145–1152.

Denham, S. A., Renwick, S., & Holt, R. (1991). Working and playing together: Prediction of preschool social–emotional competence from mother–child interaction. *Child Development, 62,* 242–249.

Denham, S. A., Zahn-Waxler, C., Cummings, E. M., & Iannotti, R. J. (1991). Social competence in young children's peer relationships: Patterns of development and change. *Child Psychiatry and Human Development, 22,* 29–43.

Dix, T. (1991). The affective organization of parenting: Adaptive and maladaptative processes. *Psychological Bulletin, 110,* 3–25.

Dodge, K. A., Pettit, G., McClaskey, C. L., & Brown, M. M. (1986). Social competence in children. *Monographs of the Society for Research in Child Development, 51(2),* 1–85.

Dodge, K. A., & Somberg, D. R. (1987). Hostile attribution biases among aggressive boys are exacerbated among conditions of threat to the self. *Child Development, 58,* 213–224.

Donaldson, S. K., & Westerman, M. A. (1986). Development of children's understanding of ambivalence and causal theories of emotions. *Developmental Psychology, 22,* 655–662.

Doyle, A.-B., & Connolly, J. (1989). Negotiation and enactment in social pretend play: Relations to social acceptance and social cognition. *Early Childhood Research Quarterly, 4(3),* 289–302.

Dunn, J., & Cutting, A. L. (1999). Understanding others, and individual differences in friendship interactions in young children. *Social Development, 8,* 201–219.

Dunn, J., & Herrera, C. (1997). Conflict resolution with friends, siblings, and mothers: A developmental perspective. *Aggressive Behavior, 23,* 343–357.

Dunn, J., & Hughes, C. (1998). Young children's understanding of emotions within close relationships. *Cognition and Emotion, 12,* 171–190.

Dunn, J., Slomkowski, C., Donelan, N., & Herrera, C. (1995). Conflict, understanding, and relationships: Developments and differences in the preschool years. *Early Education and Development, 6,* 303–316.

Eisenberg, N., Cumberland, A., & Spinrad, T. L. (1998). Parental socialization of emotion. *Psychological Inquiry, 9,* 241–273.

Eisenberg, N., & Fabes, R. A. (1994). Mothers' reactions to children's negative emotions: Relations to children's temperament and anger behavior. *Merrill–Palmer Quarterly, 40,* 138–156.

Eisenberg, N., Fabes, R. A., Bernzweig, J., Karbon, M., Poulin, R., & Hanish, L. (1993). The relations of emotionality and regulation to preschoolers' social skills and sociometric status. *Child Development, 64,* 1418–1438.

Eisenberg, N., Fabes, R. A., Guthrie, I. K., Murphy, B. C., Maszk, P., Holmgren, R., et al. (1996). The relations of regulation and emotionality to problem behavior in elementary school children. *Development and Psychopathology, 8,* 141–162.

Eisenberg, N., Fabes, R. A., Murphy, B., Maszk, P., Smith, M., & Karbon, M. (1995). The role of emotionality and regulation in children's social functioning: A longitudinal study. *Child Development, 66,* 1360–1384.

Eisenberg, N., Fabes, R. A., & Murphy, B. C. (1996). Parents' reactions to children's negative emotions: Relations to children's social competence and comforting behavior. *Child Development, 67,* 2227–2247.

Eisenberg, N., Fabes, R. A., Nyman, M., Bernzweig, J., & Pinuelas, A. (1994). The relation of emotionality and regulation to preschoolers' anger-related reactions. *Child Development, 65,* 1352–1366.

Eisenberg, N., Fabes, R. A., Shepard, S. A., Guthrie, I., Murphy, B. C., & Reiser, M. (1999). Parental reactions to children's negative emotions: Longitudinal relations to quality of children's social functioning. *Child Development, 70,* 513–534.

Eisenberg, N., Fabes, R. A., Shepard, S. A., Murphy, B. C., Guthrie, I. K., Jones, S., et al. (1997). Contemporaneous and longitudinal prediction of children's social functioning from regulation and emotionality. *Child Development, 68,* 642–664.

Eisenberg, N., Gershoff, E. T., Fabes, R. A., Shepard, S. A., Cumberland, A., Losoya, S., et al. (2001). Mothers' emotional expressivity and children's behavior problems and social competence: Mediation through children's regulation. *Developmental Psychology, 37,* 475–490.

Eisenberg, N., Valiente, C., Morris, A. S., Fabes, R. A., Cumberland, A., Reiser, M., et al. (2003). Longitudinal relations among parental emotional expressivity, children's regulation, and quality of socioemotional function. *Developmental Psychology, 39,* 3–19.

Fabes, R. A., Eisenberg, N., McCormick, S. E., & Wilson, M. S. (1988). Preschoolers' attributions of the situational determinants of others' naturally occurring emotions. *Developmental Psychology, 24,* 376–385.

Fabes, R. A., Eisenberg, N., Nyman, M., & Michealieu, Q. (1991). Young children's appraisal of others spontaneous emotional reactions. *Developmental Psychology, 27,* 858–866.

Feito, J. A. (1997). Children's beliefs about the social consequences of emotional expression. *Dissertation Abstracts International, 59*(03B), 1411.

Garner, P. W. (2003). Child and family correlates of toddlers' emotional and behavioral responses to a mishap. *Infant Mental Health Journal, 24,* 580–596.

Garner, P. W., & Estep, K. M. (2001). Emotional competence, emotion socialization, and young children's peer-related social competence. *Early Education and Development, 12,* 29–48.

Garner, P. W., Jones, D. C., & Miner, J. L. (1994). Social competence among low-income preschoolers: Emotion socialization practices and social cognitive correlates. *Child Development, 65,* 622–637.

Gilliom, M., Shaw, D. S., Beck, J. E., Schonberg, M. A., & Lukon, J. L. (2002). Anger regulation in disadvantaged preschool boys: Strategies, antecedents, and the development of self-control. *Developmental Psychology, 38,* 222–235.

Gnepp, J. (1989). Personalized inferences of emotions and appraisals: Component processes and correlates. *Developmental Psychology, 25,* 277–288.

Gnepp, J., & Chilamkurti, C. (1988). Children's use of personality attributions to predict other people's emotional and behavioral reactions. *Child Development, 59,* 743–754.

Gnepp, J., & Gould, M. E. (1985). The development of personalized inferences: Understanding other people's emotional reactions in light of their prior experiences. *Child Development, 56,* 1455–1464.

Gnepp, J., McKee, E., & Domanic, J. A. (1987). Children's use of situational information to infer emotion: Understanding emotionally equivocal situations. *Developmental Psychology, 23,* 114–123.

Gottman, J. M., Katz, L. F., & Hooven, C. (1997). *Meta-emotion: How families communicate emotionally.* Mahwah, NJ: Erlbaum.

Greenberg, M. T., Domitrovich, C., & Bumbarger, B. (2001). The prevention of mental disorders in school-aged children: Current state of the field. *Prevention & Treatment, 4,* Article 1. http://journals.apa.org/prevention/

Greenberg, M. T., & Snell, J. L. (1997). Brain development and emotional development: The role of teaching in organizing the frontal lobe. In P. Salovey & D. J. Sluyter (Eds.), *Emotional development and emotional intelligence* (pp. 93–119). New York: Basic Books.

Halberstadt, A., Denham, S. A., & Dunsmore, J. (2001). Affective social competence. *Social Development, 10,* 79–119.

Halberstadt, A. G. (1991). Socialization of expressiveness: Family influences in particular and a model in general. In R. S. Feldman & S. Rimé (Eds.), *Fundamentals of emotional expressiveness* (pp. 106–162). Cambridge, UK: Cambridge University Press.

Harter, S., & Whitesell, N. R. (1989). Developmental changes in children's understanding of single, multiple, and blended emotion concepts. In P. Harris & C. Saarni (Eds.), *Children's understanding of emotion* (pp. 81–116). Cambridge, UK: Cambridge University Press.

Honig, A. S. (1999, Spring). Creating a prosocial curriculum. *Montessori LIFE,* pp. 35–37.

Honig, A. S., & Wittmer, D. S. (1996). Helping children become more prosocial: Ideas for classrooms, families, schools, and communities. *Young Children, 51*(2), 62–70.

Howes, C. (1987). Social competence with peers in young children: Developmental sequences. *Developmental Review, 2,* 252–272.

Hughes, C., Dunn, J., & White, A. (1998). Trick or treat?: Uneven understanding of mind and emotion and executive dysfunction in "hard-to-manage" preschoolers. *Journal of Child Psychology and Psychiatry, and Allied Disciplines, 39,* 981–994.

Hyson, M. C. (1994). *The emotional development of young children: Building an emotion-centered curriculum.* New York: Teachers College Press.

Izard, C. E., Fine, S., Schultz, D., Mostow, A., Ackerman, B., & Youngstrom, E. (2001). Emotions knowledge as a predictor of social behavior and academic competence in children at risk. *Psychological Science, 12,* 18–23.

Josephs, I. (1994). Display rule behavior and understanding in preschool children. *Journal of Nonverbal Behavior, 18,* 301–326.

Keogh, B. K. (1992). Temperament and teachers' views of teachability. In W. Carey & S. McDevitt (Eds.), *Prevention and early intervention: Individual differences as risk factors for the mental health of children* (pp. 246–254). New York: Brunner/Mazel.

Kestenbaum, R., & Gelman, S. (1995). Preschool children's identification and understanding of mixed emotions. *Cognitive Development, 10,* 443–458.

Kieras, J. C., Tobin, R. M., & Graziano, W. G. (2003, April). *Effortful control and emotional responses to undesirable gifts.* Paper presented at a meeting of the Society for Research in Child Development, Tampa, FL.

Ladd, G. W., Birch, S. H., & Buhs, E. S. (1999). Children's social and scholastic lives in kindergarten: Related spheres of influence? *Child Development, 70,* 1373–1400.

Ladd, G. W., Kochenderfer, B. J., & Coleman, C. C. (1996). Friendship quality as a predictor of young children's early school adjustment. *Child Development, 67,* 1103–1118.

Lemerise, E. A., & Arsenio, W. F. (2000). An integrated model of emotion processes and cognition in social information processing. *Child Development, 71,* 107–118.

Lemerise, E. A., & Dodge, K. A. (2000). The development of anger and hostile interactions. In M. Lewis & J. M. Haviland-Jones (Eds.), *Handbook of emotions* (2nd ed., pp. 594–606). New York: Guilford Press.

Lewis, M., Alessandri, S. M., & Sullivan, M. W. (1992). Differences in shame and pride as a function of children's gender and task difficulty. *Child Development, 63*, 630–638.

Lewis, M., Stanger, C., & Sullivan, M. E. (1989). Deception in three-year-olds. *Developmental Psychology, 25*, 439–443.

Martin, R. P., Drew, D., Gaddis, L. R., & Moseley, M. (1988). Prediction of elementary school achievement from preschool temperament: Three studies. *School Psychology Review, 17*, 125–137.

Miller, A. L., & Olson, S. L. (2000). Emotional expressiveness during peer conflicts: A predictor of social maladjustment among high-risk preschoolers. *Journal of Abnormal Child Psychology, 28*, 339–352.

Miller, P. H., & Aloise, P. A. (1989). Young children's understanding of the psychological causes of behavior: A review. *Child Development, 60*, 257–285.

Mize, J., & Cox, R. A. (1990). Social knowledge and social competence: Number and quality of strategies as predictors of peer behavior. *Journal of Genetic Psychology, 151*, 117–127.

Morrison, E. F., Rimm-Kauffman, S., & Pianta, R. C. (2003). A longitudinal study of mother–child interaction at school entry and social and academic outcomes in middle school. *Journal of School Psychology, 41*, 185–200.

Murphy, B. C., Shepard, S., Eisenberg, N., Fabes, R. A., & Guthrie, I. K. (1999). Contemporaneous and longitudinal relations of dispositional sympathy to emotionality, regulation, and social functioning. *Journal of Early Adolescence, 19*, 66–97.

Nunner-Winkler, G., & Sodian, B. (1988). Children's understanding of moral emotions. *Child Development, 59*, 1323–1338.

Palinsin, H. A. (1986). Preschool temperament and performance on achievement tests. *Developmental Psychology, 22*, 766–770.

Park, K. A., Lay, K., & Ramsay, L. (1993). Individual differences and developmental changes in preschoolers' friendships. *Developmental Psychology, 29*, 264–270.

Parker, J. G., & Gottman, J. M. (1989). Social and emotional development in a relational context: Friendship interaction from early childhood to adolescence. In T. J. Berndt & G. W. Ladd (Eds.), *Peer relationships in child development* (pp. 95–131). New York: Wiley.

Payton, J. W., Wardlaw, D. M., Graczyk, P. A., Bloodworth, M. R., Tompsett, C. J., & Weissberg, R. P. (2000). Social and emotional learning: A framework for promoting mental health and reducing risk behaviors in children and youth. *Journal of School Health, 70*(5), 179–185.

Peng, M., Johnson, C. N., Pollock, J., Glasspool, R., & Harris, P. L. (1992). Training young children to acknowledge mixed emotions. *Cognition and Emotion, 6*, 387–401.

Pettit, G. S., Dodge, K. A., & Brown, M. M. (1988). Early family experience, social problem solving patterns, and children's social competence. *Child Development, 59*, 107–120.

Raver, C. C., Blackburn, E. K., Bancroft, M., & Torp, M. (1999). Relations between effective emotional self-regulation, attentional control, and low-income preschoolers' social competence with peers. *Early Education and Development, 10*, 333–350.

Roberts, W. R., & Strayer, J. A. (1996). Empathy, emotional expressiveness, and prosocial behavior. *Child Development, 67*, 449–470.

Robins, L. N., & Rutter, M. (1990). *Straight and devious pathways from childhood to adulthood.* Cambridge, UK: Cambridge University Press.

Roff, J. D. (1990). Childhood peer rejection as a predictor of young adults' mental health. *Psychological Reports, 67*, 1263–1266.

Rozek, M. K. (1987). Preschoolers' understanding of display rules for emotional expression. *Dissertation Abstracts International, 47*(12B), 5076.

Rubin, K. H., & Clark, M. L. (1983). Preschool teachers' ratings of behavioral problems: Observational, sociometric, and social-cognitive correlates. *Journal of Abnormal Child Psychology, 11*, 273–286.

Rubin, K. H., & Daniels-Beirness, T. (1983). Concurrent and predictive correlates of sociometric status in kindergarten and grade 1 children. *Merrill–Palmer Quarterly, 29,* 337–352.

Rydell, A.-M., Berlin, L., & Bohlin, G. (2003). Emotionality, emotion regulation, and adaptation among 5- to 8-year-old children. *Emotion, 3,* 30–47.

Saarni, C. (1999). *Children's emotional competence.* New York: Guilford Press.

Schultz, D., Izard, C. E., & Ackerman, B. P. (2000). Children's anger attribution bias: Relations to family environment and social adjustment. *Social Development, 9,* 284–301.

Schultz, D., Izard, C. E., Ackerman, B. P., & Youngstrom, E. A. (2001). Emotion knowledge in economically disadvantaged children: Self-regulatory antecedents and relations to social difficulties and withdrawal. *Development and Psychopathology, 13,* 53–67.

Shonkoff, J. P., & Phillips, D. A. (2000). *From neurons to neighborhoods: The science of early childhood development.* Washington, DC: National Academy Press.

Smith, M. (2001). Social and emotional competencies: Contributions to young African-American children's peer acceptance. *Early Education and Development, 12,* 49–72.

Sroufe, L. A., Schork, E., Motti, F., Lawroski, N., & LaFreniere, P. (1984). The role of affect in social competence. In C. E. Izard, J. Kagan, & R. B. Zajonc (Eds.), *Emotions, cognition, and behavior* (pp. 289–319). Cambridge, UK: Cambridge University Press.

Strayer, J. (1980). A naturalistic study of empathic behaviors and their relation to affective states and perspective-taking skills in preschool children. *Child Development, 51,* 815–822.

Strayer, J., & Roberts, W. (1997). Facial and verbal measures of children's emotions and empathy. *International Journal of Behavioral Development, 20*(4), 627–649.

Strayer, J., & Roberts, W. (2004a). Children's anger, emotional expressiveness, and empathy: Relations with parents' empathy, emotional expressiveness, and parenting practices. *Social Development, 13,* 229–254.

Strayer, J., & Roberts, W. (2004b). Empathy and observed anger and aggression in five-year-olds. *Social Development, 13,* 1–13.

Thompson, R. A. (1994). Emotion regulation: A theme in search of definition. *Monographs of the Society for Research in Child Development, 59*(2–3, Serial No. 240), 25–52.

Walter, J. L. (2002). *The emergence of the capacity for guilt in preschoolers: The role of personal responsibility in differentiating shame from guilt.* Eugene, OR: University Microfilms International.

Weissberg, R. P., & Greenberg, M. T. (Eds.). (1998). *Child psychology in practice: Vol 4. School and community competence-enhancement and prevention programs* (5th ed.). New York: Wiley.

3

Cognitive Development

AMY K. HEFFELFINGER and CHRISTINE MRAKOTSKY

Understanding a child's cognitive abilities and development is essential for accurate mental health diagnosis, especially during the preschool age. This is important in the context of two main positions. First, the development of cognitive abilities is typically tightly connected with the development of emotional and behavioral regulation (Bell & Wolfe, 2004); in that sense, a 3-year-old with the cognitive ability level (or mental age) of a 2-year-old is also likely to regulate behaviors and emotions like a 2-year-old, which has major implications for not only this child's cognitive but also his or her socioemotional development. Second, although research on the neuropsychological correlates of preschool psychopathology is sparse, older children and adults with psychiatric problems are at increased risk for specific neuropsychological difficulties. It is likely that psychopathology-specific cognitive impairments are also present in the preschool years. To determine whether a preschooler has specific cognitive difficulties, however, it is essential first to understand "typical" cognitive development.

GENERAL VERSUS SPECIFIC AREAS OF COGNITIVE FUNCTIONING

The definition of "cognition," or intelligence, has been widely debated for years and is generally based on the mature individual. Initially, intelligence was considered a unitary variable, which increased as a singular trajectory in childhood (Binet & Simon, 1908; Terman, 1916). As neuropsychological research, particularly lesion studies, revealed that certain types and locations of brain injury resulted in specific rather than global impairment in aspects of intellectual functioning, the view that general intelligence actually comprises several specific classes of intellectual functioning was adopted (Lezak, 1983).

Intelligence is viewed as stable throughout life. However, because early developmental abilities are not stable throughout the first years of life and are not predictive of future intelligence, the expression of these abilities is often referred to as "cognition." Cognition, the process of reasoning and knowing facts, is assessable in the preschool years, and includes the increasing knowledge base regarding facts (grass is green) and physical processes (gravity) in the world. Cognition subsumes both verbal and nonverbal abilities, including both problem-solving and factual knowledge. Verbal cognitive abilities refer to knowledge of verbal facts and verbal reasoning. In infants, verbal skills emerge with the development of receptive and expressive language. Nonverbal abilities typically refer to perceptual reasoning and spatial construction abilities. By definition, they should not require verbal processing or knowledge. Visual perception is demonstrated when a preschool child is capable of recognizing, matching, selecting, or differentiating objects with cognitive similarities, such as by color, shape, or size.

Neuropsychology further classifies functioning into specific ability domains based on underlying brain systems, including sensory, motor, attention, executive, language, visual spatial, and memory systems as separate but interrelated abilities. Most adults have fairly commensurate abilities across domains accented by relative strengths and weaknesses. It is believed that this is also true for children.

DEVELOPMENT OF SPECIFIC NEUROPSYCHOLOGICAL ABILITIES

Normative early development is characterized by the acquisition of age-appropriate skills within each specific cognitive domain and a steep developmental trajectory that occurs throughout the first 5 years of life. Understanding what is considered "normative" across these ages will help in determining (1) whether a child needs an evaluation and (2) whether a child's developmental level explains his or her behavior and emotional functioning. Well-intentioned parents, teachers, and medical professionals often consider a child developmentally delayed in the face of age-appropriate skills. More concerning, however, is the reverse, when true delays go undetected and untreated because of poor awareness of typical development. In this section, expected normative development of preschoolers is discussed.

Sensory Perception

Basic sensory perception, including hearing and vision, is paramount to the development of higher cortical functions. Neural systems that mediate the basic senses primarily develop prenatally through the first months of life. In fact, newborns possess the basic skills needed to perceive sights, sounds, taste, smell, and touch (for general reviews, see Spreen, Risser, & Edgell, 1995 and Nelson & Luciana, 2001). The auditory system is functional several weeks before birth, and newborns crudely localize sounds and recognize familiar sounds, with a preference for voices (Aslin & Hunt, 2001; Hecox & Burkard, 1982). All areas of auditory perception improve dramatically in the first 6 months of life, with adult-like pitch perception emerging by about 7 months (Clarkson & Clifton, 1985) but temporal perception not reaching maturity until at least the preschool years (Whiteman, Allen, Dolan, Kistler, & Jamieson, 1989).

Development of the visual systems has been studied extensively and is reviewed in detail elsewhere (Dannemiller, 2001). At birth, infants can rudimentarily perceive and orient to visual objects, reflecting basic shape and color discrimination that appears to be functional shortly following a full-term birth (Atkinson, Hood, Wattam-Bell, Anker, & Tricklebank, 1988; Dannemiller, 2001; Johnson, 1990). Newborns also can differentiate human faces (Morton & Johnson, 1991). The ability to perceive movement develops 6 to 8 weeks post-gestation (Wattam-Bell, 1991), and depth perception emerges around age 3 to 4 months (Birch, Gwiazda, & Held, 1982). In general, basic sensory perception matures in the first 6–10 months of life, setting the foundation for higher-level cognitive development to occur that requires these basic perceptual abilities.

If a child is *not* developing typically, abnormal sensory perceptual ability can be misperceived as symptoms of psychopathology. For example, a language delay, along with "not responding to one's name" is a common symptom of autism but could also result from an inability to hear. If a child cannot see, then nonverbal/perceptual ability will not develop in its regular trajectory, because the blind child's exploration of and experience with the world around him or her is very different from that of the seeing child. Similarly, deafness alters the course of the development of language. Absence of a particular sensory perception requires specific and intensive intervention to promote holistic development despite atypical sensory input.

Heightened perception of sensory stimulation, often associated with temperamental patterns, is called sensory integration disorder and decreases the child's willingness to explore the environment and novelty. This difficulty with regulating sensory input is often mistaken as the primary cause of developmental disorders, rather than as an early presenting symptom, or by-product, of atypical neural development.

Motor Skills

Basic gross motor skills, referring to ambulation and posture, often serve as a general marker for overall development. All children, however, do not acquire motor skills at the same age. Rather, there is a normative age range in which children tend to develop these skills. For example, 12 months is considered the milestone to begin walking, with the majority of children beginning to walk between the ages of 9 and 15 months. Parents are usually asked about other milestones, too, such as when their child first rolled over, sat without support, and ran. By the preschool period, gross motor abilities are highly developed, with running, jumping, and balancing usually occurring by age 2–3 years. Table 3.1 delineates the target date for several gross motor milestones.

Fine motor ability, referring to "small" motor activities such as writing and cutting, is not as easy for parents to report as gross motor skills. At 1 year of age, infants can usually pick up items with either a full-hand grasp or a pincer grasp with the thumb and forefinger. They tend to be able to use a spoon, take objects out of containers, and put one or two items back into a container with a large opening. By 2 years of age, most children consistently use a pincer grasp, can put simple shapes into shape sorters and form boards, and can place pennies into a bank oriented horizontally. By 3 years of age, the range of age-appropriate skills becomes quite broad. Many children can now draw two to three simple shapes, complete interlocking puzzles that have a border, use scissors to cut on paper, use a fork and knife for some foods, and manipulate a penny into a slot from any direction. However, some typically developing children do not achieve these skills until the end of the third year. Also during age 3–4 years, children's activities require increased visual–motor integration, or the ability to integrate what is seen with motor output, such as tracing, coloring, and drawing.

Attention

Attention encompasses the ability to direct, sustain, and select attentional focus (Posner & Petersen, 1990). The primary variables of interest include inattentiveness and distractibility, sustained attention or ability to focus attention to task, and impulsivity or acting without thinking. Directing and disengaging attention, the basic components of attention, develop to qualitatively adultlike like levels by 4 months of age (Johnson, Posner, & Rothbart, 1991). These skills are evident in infants being able to attend to faces, voices, and the environment, and are necessary for the optimal development of attachment and cognition. Distractibility, or the process of attention being disengaged from a task and directed elsewhere, is a normative behavior. At about 3 months of age, babies experience a stage called "obligatory looking," in which they are able to focus attention but have a difficult time being distracted or disengaged (Johnson, 1990). This stage is brief, because distractibility develops more over time to allow infants to explore their environment. Being highly distractible, however, is not typical, and eventually results in impaired ability to focus on activities that require sustained attention, such as eating, listening to instructions or stories, watching television programs, and completing activities of daily living, such as dressing or cleaning up toys. Level of distractibility diminishes rapidly in the first 6 months of life and then more gradually (Ruff & Capozzoli, 2003).

Sustained attention clearly improves throughout infancy and early childhood, both quantitatively and qualitatively (Ruff & Lawson, 1990). Sustained attention can be categorized into three mutually exclusive types of

TABLE 3.1. Range of Months of Typical Acquisition of Motor Milestones

Months	Gross motor	Fine motor
1–2	Holds head.	
3–5	Rolls over in one direction.	Brings rattle to mouth.
5–8	Sits with support.	Grasps with thumb/finger.
8–15	Walks.	Puts toys in.
15–21	Runs.	Builds two-block tower.
20–28	Jumps.	Grasps small things.
30–36	Climbs stairs unassisted.	Draws two objects.

sustained attention: (1) *casual attention*, looking but not being engaged; (2) *settled attention*, a pause from casual attention to engage a stimulus; and (3) *focused attention*, concentrated attention often associated with a reduction in motor movement and vocalizations (Ruff, Capozzoli, & Weissberg, 1998; Ruff & Capozzoli, 2003). Between ages 2 and 3½ years, the amount of time spent attending to stimuli casually, without clearly focusing, declines, whereas the more "settled" and "focused" attention consistently increases from ages 1–3½ years (Ruff & Capozzoli, 2003). Demonstration of focused attention, the highest level of sustained attention, is, however, relatively low at ages 1 and 2 years, with a substantial increase occurring between ages 2 and 3½ years. By the age of 4 years, attentional systems, highly governed by goal-directed behavior and impulse control, can mediate highly focused attention to tasks or activity. For example, enjoyment of play, completion of tasks, and following rules are often important goals for preschool children (Ruff & Capozzoli, 2003).

It is also important to note that distractibility and sustained attention are interrelated. Children are easily distracted during the casual phase of sustained attention but are less distractible with increased sustained attention in the focused attention phase. This phenomenon is apparent throughout infancy and childhood, and suggests that focused sustained attention reflects a state that makes young children less responsive to distractions (Richards & Cronise, 2000; Richards & Turner, 2001; Ruff & Capozzoli, 2003).

Executive Functions

"Executive functions" is an umbrella term for a wide range of regulatory and metacognitive functions that have as their core the ability to plan, organize, and control behaviors (Pennington & Ozonoff, 1996). Vygotsky and Luria suggested many years ago that language acquires directive functions that allow young children to organize and plan their behaviors (Luria, 1961; Vygotsky, 1934/1962; Zelazo, 1999). Clinical neuropsychologists have assumed that these skills do not begin to develop until early school age, but a surge of research suggests that executive functions begin to develop in the first years of life and continue to develop slowly into adulthood (Diamond, 1991; Espy, Kaufman, McDiarmid, & Glisky, 1999; Gerstadt, Hong, & Diamond, 1994; Rothbart & Posner, 2001). During the preschool age, the rapid development of three skills areas is of particular importance: (1) rule learning and following; (2) flexibility; and (3) novel problem solving.

Rules are consistently learned during the first years of life. Some of them are inherent to a task or to the environment, such as rules about gravity and size, and are acquired by attending to the environment. Other rules have to be taught, including those about appropriate behaviors specific to situations. It is widely acknowledged that by 8 to 12 months of age, infants are capable of understanding basic rule concepts, and their memory can support remembering these rules at least briefly over time. For example, at this age, infants understand object permanence, remembering that an object of interest still exists if it is hidden or out of sight (Piaget, 1954). Between ages 2 and 3 years, children can learn to search in alternating patterns for a reward, relying on their memory for the alternation rule and for the place the rewards have been hidden previously (Espy et al., 1999). In the fourth year, children are able to learn two rules that interfere with previously learned rules and apply those to their behavior (Diamond & Taylor, 1996). An example of this is playing Simon Says. As this skill is developing, there is an amazing and often exasperating phase wherein a child can verbalize the rules but cannot apply them to behavior, demonstrating a disparate skill level between impulse control and cognitive knowledge. Siegler (1998) demonstrated that 4- to 6-year-olds are only able to apply one rule to a problem. Once children are able to learn and follow several new rules for one problem, they begin to develop the ability to switch between competing rule sets based on an additional rule. For example, if the sign says "go," red = stop and green = go, but if the sign says "stop," red = go and green = stop. This ability to switch readily between rule sets appears to develop in the fifth and sixth years (Frye, Zelazo, & Palfai, 1995).

The example just described also represents the increase in flexibility of behaviors as a child approaches school age. "Flexibility" refers to the ability to switch between various rules, behaviors, and routines with little preparation or emotional distress. It develops throughout childhood and into adulthood (Siegler, 1998), but it is now clear that it develops at more basic levels in preschool age. Flexibility, also viewed as an aspect of temperament, is essential for children's experiential learning, behaving adaptively as they enter school, and functioning more independently.

Earlier in the preschool years, around ages 2 and 3 years, being "perseverative," or needing to repeat certain behaviors, is often adaptive. During this stage, children thrive on watching the same television program, hearing the same songs, reading the same books; and they happily repeat them frequently. Although these behaviors may bore the adults or siblings involved, they promote the child's learning of these events. In the same manner, this is the age where having a tendency to perseverate on behaviors is useful for developing the young child's routines, such as the order of steps in toileting or brushing teeth. Around age 4 years, many preschool children become more flexible and require less repetition. This skill likely develops in conjunction with increased ability to learn quickly and follow new rules, and facilitates the remarkable amounts of new cognitive skills that children acquire in this later preschool period.

Finally, novel problem solving develops at a rapid trajectory during the preschool period. Problem solving requires several processes to attain the final goal, including planning, analogical reasoning, causal inference, tool use, scientific reasoning, and deductive reasoning (Siegler, 1998). Between ages 1 and 2 years, it is often evident that infants struggle to think in novel ways but do intend to try to solve problems. They approach tasks in the same way over and over, even if it does not work. For example, they can easily place objects into the top of a container (Diamond, 1991). If the container is turned on its side, the infant is typically not able to place objects in it, because the opening is now on the side. By age 2 years, children are able to generate several solutions to this simple search problem. Another example presented by a 2-year-old's parent regarded the child's strategy to get to the other side of a gate in their house. The little boy first took a stool and placed it on the other side of the gate, then proceeded to turn a toy on its side on his side of the gate. He then stepped on the toy, over the gate, onto the stool, and he was free! Furthermore, complex pretend play often represents underlying novelty, especially as the preschooler is acting out different endings to the same scenario. The abilities to learn and apply rules, to be flexible, and to engage in novel problem solving are present and established by the end of the preschool period, allowing for higher-order executive functions to develop during the school years.

Language

Language includes the abilities to understand spoken language (receptive language), use words to express oneself (expressive language), and to understand and use nonverbal social communication and pragmatics. From shortly after birth, neonates respond differently to speech versus nonspeech sounds (Dehaene-Lambertz, 2000). It appears that the auditory perceptual system is set up, in part, to focus on speech and on the native language. Although this preference is at least partially experience driven, the human brain is structured such that the development of speech perception occurs early and can then be finely tuned through neural development and experience to gain language (Werker & Vouloumanos, 2001).

Expressive language typically develops in a predictable set of steps, regardless of whether a child develops spoken language earlier or later within the expected time frame, from around 4–8 months through 18–30 months. Most infants begin to make cooing sounds (vowel sounds) first; then they begin to make single-syllable consonant–vowel sounds (i.e., *da*). Sounds made are typically an expression of their state and an exploration of sounds, but individual utterances do not have a singular meaning. Next, they begin to use "reduplicate babbling," or the repetition of consonant–vowel sounds (*dada*) and other word-like sounds. It is important for professionals to recognize that this does not represent the infant's first word, because it likely does not yet contain meaning. Shortly thereafter, the first word appears, and it is often the same as one of the commonly used consonant–vowel sounds, such as *dada* when looking at the father (11–13 months). At this time, the single word is used to label and to communicate. From here, the infant typically develops a set of consistently used nouns, usually referring to very important people (*mama, dada, nana*) and objects (*ball, juice, bottle*). These first words are unstable and will likely come and go from use until the vocabulary reaches about 10 words. Next there is a gradual and steady building of vocabulary to about 50–75 words. Often consistent with the increase in vocabulary, the young child begins to use two to three phrases that contain nouns and verbs. Then, the explosion in vocabulary typically occurs, increasing average vocabulary to about 300 words at 24 months and 500 words by 30 months (Fenson et al., 1994). Table 3.2 presents a general list of language milestones.

Grammar also experiences a burst in development between ages 20 and 36 months (Bates & Roe, 2001; Fenson et al., 1994). Young children tend to speak in complete sentences, but they make many grammatical and syntactical errors. In fact, sometime between two and three years of age, children often speak using correct verb tenses and adjectives, only to be followed by 1–2 years of using them incorrectly. As a child first learns to use sentences, the sentences are often used as rote strings of words, with the same words used in the same sequence. For example, a 2-year-old may say, "Daddy went to work" and "I am going to school," both of which are used regularly in correct syntactical form. At this age, however, the child tends not to create novel sentences. When children begin to put new sentences together from thoughts, they have to practice word rules, such as past, present, and future tense. During this time, the child often misuses verbs, particularly those with irregular tense, in order to follow the most general language rules, such as "Daddy goed to work." This does not reflect a regression, but rather a perseveration to the basic, concrete rules of language. Also around age 3, children develop increased fluency, including coarticulation, when children anticipate the next utterance and move the mouth in position on an earlier speech sound. By the time a child is 4 years old, most expressive language is developed and used appropriately (Bates & Roe, 2001). From ages 4–6 years, children begin to use sentences that are clearly connected to the other sentences around it (Bates & Roe, 2001).

The other primary components of language are receptive and pragmatic language, which will only be discussed briefly here. Although a newborn can recognize the parents' voices at birth, this reflects sound perception and social recognition, not processing of language meaning. Receptive language develops in conjunction with expressive language, although the ability to understand word meanings develops slightly earlier than ability to use them. Under-

TABLE 3.2. Range of Months of Typical Acquisition of Language Milestones

Months	Expressive language	Receptive language
5–9	Makes and mimics sounds.	Responds to "No."
10–14	Utters single words, mimics single words.	Follows "Give me the . . . " and "Show me" commands.
15–21	Says 10 words and first two- to three-word phrases.	Identifies body parts, follows one-step commands.
21–27	Says some three-word sentences and questions.	Follows commands that include prepositions.
27–33	Uses pronouns and prepositions.	Understands adjectives, pronouns, and prepositions.
33–39	Answers logical questions.	Understands negatives.

standing of actual single words begins at around 8–10 months, followed by an explosion of single-word, receptive vocabulary over the next 6–12 months (Fenson et al., 1994). Prior to saying two- to three-word phrases, and later sentences, a child can understand their meaning. Comprehension of grammar and syntax develops in the 3- to 4-year time period.

"Pragmatic language" refers to the ability to communicate based on knowledge and awareness of basic social and cultural norms (i.e., greeting) and "social-inferential language" refers to ability to use and perceive puns, sarcasm, and jokes (Bates & Roe, 2001). According to Vygotsky (1934/ 1962), it is the exposure to social practices and interactions that precedes language, and particularly pragmatic language, development. Both pragmatic language and social-inferential language rely to some degree on more subtle social cognition. There is limited research on the development of these abilities in preschoolers, but they clearly begin to develop during this period. Use of socially appropriate greetings begins toward the end of the first year by infants waving appropriately as someone approaches or departs. Young preschoolers can already find humor or mixed meaning in communication involving highly exaggerated facial movements and voice intonation, but sarcasm and jokes confuse them, because their minds are still anchored in very literal thinking. Also, young preschoolers can often understand metaphors using concrete objects, such as "You are as fast as a car," but cannot understand metaphors using higher conceptual concepts, such as "You are as fast as the wind." Development of such social language skills involves not only basic language skills but also social and cognitive skills.

Visual–Spatial Abilities

Visual–spatial abilities describe a wide range of skills such as object recognition, recognition and copying of two-dimensional designs, and actual localization, navigation, and rotation in space. The first "spatial" abilities to emerge in infancy are those linked with the concept of objects and their localization in space. In his stage theory, Piaget (1952) suggested that infants do not differentiate between space and their own actions in the space during the first 4 months. The infant does not yet distinguish between changes in position and changes in state; thus, he or she does not yet understand positions of objects. Following this, at around 4 to 8 months, the infant begins to observe his or her own actions, and through coordination of vision is able to understand rudimentarily the existence of external objects. Objects are assigned positions in space but are still dependent on self-reference. For example, the infant does not search for an object hidden under a cover, indicating that the object's position is only related to a subject and not to other objects. Concepts of space and objects develop further toward the end of the first year (8–12 months). The emergence of searching for a hidden object is critical; that is, the child is now able to watch an object being hidden and retrieve the object from the place of hiding. Besides the implication for the emergence of object permanence, this new ability is seen as a significant factor of understanding spatial relations. From ages 12 to 18 months, infants are able to view space in an objective manner, separating objects from their activities. They are, however, not yet able to understand their own position in space, but begin to gain this experience and knowledge through their increasing mobility and exploration of space. At this age, infants are only able to search for hidden objects when they can actually see the place of hiding. Toward the end of the second year (18–24 months), they become increasingly able to solve invisible displacement of objects (without seeing the place of hiding) and also become aware of their own position in space.

From about 1 to 4 years of age, spatial perception and constructional abilities develop rapidly. At about 12 months, children are able to build a tower of two blocks and place circle pieces into a formboard, reflecting early understanding of spatial concepts. Next children can build higher towers, place several shapes in formboards, and scribble with a crayon. During the third year, more complex constructional skills emerge, with the building of basic three-dimensional structures. Children can then discriminate visual–spatial differences in patterns and size. Later, in the preschool age, children are able to build complex block structures, both from their imagination and by copying, such as houses or even cities. They can also draw several shapes and possibly even some letters in the fourth year of life.

The ability to draw and copy more complex designs depends on planning and organization abilities but is also highly related to the ability to judge the angulation and orientation of lines, which together contribute to the construct "visual–spatial abilities." At age 4–5 years, preschoolers are well able to copy simple patterns and identify, draw, and walk oblique lines (Rudel, Holmes, & Pardes, 1988), reflecting the understanding of spatial relations. At this age children are also able to construct configurational maps of familiar areas, and right–left discrimination is emerging. All of these are related to the later, more advanced spatial abilities.

Memory Abilities

Memory and learning are the basic fundaments of a child's cognitive development and later achievement. Memory abilities include short-term memory span, immediate and delayed recall of information, and recognition of information. In children, the ability to encode and recall novel information is essential for cognitive development. Short-term memory, referring to events that occurred in the recent past, usually involves recall within seconds or minutes of exposure. One way to assess this is to have a child repeat a series of digits. At about 4 years old, a child can recall two to three items, but a 12-year-old can recall about six digits (Gathercole, 1998). Subvocal rehearsing is a strategy commonly used by older children, but it is not used by preschool children without coaching. In all areas of short-term memory, including visual–spatial and auditory information, there is a steep and linear increase in short-term memory ability that does not reach adult-like levels until middle school age.

A preexplicit, or predeclarative, memory exists in infants as young as 2 months, as demonstrated on recognition memory tasks in which infants look longer at familiar faces and objects (Nelson, 1994; Nelson & Xu, 1995; Nelson, 1997). Adult-like declarative memory begins to emerge at around 1 year and long-term storage at around 2 years of age (Nelson, 1997). The declarative memory system then matures throughout the preschool years (Gathercole, 1998; Luciana & Nelson, 1998) and childhood. Although preschool children are limited by immature memory strategies, their rapid acquisition of cognitive concepts and vocabulary demonstrates functional, and in some respects, advanced, declarative memory abilities. Memory continues to be a neglected set of skills in assessment during the preschool period. Although it is logical that these skills underlie all knowledge and skills growth during childhood, it remains unclear whether memory skills are predictive of future abilities.

INTERRELATIONSHIPS OF NEUROPSYCHOLOGICAL FUNCTIONS

It is essential to recognize that neuropsychological functions are interrelated and likely have a hierarchical relationship with each other. Traditional neuropsychological assessment of adults within the Boston process approach emphasized that basic functions, such as sensory and motor, are necessary for successful performance of higher-order skills, including executive and language (Kaplan, 1988). From early in gestation, functional systems of the brain are developing together, relying on shared trophic growth factors, genetic factors, and experiences. Although interconnected, however, these functional neural systems are based on unique neural networks, each with individual timelines for development (Johnson, 2003). Understanding a child's neuropsychological abilities, then, requires both awareness of the independence of the functional systems and acknowledgment of the interdependency of these functions.

For example, sensory and motor skills need to be grossly intact for accurate assessment of all other abilities. A person who has limited vision cannot complete visual attention tasks, and a person who has spastic diplegia affecting his or her upper extremities will not be able to complete visual spatial tasks requiring fast hand–eye coordination. Consistent deployment of attention is needed to complete successfully tasks of all areas of functioning, especially including executive functioning, language, visual–spatial, and memory tasks. Spatial perception heavily depends on the intact development of visual, attention, and orienting systems, which go hand in hand with the development of planning, problem solving, and visual–motor integration behaviors.

Finally, a child's level of functioning results from a combination of three factors: the brain, the child's context, and development (Bernstein, 2000). Other theories of the basis for assessment have included primary focus on the development or the brain but have not integrated knowledge of developmental principles, environment, and neural systems (Taylor & Fletcher, 1990; Rourke, 1989). In Bernstein's (2000) theory, each factor has to be considered when thinking about each individual child. The brain is owned by the child and is his or her organ of learning. It accounts for all aspects of this child's functioning. Neural systems, however, operate within the "context" of the individual. This context includes all aspects of the child at that time in life: demographic, emotional, and situational. The child's brain and context cannot adequately be understood without equal consideration of "development." Bernstein states, "The cardinal feature of the child is that he or she is developing" (p. 425). Understanding the child's developmental trajectory within functional systems, including current and previous repertoire of skills, is essential. Because of the high rate of developmental progress during the preschool years, specific neuropsychological functions, as well as the underlying neural systems and the child's environment, are constantly changing.

SUMMARY

In summary, when working with a preschool child with possible developmental, behavioral and emotional problems, it is essential to have a gross understanding of his or her cognitive functioning, environment, and history of developmental milestones. First of all, delayed cognitive development may reflect global delays that have resulted in slowed development of emotional and behavioral control. Second, understanding a child's specific strengths and weaknesses in cognitive functioning may help to explain the concerning symptoms. For example, a child with higher cognitive and language abilities but lower attention and executive functions is likely to have difficulty controlling impulsive behavior despite complete understanding of the inappropriateness of the behavior. Table 3.3 provides a list of domain-specific functions

TABLE 3.3. Indications for Neuropsychological Testing

12 months	24 months	36 months	48 months

Sensory perception

(At all ages) Vision as evidenced by attending to objects near and far.
Differentiate colors by matching. Hearing as evidenced by orienting to environmental sounds and soft voices, especially own name, names like Mama, and objects like "cookie" or "ball."

Motor

12 months	24 months	36 months	48 months
Sit without support, pick up small objects like a Cheerio, reach and bang at midline.	Walk independently and smoothly, feed self with spoon.	Use stairs with same foot first on each step; jump; use coordinated pincer grasp; draw single shape.	Pedal, run smoothly, draw several shapes, dress self, easily insert pennies into banks.

Attention

12 months	24 months	36 months	48 months
Focus on visual objects, novel sounds, and touch as evidenced by change in motor activity.	Stop momentarily to focus on a single object during exploration or play.	Focus attention for at least 5 minutes on single play activity (not only TV and computer).	Focus attention for at least 10 minutes on single play activity (not only TV and computer).

Executive

12 months	24 months	36 months	48 months
Look for desired object that has been hidden, lost, or moved within moments of disappearance.	Generate solutions to search tasks, even if the task is altered or oriented differently.	Use single rule to sort or match, inhibit briefly from taking candy, toy, present.	Follow two-step rule games such as Red Light–Green Light, inhibit behavioral impulses in games like Don't Spill the Beans.

Language

12 months	24 months	36 months	48 months
Make consonant–vowel sounds, understand own name.	Use vocabulary of 20 words; identify body parts, common objects; follow one-step commands.	Comprehend two- to three-word phrases; use vocabulary of 300 words.	Ask and answer questions; use several sentences to express thoughts; use vocabulary of 500 words.

Visual–spatial

12 months	24 months	36 months	48 months
Take objects out of container, drop objects on purpose.	Place circle in formboard.	Complete shape formboard.	Complete interlocking puzzles of at least six pieces.

Note. If a child is *not* performing skills at the age listed, then the parent may want to consult the pediatrician regarding referral.

that a child should be able to perform at each age. If a child cannot perform these functions, then the parent may want to consult the pediatrician regarding a possible referral for a neuropsychological evaluation.

One final caution is also important to emphasize. Each of these specific functions is undergoing its own development, and the trajectory for these functions can differ widely within one individual and even more so between individuals. A child having one area of functioning that is slightly delayed could very well be normative, just as having one area developing faster than that of peers could also be normative. Parents often worry if their child is developing slowly in a particular area. These parents will be assured to know that slightly delayed development does not mean long-term delays, and the delay is likely not problematic if it is an isolated difficulty. On the other hand, if a preschool child is delayed in more than one area, such as not walking or talking by the end of the second year, then an evaluation to help determine etiologies and appropriate educational and therapy services is strongly advised. Similarly, if a preschool child is having difficulties functioning due to concerning behaviors and emotions, and also has specific or global cognitive difficulties, an evaluation is warranted.

REFERENCES

Aslin, R. N., & Hunt, R. H. (2001). Development, plasticity, and learning in the auditory system. In C. Nelson & M. Luciana (Eds.), *Handbook of developmental cognitive neuroscience* (pp. 205–220). Cambridge, MA: MIT Press.

Atkinson, H., Hood, B., Wattam-Bell, J., Anker, S., & Tricklebank, J. (1988). Development of orientation discrimination in infancy. *Perception, 17,* 587–595.

Bates, E., & Roe, K. (2001). Language development in children with unilateral brain injury. In C. Nelson & M. Luciana (Eds.), *Handbook of developmental cognitive neuroscience* (pp. 281–308). Cambridge, MA: MIT Press.

Bell, M. A., & Wolfe, C. D. (2004). Emotion and cognition: An intricately bound developmental process. *Child Development, 75,* 366–370.

Bernstein, J. H. (2000). Developmental neuropsychology assessment. In K. O. Yeates, M. D. Ris, & H. G. Taylor (Eds.), *Pediatric neuropsychology: Research, theory, and practice* (pp. 405–438). New York: Guilford Press.

Binet, A., & Simon, T. (1908). Le development de l'intelligence chez les enfants [The development of intelligence in children]. *L'Année Psychologique, 14,* 1–94.

Birch, E., Gwiazda, J., & Held, R. (1982). Stereoacuity development for crossed and uncrossed disparities in human infants. *Vision Research, 22,* 507–513.

Clarkson, M. G., & Clifton, R. K. (1985). Infant pitch perception: Evidence for responding to pitch categories and the missing fundamental. *Journal of the Acoustic Society of America, 77,* 1521–1528.

Dannemiller, J. L. (2001). Brain–behavioral relationships in early visual development. In C. Nelson & M. Luciana (Eds.), *Handbook of developmental cognitive neuroscience* (pp. 221–236). Cambridge, MA: MIT Press.

Dehaene-Lambertz, G. (2000). Cerebral specialization for speech and non-speech stimuli in infants. *Journal of Cognitive Neuroscience, 12,* 449–460.

Diamond, A. (1991). Neuropsychological insights into the meaning of object concept development. In S. Carey & R. Gelman (Eds.), *The epigenesis of mind: Essays on biology and cognition* (pp. 67–110). Hillsdale, NJ: Erlbaum.

Diamond, A., & Taylor, C. (1996). Development of an aspect of executive control: Development of the ability to remember what I say and to "Do as I say, not as I do." *Developmental Psychobiology, 29*, 315–334.

Espy, K. A., Kaufman, P. M., McDiarmid, M. D., & Glisky, M. L. (1999). Executive functioning in preschool children: Performance on A-not-B and other delayed response format tasks. *Brain and Cognition, 41*, 178–199.

Fenson, L., Dale, P. S., Reznick, J. S., Bates, E., Thal, D., & Pethnik, S. J. (1994). Variability in early communicative development. *Monographs of the Society for Research in Child Development, 59*(5).

Frye, D., Zelazo, P. D., & Palfai, T. (1995). Theory of mind and rule-based reasoning. *Cognitive Development, 10*, 483–527.

Gathercole, S. E. (1998). The development of memory. *Journal of Child Psychology and Psychiatry, 39*(1), 3–27.

Gerstadt, C. L., Hong, Y. J., & Diamond, A. (1994). The relationship between cognition and action: Performance of children 3½–7 on a Stroop-like Day–Night Test. *Cognition, 53*, 129–153.

Hecox, K., & Burkard, R. (1982). Developmental dependencies of the human auditory evoked response. *Annals of the New York Academy of Science, 388*, 538–556.

Johnson, M. H. (1990). Cortical maturation and the development of visual attention in early infancy. *Journal of Cognitive Neuroscience, 2*, 81–95.

Johnson, M. H. (2003). Development of human brain functions. *Biological Psychiatry, 54*, 1312–1316.

Johnson, M. H., Posner, M. I., & Rothbart, M. K. (1991). Components of visual orienting in early infancy: Contingency learning, anticipatory looking, and disengaging. *Journal of Cognitive Neuroscience, 3*, 335–344.

Kaplan, E. (1988). A process approach to neuropsychological assessment. In T. Boll & B. K. Bryant (Eds.), *Clinical neuropsychology and brain function*. Washington, DC: American Psychological Association.

Lezak, M. D. (Ed.). (1983). *Neuropsychological assessment*. (2nd ed.). New York: Oxford University Press.

Luciana, M., & Nelson, C. A. (1998). The functional emergence of prefrontally-guided working memory systems in four- to eight-year-old children. *Neuropsychologia, 36*(3), 273–293.

Luria, A. R. (1961). *The role of speech in the regulation of normal and abnormal behaviour* (J. Tizard, Ed.). New York: Pergamon Press.

Morton, J., & Johnson, M. H. (1991). Conspec and Conlern: A two-process theory of infant face recognition. *Psychological Review, 98*, 164–181.

Nelson, C., & Luciana, M. (Eds.). (2001). *Handbook of developmental cognitive neuroscience*. Cambridge, MA: MIT Press.

Nelson, C. A. (1997). The neurobiological basis of early memory development. In N. Cowan (Ed.), *The development of memory in childhood* (pp. 41–82). Hove, East Sussex, UK: Psychology Press.

Nelson, D. L., & Xu, J. (1995). Effects of implicit memory on explicit recall: Set size and word-frequency effects. *Psychological Research, 57*(3–4), 203–214.

Nelson, K. (1994). Long-term retention of memory for preverbal experience: Evidence and implications. *Memory, 2*(4), 467–475.

Pennington, B. F., & Ozonoff, S. (1996). Executive functions and developmental psychopathology. *Journal of Child Psychology and Psychiatry, 37*(1), 51–87.

Piaget, J. (1952). *The origins of intelligence in children*. Oxford, UK: International Universities Press.

Piaget, J. (1954). *The construction of reality in the child*. New York: Basic Books.

Posner, M. I., & Petersen, S. E. (1990). The attention system of the human brain. *Annual Review of Neuroscience, 13*, 25–42.

Richards, J. E., & Cronise, K. (2000). Extended visual fixation in the early preschool years: Look duration, heart rate changes, and attentional inertia. *Child Development, 71*, 602–620.

Richards, J. E., & Turner, E. (2001). Extended visual fixation and distractibility in children from six to twenty-four months of age. *Child Development, 72*(4), 963–972.

Rothbart, M., & Posner, M. (2001). Mechanisms and variation in the development of attentional networks. In C. Nelson & M. Luciana (Eds.), *Handbook of developmental cognitive neuroscience* (pp. 353–364). Cambridge, MA: MIT Press.

Rourke, B. P. (1989). *Nonverbal learning disabilities: The syndrome and the model*. New York: Guilford Press.

Rudel, R. G., Holmes, J. M., & Pardes, J. R. (1988). *Assessment of developmental learning disorders: A neuropsychological approach*. New York: Basic Books.

Ruff, H. A., & Capozzoli, M. (2003). Development of attention and distractibility in the first 4 years of life. *Developmental Psychology, 39*(5), 877–890.

Ruff, H. A., Capozzoli, M., & Weissberg, R. (1998). Age, individuality, and context as factors in sustained visual attention during the preschool years. *Developmental Psychology, 34*, 454–464.

Ruff, H. A., & Lawson, K. R. (1990). Development of sustained, focused attention in young children during free play. *Developmental Psychology, 26*(1), 85–93.

Siegler, R. S. (1998). *Children's thinking* (3rd ed.). Upper Saddle River, NJ: Prentice-Hall.

Spreen, O., Risser, A. T., & Edgell, D. (1995). *Developmental neuropsychology*. New York: Oxford University Press.

Taylor, H. G., & Fletcher, J. M. (1990). Neuropsychological assessment of children. In G. Goldstein & M. Hersen (Eds.), *Handbook of psychological assessment* (2nd ed.). New York: Pergamon Press.

Terman, L. M. (1916). *The measurement of intelligence*. Boston: Houghton Mifflin.

Vygotsky, L. S. (1962). *Thought and language* (E. Hanfmann & G. Vakar, Trans.). Cambridge, MA: MIT Press. (Original work published 1934)

Wattam-Bell, J. (1991). Development of motion-specific cortical responses in infancy. *Vision Research, 31*, 287–297.

Werker, J. F., & Vouloumanos, A. (2001). Speech and language processing in infancy: A neurocognitive approach. In C. Nelson & M. Luciana (Eds.), *Handbook of developmental cognitive neuroscience* (pp. 269–280). Cambridge, MA: MIT Press.

Whiteman, F., Allen, P., Dolan, T., Kistler, D., & Jamieson, D. (1989). Temporal resolution in children. *Child Development, 60*, 611–624.

Zelazo, P. D. (1999). Language, levels of consciousness, and the development of intentional action. In P. D. Astington, J. W. Olson, & D. R. Zelazo (Eds.), *Developing theories of intention: Social understanding and self-control* (pp. 95–118). Mahwah, NJ: Erlbaum.

Part II

Mental Disorders Arising in the Preschool Period

4

Attention-Deficit/Hyperactivity Disorder

KENNETH W. STEINHOFF, MARC LERNER, AUDREY KAPILINSKY, RON KOTKIN,
SHARON WIGAL, ROBIN STEINBERG-EPSTEIN, TIM WIGAL, and JAMES M. SWANSON

Historically, attention-deficit/hyperactivity disorder (ADHD) has been viewed as a disorder of elementary school–age children. Only recently has the persistency of this disorder, especially its morbidity, come to be appreciated. Consequently there is a relative wealth of data for the school-age child, some for adults, little for adolescents, and almost none for preschool children (Dulcan, 1997). For example, as of 2002, a review of all psychopharmacological studies of ADHD stratified by age (Wilens, Biederman, & Spencer, 2002) discovered only seven studies for preschoolers compared to 171 studies for school-age children. Further review (Connor, 2002) revealed a total of 206 3- to 6-year-olds in controlled stimulant studies of ADHD. Prompted by a desire to decrease overall morbidity, increase understanding of the developmental course of disorders, interest in early gene–environment interactions, and notions of kindling and possible critical periods; there has been greater attention to detection and intervention as early as possible for disorders. Given this interest, coupled with a paucity of data, this chapter compares and contrasts existing preschool data with a well-established body of work for school-age ADHD. In addition, a multicenter, National Institute of Mental Health (NIMH)-funded Preschool ADHD Treatment Study has recently been completed, and some initial findings are presented in this chapter.

EPIDEMIOLOGY: APPROACHES IN THE PRESCHOOL AGE GROUP

The prevalence for school-age ADHD is well established to be 4–12% (American Academy of Pediatrics, Subcommittee on ADHD, Committee on Quality

Improvement, 2001), with some variation depending on the socioeconomic status and location of the community sampled (Goldman, Genel, Bezman, & Slanetz, 1998). Epidemiological evaluation of incidence and prevalence of ADHD in the preschool-age group is early in its development. Most data derive from clinic and referred samples rather than from community-wide study. Available community samples are typically restricted to specific, isolated geographic areas (Connor, 2002) and therefore cannot accurately inform general population prevalence estimates. To date, no large multicommunity sample studies of prevalence in the preschool-age group have been completed.

Compared with community-based epidemiological studies that typically rely on checklists and lay interviewers, the advantage of clinic-based studies is the presumption of careful diagnostic evaluation. A disadvantage of the clinic-based sample is the absence of systematic sample ascertainment. Also selection factors, such as the tendency to seek treatment and referral bias, can influence prevalence rates determined by clinic-based samples.

In one of the larger primary care pediatric samples, 2% of 510 2- to 5-year-olds in a Chicago metropolitan area practice were diagnosed with ADHD (Lavigne et al., 1996). In contrast, an academic center specialty behavioral clinic in the Boston metropolitan area characterized 200 sequentially referred (for general psychiatric evaluation) children under age 6, and found that the prevalence of ADHD in a specialty clinic sample was 86% (Wilens, Biederman, Brown, Tanguay, et al., 2002)

DIFFICULTIES IN DIAGNOSIS OF PRESCHOOL CHILDREN

The diagnosis of ADHD in children ages 6–12 has been the subject of much investigation. DSM (*Diagnostic and Statistical Manual of Mental Disorders*) criteria for ADHD have been repeatedly demonstrated to be clinically consistent, reliable in school-age children. The diagnosis of preschool children has not been systematically investigated and must address a number of inherent ambiguities unique to this age group.

DSM diagnostic criteria for ADHD are designed specifically for children ages 6–12. Application to younger children is subject to the clinician's individual interpretation of how to interpret these criteria in 3- to 6-year-olds. "Often leaves seat in classroom" may be easily translated to "Often leaves seat at dinner table," but other translations are more difficult to operationalize with certainty. For instance, what does "Often does not follow through on instructions and fails to finish schoolwork, chores, or duties in the workplace" look like in a 3-year-old? How can this be distinguished from "normal" behavior, especially if the child is not attending preschool, or some other structured setting? What "chores" are reasonable for a parent to expect a 3-year-old to complete? And would the finding that a particular child was unable to complete a chore signify a clinical symptom?

Answers to these questions await systematic investigation of a preschool nosology for ADHD. Further elucidation will arise from field trials and psychometric analyses of alternative and/or more age-specific probes. In the meantime, however, most clinicians rely on a best approximation strategy and look for significant impairment arising from the symptoms.

Our current DSM-IV-TR (American Psychiatric Association, 2000) diagnostic ADHD paradigm is predicated on the notion that symptoms are sensitive and specific indicators of discreet, stable disorders. As this paradigm is applied to younger and younger children, at some point the predicate may not hold. Younger children are undeveloped in their use of language, especially in descriptions of their internal emotional state. Preverbal children must rely on a strictly behavioral "vocabulary" to express symptoms. In the preschool-age group, it may be that ADHD symptoms could in some cases serve as the "final common pathway" for symptom expression of a number of learning, anxiety, mood, and aggressive disorders.

For example, although the Conners' (2001) Rating Scales have been normed for ages 3–6, with credible psychometric properties, this information has been obtained in a cross-sectional fashion from 198 males and 177 females ages 3–5 years and combined with data from older children for validity and reliability analysis. Children diagnosed in such a manner have not been followed longitudinally to determine whether these symptom clusters or patterns of rating scale responses demonstrate continuity with the disorder in 6- to 12-year-olds, or represent early, less specific symptom clusters.

"Hyperactivity" and "Inattention" as a Developmental Stage

It is common wisdom that the ability to "sit still and pay attention" generally increases with age. What is unclear is the amount and breadth of normative developmental variability in the general population. If in fact development of attention grows in fits and starts, a 3-year-old who meets population distribution–determined cutoff criteria for ADHD may offset at age 4 after a developmental burst. Such a child should be considered a variant of normal development and not have "true" ADHD.

On the other hand, suggesting that a child will, "grow out of" early attentional problems is equally unjustified in the absence of clear data. In the absence of well-elucidated determinants of normal developmental pathways for hyperactivity and inattention, most clinicians regard overall impairment as a guide to the need for treatment (see Heffelfinger & Mrakotsky, Chapter 3, this volume, for general guidelines on normative development of attention).

The primary impairment measure in the DSM-IV-TR is the Global Assessment of Functioning (GAF), which is typically worded and designed for adults rather than children. In addition, when specifically targeted for children (e.g., estimates of school functioning), the anchor points are more specific to adolescents (questions of suicidality and self-harm) or school-age children (questions of school functioning) than to the preschool-age group. In a similar fashion, the Clinical Global Index of Severity (CGI-S) is also limited in its structure by requiring difficulty in multiple areas (family, social, work or school). Since many preschool children interact primarily with their families, these other domains frequently are difficult to evaluate.

As expectations shift for preschool children (e.g., greater numbers of children are attending preschool programs) and demands increase in both amount and diversity, definitions of disability must also change. Although it is clear that many children can function extremely well in what 20 years ago would have been deemed a demanding and rigorous preschool environment, it is not clear what the implications of being unable to function in such an environment might mean. Trends in kindergarten readiness recommendations have oscillated between early entry and holding children back, without fear that long-term disability is signaled in children who might not yet be mature enough to enter school. This quandary is even sharper for the 3-year-old who is intolerant of the preschool structure or social demands. Although children with dramatic, repeated failures are clearly disabled, there is currently no accepted fine-grained tool for estimating the degree of moderate or slight disability, let alone one with predictive value.

Informant Limitations

Parents as Informants

In some respects parents of the preschoolers have more information available to them than do parents of school-age children. Frequently the child may spend the day with his or her caretaker—a parent, relative, or an employee—who can provide easier access to information about the child's behaviors than a schoolteacher. Typically, preschool children are not forced to accommodate to external structure to the extent that school-age children must. Parents frequently compensate for many behavioral limitations in their children with ADHD. These so-called "helicopter" parents (because they must hover over their children) provide auxiliary impulse control, as well as assistance for expediency sake (tying a child's shoes, organizing and cleaning the child's room, etc.). In the preschool-age group, where developmental rates vary, this is often considered in the range of normal. However, simple inquiry that does not measure the amount of parental input required will likely underreport the severity of a symptom (e.g., Question: "Is [the child] organized?" Answer: "We are very organized" or Question: "Does [the child] lose things often?" Answer: "No . . . [the child] is only 3, so we keep track of things").

In the absence of preschool or day care, social activities outside the home may be limited to play groups, religious activities, and family gatherings. In these cases, aside from only seeing their children in less structured activities, parents may have limited observation of other children of the same age as a reference point for developmentally appropriate expectations.

Preschool Teachers as Informants

Depending on the level of professional training, preschool teachers may be less likely to be aware of behavioral symptoms of ADHD. Additionally, in private settings, preschool teachers are more likely to be influenced by the family as a "customer," which may limit the flow of critical feedback. Out of respect for individual differences, anticipation of variations in developmental trajectories, and a wish to avoid premature labeling, many of these teachers avoid descriptions of problem behavior until the situation becomes unbearable and the child is abruptly asked to leave a child care placement. In extreme, this underrating of symptom severity can present as symptoms rated *just a little* on structured forms, despite the parents being told their child *just doesn't fit in.*

Adults in General as Informants

Adults are generally more inclined to give behavioral leeway to younger children. For instance, oppositional behavior at young ages is at times considered "cute" as the child develops a sense of independence, and may be tacitly indulged, if not openly fostered. In addition, given the notion that behavioral development is variable and may be the product of "stage" rather than a comment on the person per se, many adults are reluctant to "label" children at such a young age. Adults often fear a self-fulfilling effect if they mislabel a child.

Preschoolers as Informants

Restlessness is the only ADHD symptom that requires a patient to report on his or her inner state. Young children typically are not good reporters of their symptoms in externalizing disorders. Not until adolescence or adulthood are symptom self-reports sometimes considered reliable.

DIFFERENTIAL DIAGNOSTIC CONSIDERATIONS

Disorders Presenting in the Preschool Years

Speech–Language Disorders, Poor Auditory Acuity, and Otitis Media

Speech and language development is complex and dramatic during the preschool period. Many symptoms of ADHD, particularly those of inattentive type, may appear as either a direct or indirect result of a language disorder. For instance, a receptive language delay may account directly for "does not seem to listen when spoken to directly" and "does not follow through on instructions," and indirectly for "makes careless errors" (due in reality to poor comprehension), "difficulty sustaining attention," "avoids tasks with sustained mental effort," and "is easily distracted" (due in reality to boredom secondary to poor comprehension).

In a broader sense, language both organizes behavior and is reflective of that organization. Without the age-appropriate development of language to organize and plan impulse gratification internally or to negotiate with care-takers externally, a child may present as impulsive and oppositional. In a similar sense, children who cannot use language to organize their thinking and memory may present as inattentive and forgetful.

Closely related to the development of language is the presence of poor auditory acuity, which may arise for several reasons. Although there is controversy as to how commonly chronic otitis media is associated with delayed development of speech (Roberts, Rosenfeld, & Zeisel, 2004), such conditions are easily screened.

In the case of either "pure" speech disorders or combined speech and language disorders, it has been empirically established (Baker, Cantwell, & Mattison, 1980; Cantwell & Baker, 1987) that their presence predicts much higher rates of psychiatric and learning disorders. More than half of children with these communication difficulties do not recover within 4 years, and the presence of these problems also predicts poor psychiatric outcome 4 years later. Therefore, clinicians assessing for the presence of ADHD in the young child should be alert to speech, language, and hearing problems.

Obstructive Sleep Apnea

The interplay between alertness and attention is complex but synergistic. Attention typically suffers with fatigue or boredom, so it is not surprising that children with sleep disordered breathing are at increased risk for "hyperactivity and learning problems" (Schechter, 2002). In a meta-analytic review the combined odds ratios for attention and hyperactivity problems in children who snore was found to be 2.93 compared with controls. Likewise, school-age children with ADHD frequently have sleep difficulties that include increased nighttime activity, reduced rapid eye movement (REM) sleep, daytime somnolence, and possibly periodic limb movements (Cohen-Zion & Ancoli-Israel, 2004).

Although sleep disordered breathing is more prevalent in children with mild hyperactivity and attention, reduced REM sleep is more prevalent in children with severe symptoms of ADHD (O'Brien et al., 2003). This suggests that although sleep disordered breathing can have an impact on the attention/activity system, changes in the sleep architecture may be reflective of the underlying neurological problems of ADHD.

Pervasive Developmental Disorder

Some children with pervasive developmental disorder have difficulty with attention. It is at times hard to distinguish between lack of attention (especially to social cues) and lack of interest. In addition, many children with ADHD are socially ostracized for aggressively and impulsively demanding rather than collaborating, which can also be viewed as a failure of social reciprocity.

Oppositional Disorder, Conduct Disorder, and Aggression

About half (50–70%) of the school-age children diagnosed with ADHD meet diagnostic criteria for oppositional defiant disorder (ODD) or conduct disorder as well (Reeves, Werry, Elkind, & Zametkin, 1987; see Rockhill, Collet, McClellan, & Speltz, Chapter 5, this volume, for details of preschoolers with ODD). It also appears that about half (40–70%) of the school-age children with ODD meet criteria for ADHD (Anderson, Williams, McGee, & Silva, 1987). Although aggression in the preschool-age group is one of the most stable early symptoms (McKay & Halperin, 2001), it is not clear whether early childhood aggression specifically predicts ADHD, more severe ADHD later, or bipolar disorder. What is clear is that early childhood aggression can load onto several symptoms of ADHD (difficulty awaiting one's turn, interrupting, blurting out, etc.) especially when the aggression is impulsive rather than planned. In a more indirect manner, children with ADHD who have poor impulse control and planning ability are less likely to see the value of restrictive rules and more likely to be in increasingly frustrating situations.

Developmental Confounds to Inattention/Hyperactivity in the Preschool Years

Developmentally Appropriate Anxiety

Symptoms of anxiety directly impact children's ability to sit still, pay attention, and perform to their cognitive ability. In classic psychosexual development, 4 to 6 years of age is classified as the oedipal period, marked with castration anxiety, which typically manifest as fears for body integrity, dreams of monsters, and occasionally obsessional defenses. More modern empirical studies demonstrate that anxiety severe enough to impact behavior is relatively uncommon (Bell-Dolan, Last, & Strauss, 1990) in nonreferred patients.

Developmentally Appropriate Opposition

Episodic unwillingness to comply with adult requests is common in the preschool-age group. Although some opposition is essential to the development of self-control and autonomy, it can be difficult to differentiate whether a child "cannot" or "will not" comply with expected behaviors. Children with ADHD more commonly are not able to "behave" because of impulsivity and poor planning.

NATURAL COURSE

Persistency

It is generally believed that preschool children diagnosed with ADHD have the same biological, chronic, and disabling condition as school-age children with ADHD. In one longitudinal study, children identified with a full diagnosis of ADHD at age 3 have at follow-up demonstrated a positive predictive value of 50% at age 6 and 48% at age 9. Symptoms of hyperactivity, poor attention, and disobedience present in the context of peer problems (not liked, does not share) and aggression (destructive, tells lies, fights) were more likely to persist (Campbell & Ewing, 1990).

In a more recent study (Lahey et al., 1994) based on 96 children from two different cities, ages 3 years, 8 months to 7 years old, meeting full diagnostic criteria for ADHD predicted a full diagnosis 4 years later, with a positive predictive value of 0.75 and a negative predictive value of 0.86. Interestingly, this study also tracked 29 children who met criteria in only one setting (e.g., school or home), thereby not meeting the full diagnostic criteria. This group with "situational ADHD" was significantly less likely to meet full diagnostic criteria 4 years later, but 34% did meet full criteria eventually, compared with 3.1% for comparison children. Together these studies suggest a general pattern of persistence of symptoms and impairment in carefully diagnosed cases, as well as a more progressive course with a substantial minority of young children demonstrating symptoms in only some environments.

Predominance of Hyperactive–Impulsive Symptoms in the Early Years

In DSM-IV field trials, 18% (50/276) of children with ADHD were diagnosed as hyperactive–impulsive subtype (Lahey et al., 1998). However, 75% of these children were less than 6 years old. The mean age for this group was 5 years, 7 months younger than either the inattentive or the combined subtype groups. On the older end of the school-age group spectrum, 26% of the inattentive type children first exhibited their symptoms after 7-years of age, compared to 13% of those with combined type, and 8% of hyperactive–impulsive type children. Together, these result suggests that hyperactivity is more prominent in the younger years, whereas inattention becomes more preeminent in later years. However, this and similar studies use a clinic-based, nonepidemiological patient ascertainment strategy, so these rates may be confounded by a tendency to refer preschool children who have more externalizing symptoms. Also, hyperactive symptoms overshadow, or mask, inattentive symptoms. For example, when children are constantly "on the go," and "cannot remain seated," it is difficult to assess their attention to detail or their forgetfulness. When both sets of symptoms are present, parents and teachers seem to be more concerned with the active and oppositional symptoms.

IMPACT ON GROWTH

Historically, there have been concerns that stimulant medication may suppress growth in children with ADHD. A careful review (Spencer, Biederman, & Wilens, 1998) has suggested that any growth delays are more likely due to the illness itself (perhaps due to a co-located gene or a common physiological process). The NIMH Multimodal Treatment Study of Children with ADHD (MTA) study has once again raised concerns that stimulant treatment may suppress growth. However, it was noted in the MTA study that children with ADHD grew at a faster than normal rate whenever they were not taking stimulant medication (MTA Cooperative Group, 2004).

In the Preschool ADHD Treatment Study (PATS), children were much larger than average. Although this is again consistent with the hypothesis that children with ADHD grow faster, it may be that larger, hyperactive children are more likely to be referred (due to greater concern about the potential for destructive effects of impulsive behavior and the effect of their size on peer interaction).

TREATMENT

Perhaps the richest source of information for the treatment of school-age children with ADHD is the NIMH MTA study, which underscored the value of both well-done psychosocial intervention and medication management as treatment interventions; however, the MTA did not study preschool children.

Parent Training

Much has been written about instructing parents of preschool children in the use of behavioral techniques. However, the bulk of this work focuses on children with general "behavioral" problems and has not been specifically applied to children for whom homogeneous diagnostic criteria have been applied. In addition, most studies include only small numbers of families, which makes results difficult to generalize.

Community-Oriented Parent Educational System

The Community-Oriented Parent Educational System (COPE) program is one of the few training programs for parents of preschool children with behavioral disorders which has been studied with sizable numbers of children. A total of 3,564 families completed a 12-week course of individual family therapy, the COPE program, or wait-list control. Measuring via symptom checklists, the COPE group sustained significantly more improvement immediately and 6-months after treatment (Cunningham, Bremner, & Boyle, 1995).

Unlike traditional parent education, the COPE program is designed for large groups of parents who interact and problem-solve. Each session is organized around a behavioral management problem introduced to the group at large by the therapist, commonly with a video of a child in a moderately provocative behavioral situation (e.g., ignoring his or her parents' directions). The child's behavior in the video is always moderate (to shift focus from what the child is doing to parents' choices in managing the child's behavior). Parents then problem-solve interactively in small groups, whose activities are directed by the therapist and include practicing and didactic elements, as well as adhering to the principles of behavioral therapy.

ADAPTING COPE TO FAMILIES OF CHILDREN WITH ADHD

This model has been further evaluated in the PATS (Greenhill, Kollins, Swanson, Abikoff, & Wigal, 2004) for families of preschool children specifically diagnosed with ADHD. In the PATS, 10 modules from the COPE training manual were selected for use in once weekly 2-hour classes.

In addition to the parenting class a simultaneous child training/child care program was offered. Frequent prompts and praise, as well as a token system pairing primary reinforcers (food) with tokens (marbles in a jar), were used to shape each child's behavior and to practice a positive response to parents' effort. The focus of the child sessions was designed to parallel topics in the parenting sessions. For example, parents were taught to give clear and concise directions to increase the likelihood that their child would comply with them. The children were taught in the same evening to follow adult directions.

In addition to the standard COPE program, parents were given weekly phone calls to allow them to ask questions. Parents were asked how their home practice was going, which added an additional prompt to complete homework assignments and problem-solve with the Parent Trainer on an individual basis, thereby improving adherence to treatment.

ADAPTING COPE AS A POSITIVE SCREEN/COMMUNITY-BASED INTERVENTION

Utilizing a unique health care delivery model, COPE has been used at the University of California, Irvine (UCI; Tamm et al., 2005) to deliver service prior to diagnosis. Families are self-referred to a COPE program administered within local communities (and in three different languages) across the county. If they are not satisfied with the results, parents are provided with a full diagnostic evaluation in a multidisciplinary, developmental pediatrics clinic. Thus, early and easily accessible treatment provides a positive screen, providing specialty diagnosis and care for the treatment nonresponders.

Over 1,500 families have been treated in 333 combined "Parenting Strategy" and "Social Skills" sessions. The program is successful by a number of measures. Systematic evaluation of parent satisfaction is high, and parent-rated behavioral changes show significant improvement in ADHD and ODD behavior ratings. From a public health perspective, only 30% of families elect to seek further evaluation in the multispecialty clinic, and the cost of COPE treatment is relatively small, suggesting that this approach also provides an economical, combined screening and treatment tool.

Medication

History of Stimulant "Labels"

Stimulant treatment is the mainstay of ADHD treatment in all age groups. The only nonstimulant medications to date that have received U.S. Food and Drug Administration (FDA) approval for the indication of ADHD treatment is atomoxetine (6 years old to adult) and modafinil (6–18 years old).

Historically, the amphetamines were approved by the FDA for ADHD in children age 3 years old and up, before there were general public concerns about the use of stimulants. In the late 1960s, based on an epidemic of overuse in Sweden rather than any specific data, an FDA advisory panel encouraged limiting the age range of the use of stimulants. Thus, when methylphenidate (MPH) was created and brought to market, the FDA allowed the label to indicate use only for individuals age 6 years and older (Greenhill et al., 2004).

Yet, the American Academy of Child and Adolescent Psychiatry (AACAP) Stimulant Practice Parameters report that although there are eight published studies of MPH in the under 6 age range, there are none for pemoline, dextroamphetamine, or mixed amphetamine salts (Greenhill et al., 2001). Clearly the bulk of the data for medication intervention in younger children lies with MPH.

Reports of the use of psychoactive medication (Zito et al., 2000) suggest a dramatic increase in the use of MPH in preschool children. This is consistent with the fact that it is the most studied medicine for this age group, but it is concerning in view of the lack of large systematic trials or longitudinal follow-up data.

Preschool ADHD Treatment Study

Out of concern that increasing numbers of preschool children are being treated "off-label" with MPH for ADHD, a consortium of researchers funded by the NIMH, and in consultation with the FDA, Drug Enforcement Administration (DEA), and AACAP research forum (Greenhill et al., 2003), set about to study carefully issues of safety in the use of MPH in this age group. In addition, questions of diagnosis, efficacy, and long-term effects were addressed.

DESIGN

Children entering the study were between ages 3 years and 5 years, 5 months, and had severe ADHD, hyperactive–impulsive or combined type diagnoses.

All children were required to be actively enrolled and participating in a pre-school to provide teacher ratings. It is important to realize these children were extremely impaired (< 55 on Children's Global Assessment Scale) and averaged 1.5 standard deviations away from the average on symptom ratings. Many had failed in at least one preschool setting, and several had failed in more than one.

The study was organized into the following sequential phases:

1. *Screening and diagnosis.* The phase comprised 8 hours of testing and interviews, culminating with a written and verbal cross-site conference call requiring unanimous approval for the subject to enter the study. Of the 553 patients initially screened in the clinics, 303 met criteria for enrollment.

2. *Nonmedication intervention.* This phase was added after scientific re-view on ethical and safety grounds to ensure minimal exposure to medication in children who might respond to other treatments. A 10-week parent train-ing program with empirical validation (COPE) was employed for this pur-pose. If the children improved (by 30% on both parent and teacher Conners' ADHD symptom ratings), they were excluded from the controlled medication portion of the study. Of the 279 patients who entered this phase, 261 com-pleted the study, with 19 patients improving enough on dimensional behav-ioral ratings that they were not allowed to participate in the medication phase of the study.

3. *Medication tolerability.* An open-label, forced, upward dose titration with MPH from 1.25 mg once daily to 7.5 mg three times per day. Of the 183 children who entered this phase, 11 terminated due to medication side effects, none of which were dangerous, demonstrating a high degree of tolerability.

4. *Crossover titration.* To determine each child's best dose, children were randomly assigned in a double-blind fashion to each of five dosing conditions (placebo, 1.25 mg, 2.5 mg, 5 mg, and 7.5 mg, all delivered three times per day), one dosing condition for each of 5 weeks. Parent and Teacher Conners' Rating Scales and side effects ratings were compared blindly for each week to determine the patient's best week and thereby the best dose. Of the 165 pa-tients who entered, five discontinued due to side effects or MPH nonresponse, demonstrating a remarkable degree of responsiveness.

5. *Efficacy.* In a double-blind, parallel group fashion, children then re-ceived either their best dose or placebo for 4 weeks. Of the 114 children who entered this phase, 33 left early due to behavioral deterioration.

6. *Open-label maintenance.* To provide for long-term follow-up, pa-tients were followed in a clinical fashion for 10 months, during which there was flexibility for the physicians to change the dose.

INTENT-TO-TREAT ANALYSIS OF CONTROLLED PORTIONS OF THE STUDY

Crossover portion of the study. The "crossover titration" phase of the study was a within-subjects design, allowing each child to act as his or her own control. This provided the ability to calculate effect sizes at each dose and to create a dose–response curve. It also allowed identification of a child's best dose. Based on a combination of parent (Conners, Loney, & Milch; CLAM) and teacher (Swanson, Kotkin, Alger, Flynn, & Pelham; SKAMP) ratings (Wigal, Gupta, Guinta, & Swanson, 1998), 85% of the children responded to MPH, 10% responded to placebo, and 5% were determined to be nonresponders to MPH. The total daily dose averaged slightly more than 14 mg, with a broad distribution. The effect size was in proportion to the dose and about one half of those in the MTA study of school-age children, where the doses were on average twice as high (MTA Cooperative Group, 1999).

Efficacy Portion of the Study. The second controlled phase operated as a parallel group (best dose vs. placebo) design. The primary outcome measure for this phase was the SNAP (Swanson–Nolan–Pehlam, Rating, an 18-item Likert rating scale of DSM-IV ADHD symptoms: 0, none, 1, just a little, 2, often, 3, all the time). The placebo group average score was 1.8, whereas the group receiving individuals best dose average score was 1.5, which is a significant difference at a p value of .02.

The effect sizes in this phase were also in proportion to dose (which ranged up to 0.9 for 7.5 mg, three times per day). Interestingly, by the end of the open-label maintenance phase, in which dosing was determined in a more common clinical fashion, the average dose increased to 20 mg total daily dose, only some of which was accounted for by growth.

SIDE EFFECTS

Overall, the pattern of side effects was consistent with that of older children. Analysis of the reasons for discontinuation of the study demonstrated that 9% dropped from the study due to medication adverse events, primarily due to crying, irritability, and insomnia.

Analysis of growth parameters demonstrated that, on average, these patients started the study at 0.4 standard deviations above their Centers for Disease Control and Prevention (CDC) growth curve (Greenhill et al., 2004) means for height and 0.7 for weight. Analysis of height changes based on the amount of time on medication yielded a suppression of height at the rate of 1.4 cm/year (compared to CDC normal growth curves). This result is larger but still similar to that noted in the MTA. Coupling this "suppression" with the fact that these children were already above average height and weight, it has been suggested that stimulant medication may be "normalizing" height and weight rather than purely "suppressing" it (MTA Cooperative Group, 2004). Definitive answers await long-term follow-up studies, but in practical terms, the average "suppression" is small at worst, since its rate decreases over time.

STRENGTHS, WEAKNESSES, AND SUMMARY

In summary, the PATS is the longest controlled trial with the largest sample to date to investigate the treatment of ADHD in the preschool-age range. Although highly structured and comprehensive, it is limited by the numerous accommodations engineered to minimize exposure to medication and to maximize safety (e.g., the requirement for initial rather than concurrent parent training, the flexibility of allowing patients to skip over placebo sections yet still receive treatment, the emphasis on small doses with a restricted dose range, and the large time investment required from the families). These limitations biased the study toward a higher attrition rate, which was already likely to be high because of general fears of medicating preschool children. However, given that MPH was found to be well tolerated, safe, and effective, the PATS will have served to pave the way for future, less restricted study.

Pharmacokinetics of MPH in Preschool Children

The UCI-Lab School (Swanson et al., 1999) is a paradigm for the study of the time course of blood levels and effects of ADHD medications across the day (Swanson et al., 2002). Typically, children are brought in early on a Saturday and kept the whole day. After initial catheter insertion, the study day is highly structured and includes many naturalistic activities, as well as measurement of attention and activity at various times during the day.

Designed as an add-on study to the PATS at the UCI site, 14 preschool children and 9 school-age children were brought into the UCI-Lab School (Greenhill et al., 2004). Children were enrolled after they had been on a stable MPH dose in the open-label maintenance phase of the PATS. This dose, considered the child's optimal dose, ranged from 2.5 mg three times a day to 10 mg three times a day for both age groups. On the study day, only one morning dose was given, and blood samples were taken at predose, 1 hour, 2 hours, 4 hours, and 6 hours after dosing. Surprisingly, the preschool-age group was found to be significantly slower in clearance and elimination than the school-age group, even when weight was taken into account. Assuming that each child is correctly, optimally dosed, this implies that preschool children are about 25% less sensitive to MPH serum concentrations. Overall, this suggests that preschool children would be more tolerant, and likely require higher average weight-corrected doses than school-age children.

RECOMMENDATIONS FOR THE MENTAL HEALTH PRACTITIONER

Diagnosis

As with school-age children, the diagnosis of ADHD in preschool children is based largely on history. Therefore, it is especially important that this history be supplied by multiple informants across multiple settings. Symptoms are most likely to be observed in situations where children are expected to adhere to some external structure and tend to be more obvious when a group of peers is present to serve as contrast. While generally helpful, the use of scales with good psychometric properties for preschool populations (such as the Conners' Rating Scale) is clearly in order when observation of the patient among his or her peers is not possible. Capturing ratings from numerous sources is essential, but one must be careful to "rate the rater," by including a direct conversation with each rater to determine his or her bias in rating a very young child. The absence of standardized age-appropriate probes, tolerance for developmental variation, and concerns for lack of specificity of symptoms should be mitigated by data suggesting that these symptoms and their associated impairment are generally stable over time and should not preclude diagnosis.

Treatment

The existing follow-up data demonstrate stability of full diagnosis and its associated impairment, suggesting the need for aggressive treatment.

Parent Training

Parent training is an essential part of treatment for young children. Although verbal, psychodynamically oriented therapies can be useful for preschoolers with ADHD on occasion, the bulk of the evidence for effective treatment lies with active, direct coaching and practice models that rely on behavioral techniques. Whereas direct effect on core ADHD symptoms is often small, effects on family satisfaction and compliance with other forms of treatment run high. In addition, parent training can function as a positive screen, given that severe ADHD will continue to surface even after the parents have mastered the parenting techniques. This can be especially useful and economical in large, community-based training models such as COPE.

Medication

The bulk of data lies with MPH treatment, which appears safe and reasonable. Although average dosage was 20 mg/day in the open-label phase of PATS, a broad range of optimal dose was encountered, suggesting that, as with school-age children, clinicians should conduct a titration trial exploring the effectiveness of higher doses as tolerated in an attempt to optimize treatment. Whether the reduced clearance rates in preschool children will influence the effect or duration of action of longer-acting MPH preparations remains to be seen.

REFERENCES

American Academy of Pediatrics, Subcommittee on ADHD, Committee on Quality Improvement. (2001). Clinical practice guidelines: Treatment of the school-aged child with attention deficit hyperactivity disorder. *Pediatrics, 108*(4), 1033–1044.

American Psychiatric Association. (2000). *Diagnostic and statistical manual of mental disorders* (4th ed., text rev.). Washington, DC: Author.

Anderson, J. C., Williams, S., McGee, R., & Silva, P. A. (1988). DSM-III disorders in preadolescent children: Prevalence in a large sample from the general population. *Archives of General Psychiatry, 44*(1), 69–76.

Baker, L., Cantwell, D. P., & Mattison, R. E. (1980). Behavior problems in children with pure speech disorders and in children with combined speech and language disorders. *Journal of Abnormal Child Psychology, 8*(2), 245–256.

Bell-Dolan, D. J., Last, C. G., & Strauss, C. C. (1990). Symptoms of anxiety disorders in normal children. *Journal of the American Academy of Child and Adolescent Psychiatry, 29*(5), 759–765.

Campbell, S. B., & Ewing, L. J. (1990). Follow-up of hard-to-manage preschoolers: Adjustment at age 9 and predictors of continuing symptoms. *Journal of Child Psychology and Psychiatry and Allied Disciplines, 31*(6), 871–889.

Cantwell, D. P., & Baker, L. (1987). Clinical significance of childhood communication disorders: Perspectives from a longitudinal study. *Journal of Child Neurology, 2*(4), 257–264.

Cohen-Zion, M., & Ancoli-Israel, S. (2004). Sleep in children with attention-deficit hyperactivity disorder (ADHD): A review of naturalistic and stimulant intervention studies. *Sleep Medicine Reviews, 8*(5), 379–402.

Conners, C. K. (2001). *Conners' Rating Scales—Revised: Instruments for use with children and adolescents.* North Towanda, NY: Multi-Health Systems.

Connor, D. F. (2002). Preschool attention deficit hyperactivity disorder: A review of prevalence, diagnosis, neurobiology, and stimulant treatment. *Developmental and Behavioral Pediatrics, 23*(1, Suppl.), S1–S9.

Cunningham, C. E., Bremner, R., & Boyle, M. (1995). Large group community-based parenting programs for families of preschoolers at risk for disruptive behavior disorders: Utilization, cost, effectiveness, and outcome. *Journal of Child Psychology and Psychiatry and Allied Disciplines, 36,* 1141–1159.

Dulcan, M. (1997). Practice parameters for the assessment and treatment of children, adolescents, and adults with attention-deficit/hyperactivity disorder. *Journal of the American Academy of Child and Adolescent Psychiatry, 36*(10, Suppl.), 85S–121S.

Goldman, L. S., Genel, M., Bezman, R. J., & Slanetz, P. J. (1998). Diagnosis and treatment of attention-deficit/hyperactivity disorder in children and adolescents. *Journal of the American Medical Association, 279,* 1100–1107.

Greenhill, L. L., Jensen, P. S., Abikoff, H., Blumer, J. L., Deveaugh-Geiss, J., Fisher, C., et al. (2003). Developing strategies for psychopharmacological studies in preschool children. *Journal of the American Academy of Child and Adolescent Psychiatry, 42*(4), 406–414.

Greenhill, L., Kollins, S., Swanson, J. M., Abikoff, H., & Wigal, S. (2004). *Preschool Attention Deficit Hyperactivity Disorder Treatment Study preliminary results.* Symposium presented at the 51st Annual Meeting of the American Academy of Child and Adolescent Psychiatry.

Greenhill, L. L., Pliszka, S., Dulcan, M. K., Bernet, W., Arnold, V., Beitchman, J., et al. (2001). *Practice parameter for the use of stimulant medications in the treatment of children, adolescents and adults.* Washington, DC: AACAP Communications.

Lahey, B. B., Applegate, B., McBurnett, K., Biederman, J., Greenhill, L., Hynd, G. W., et al. (2004). DSM-IV field trials for attention-deficit hyperactivity disorder in children and adolescents. *American Journal of Psychiatry, 151,* 1673–1685.

Lahey, B. B., Pelham, W. E., Stein, M. A., Loney, J., Trapani, C., Nugent, K., et al. (1998). Validity of DSM-IV attention-deficit/hyperactivity disorder for younger children. *Journal of the American Academy of Child and Adolescent Psychiatry, 37*(7), 695–702.

Lavigne, J. V., Gibbons, R. D., Christoffel, K. K., Arend, R., Rosenbaum, D., Binns, H., et al. (1996). Prevalence rates and correlates of psychiatric disorders among preschool children. *Journal of the American Academy of Child and Adolescent Psychiatry, 35,* 204–214.

McKay, K. E., & Halperin, J. M. (2001). ADHD, aggression, and antisocial behavior across the lifespan, interactions with neurochemical and cognitive function. *Annals of the New York Academy of Science, 931,* 84–96.

MTA Cooperative Group. (2004). National Institute of Mental Health Multimodal Treatment Study of ADHD follow-up: Changes in effectiveness and growth after the end of treatment. *Pediatrics, 113*, 762–769.

MTA Cooperative Group. (1999). A 14–month randomized clinical trial of treatment strategies for attention deficit hyperactivity disorder. *Archives of General Psychiatry, 56*(12), 1073–1086.

O'Brien, L. M., Holbrook, C. R., Mervis, C. B., Klaus, C. J., Bruner, J. L., Raffield, T. J., et al. (2004). Sleep and neurobehavioral characteristics of 5– to 7–year-old children with parentally reported symptoms of attention-deficit/hyperactivity disorder. *Pediatrics, 111*(3), 554–563.

Reeves, J. C., Werry, J. S., Elkind, G. S., & Zametkin, A. (1987). Attention deficit, conduct, oppositional, and anxiety disorders in children: II. Clinical characteristics. *Journal of the American Academy of Child and Adolescent Psychiatry, 26*, 144–155.

Roberts, J., Rosenfeld, R., & Zeisel, S. (2004). Otitis media and speech and language: A meta-analysis of prospective studies. *Pediatrics, 113*, 238–248.

Schechter, M. S., & Section on Pediatric Pulmonology, Subcommittee on Obstructive Sleep Apnea Syndrome. (2002). Technical report: Diagnosis and management of childhood obstructive sleep apnea syndrome. *Pediatrics, 109*(4), 1–20.

Spencer, T., Biederman, J., & Wilens, T. (1998). Growth deficits in children with attention deficit hyperactivity disorder. *Pediatrics, 102*(2, Part 3), 501–506.

Swanson, J. M., Alger, D., Fineberg, E., Wigal, S., Flynn, D., Fineberg, K., et al. (1999). UCI Laboratory School protocol for PK/PD studies. In L. Greenhill & B. Osman (Eds.), *Ritalin: Theory and practice* (2nd ed., pp. 405–430). Larchmont, NY: Mary Ann Liebert.

Swanson, J. M., Lerner, M., Wigal, T., Steinhoff, K., Greenhill, L., Posner, K., et al. (2002). The use of a laboratory school protocol to evaluate concepts about efficacy and side effects of new formulations of stimulant medications. *Journal of Attention Disorders, 6*(Suppl.), 73–88.

Tamm, L., Swanson, J. M., Lerner, M., Childress, C., Patterson, B., Lakes, K., et al. (2005). Intervention for preschoolers at risk for attention-deficit/hyperactivity disorder (ADHD): Service before diagnosis. *Clinical Neuroscience Research, 5*, 247–253.

Wigal, S. B., Gupta, S., Guinta, D., & Swanson, J. M. (1998). Reliability and validity of the SKAMP Rating Scale in a laboratory school setting. *Psychopharmacology Bulletin, 34*(1), 47–53.

Wilens, T. E., Biederman, J., Brown, S., Tanguay, S., Monuteaux, M. C., Blake, C., et al. (2002). Psychiatric comorbidity and functioning in clinically referred preschool children and school-age youths with ADHD. *Journal of the American Academy of Child and Adolescent Psychiatry, 41*(3), 262–268.

Wilens, T. E., Biederman, J., & Spencer, T. (2002). Attention deficit/hyperactivity disorder across the lifespan. *Annual Reviews in Medicine, 53*, 113–131.

Zito, J. M., Safer, D. J., Reis, S. D., Gardner, J. F., Boles, M., & Lynch, F. (2000). Trends in the prescribing of psychotropic medications to preschoolers. *Journal of the American Medical Association, 283*(8), 1025–1030.

5

Oppositional Defiant Disorder

Carol M. Rockhill, Brent R. Collett,
Jon M. McClellan, and Matthew L. Speltz

Along with hyperactivity and attention deficits, the externalizing behavior problems associated with oppositional defiant disorder (ODD; e.g., defiance, anger, and noncompliance) are the primary reasons for referral of preschool children to mental health programs (e.g., Gadow, Sprafkin, & Nolan, 2001; Thomas & Clark, 1998). Parents, health providers and educators often hold two seemingly contradictory views of ODD among children of this age: On the one hand, significant oppositional behavior during the preschool years is viewed as normal and developmentally expected. During this period, it is believed that a key developmental task for all families is to resolve conflicts associated with parents' attempts to contain their child's ventures into "forbidden space," and the child's negative and sometimes aggressive reactions to this prohibition. On the other hand, it is becoming clear to many clinicians that roughly half of preschool children referred to clinical programs for externalizing problems—often leading to the diagnosis of ODD—show remarkable persistence of such problems in the elementary school years and well beyond (e.g., Campbell, 2002). From this perspective, the diagnosis of ODD early in life cannot be taken lightly, despite the fact that the problems typically leading to its diagnosis may represent the extreme of a normal developmental tendency.

Several questions and issues are of intense interest to those who study or provide treatment to toddlers and preschoolers with ODD and related externalizing problems: Are there reliable methods of defining the problem; that is, distinguishing normal defiance from clinically meaningful oppositional behavior? Can we reliably distinguish referred preschoolers who outgrow their problems from those showing long-term persistence? Among preschoolers showing persisting problems, do externalizing problems simply continue and predominate (homotypical continuity), or does early ODD function as a "gateway" to more diverse psychopathology (e.g., bipolar disorder)? Does an early diagnosis of ODD have practical benefit, leading to interventions with proven, long-term effects?

This chapter attempts to provide at least tentative answers to these and other questions regarding preschool ODD, with an emphasis on areas of interest to clinicians. The chapter is divided into three major sections: Diagnosis and Clinical Course, Etiology, and Clinical Intervention, followed by a brief discussion of Future Directions. Throughout the chapter, we have tried to focus on ODD topics as they pertain to toddlers and preschoolers. However, most of what is currently known about ODD (and related disorders, and problem areas such as "conduct disorder" and "aggression") is based on the study of older children and adolescents. Our discussion therefore includes these age groups to the extent that they inform the conceptualization of preschool-age predictors and outcomes.

DIAGNOSIS AND CLINICAL COURSE OF ODD

History of DSM Classification

Oppositional disorder (OD) first appeared in the third edition of the *Diagnostic and Statistical Manual of Mental Disorders* (DSM-III; American Psychiatric Association, 1980). OD symptoms included violations of minor rules, temper tantrums, argumentativeness, defiance, provocativeness, and stubbornness. Two of the five symptoms were required for diagnosis, and had to occur more frequently than in other children of the same mental age. Onset had to be after age 3, and symptoms had to endure for 6 months or longer. These diagnostic criteria were revised for DSM-III-R (American Psychiatric Association, 1987), and the condition was renamed oppositional defiant disorder (ODD). Due to concerns about overdiagnosis, stubbornness was eliminated from DSM-III-R (American Psychiatric Association, 1987), "often" was added to each criterion, and the diagnosis was changed to require five symptoms from a list of nine (Angold & Costello, 1996; Schwab-Stone & Hart, 1996). The requirement that onset occur after age 3 was eliminated, and no age minimum was set. A clarification was added noting that oppositional and defiant behaviors are common among typically developing preschoolers and that diagnosis requires symptoms that are more frequent or intense than usual, or symptoms that endure longer than expected. Debate about the utility of the diagnosis ensued (Loeber, Lahey, & Thomas, 1991; Rey, 1995), and ODD received more rigorous study during the DSM-IV field trials (Lahey et al., 1994).

DSM-IV (American Psychiatric Association, 1994) and DSM-IV-TR (American Psychiatric Association, 2000) retained a very similar description of ODD and list of requisite symptoms. The DSM-III-R symptom "frequently swears or uses obscene language" showed weak diagnostic utility and was dropped, leaving eight symptoms. A diagnostic cutoff of four symptoms in the last 6 months was found to maximize the identification of impaired youth, agreement with clinician diagnoses, and test–retest reliability (Lahey et al., 1994). Perhaps the most important addition was the requirement of clinically significant impairment in psychosocial functioning.

DSM-IV criteria for ODD and conduct disorder (CD)—as reported by parents in semistructured interviews—can reliably distinguish referred from nonreferred preschool children (Keenan & Wakschlag, 2004). Several studies have provided support for the concurrent validity of the ODD diagnosis in preschool boys. For example, in comparison with case-matched normal peers, boys with ODD had higher ratings of behavior problems from parents and teachers (Speltz, McClellan, DeKlyen, & Jones, 1999), lower Verbal IQ (Speltz, DeKlyen, Calderon, Greenberg, & Fisher, 1999), higher probability of insecure attachments to parents (e.g., DeKlyen, Biernbaum, Speltz, & Greenberg, 1998), and more conflicted family interactions during clinic interviews (Stormschak, Speltz, DeKlyen, & Greenberg, 1997).

An issue of debate is whether ODD and CD ought to be considered distinct diagnostic entities, or whether they reflect variants of the same disorder (e.g., Loeber, Green, Lahey, Frick, & McBurnett, 2000). In their review of the literature, Loeber et al. concluded that the empirical evidence supports distinctions between ODD and CD, but that we still have much to learn about subgroups and prognosis. Furthermore, other authors have argued that the developmental relationship between these diagnoses may be less straightforward than previously proposed, especially for girls (Rowe, Maughan, Pickles, Costello, & Angold, 2002). A few authors have proposed new diagnostic subtypes, including combining ODD and CD diagnoses (Eaves et al., 2000). Angold and Costello (1996) suggested adding "mild," "moderate," and "severe" specifiers to describe children diagnosed with ODD and have two to three, four to five, or more than five symptoms, respectively.

Finally, and of particular relevance for preschoolers, there is concern that the DSM-IV leaves open to interpretation how frequently a child has to demonstrate a behavior for it to be considered "often." In the absence of epidemiological data, it is difficult to establish in any standardized fashion what an average rate of oppositional and defiant behavior might be, let alone establish such normative data for specific subgroups based on age, gender, and/or developmental status.

Prevalence of ODD in Preschool Children

Current estimates suggest that 2–3% of children across the age span meet DSM-IV symptom criteria and show significant psychosocial impairment (Canino et al., 2004; Costello, Mustillo, Erkanli, Keeler, & Angold, 2003; Maughan, Rowe, Messer, Goodman, & Meltzer, 2004). Based on DSM-III-R criteria, prevalence of ODD in preschool children from community samples ranged from 8% among low-income families (Keenan, Shaw, Walsh, Delliquadri, & Giovannelli, 1997) to 17% among preschoolers in a primary care pediatrics clinic (Lavigne et al., 1996). As might be expected, rates of ODD have declined with the increasing stringency of diagnostic criteria across successive versions of DSM (from DSM-III to DSM-IV), especially with the requirement of functional impairment (Angold & Costello, 1996; Canino et al., 2004). ODD is more common in boys (roughly 2:1 male:female ratio), particularly when teacher-report data are used to establish diagnosis (Maughan et al., 2004). Some data indicate variation across ethnic groups (e.g., Bird et al., 2001), though this issue requires further study.

Comorbidity

Comorbidity with other psychiatric disorders is extremely common. In population-based studies, one-fourth to one-half of children meeting diagnostic criteria for ODD also meet criteria for one or more other DSM-IV diagnoses, most commonly ADHD (Angold & Costello, 1996; Maughan et al., 2004). Conversely, examination of preschool children diagnosed with ADHD reveals that approximately 60% also meet criteria for ODD (Kadesjo, Haggloff, Kadesjo, & Gillberg, 2003; Lavigne et al., 1996). Not surprisingly, several research groups have found that youth meeting criteria for both ODD and ADHD show more impairment than those having either disorder alone (Biederman et al., 1996; Gadow & Nolan, 2002). Findings are mixed regarding the possibility that these children (with both disorders) are also at heightened risk for engaging in antisocial behavior and/or developing CD (Loeber et al., 2000; Moffitt, 1990; Moffitt & Caspi, 2001; Sonuga-Barke, Thompson, Stevenson, & Viney, 1997).

Co-occurrence of internalizing and externalizing symptoms (e.g., ODD comorbid with depressive disorders or anxiety disorders) is also very common in preschool children (Kadesjo et al., 2003; Keenan, Shaw, Walsh, Delliquadri, & Giovannelli, 1997; Lavigne et al., 1998; Maughan et al., 2004; Shaw, Keenan, Vondra, Delliquadri, & Giovannelli, 1997; Speltz, McClellan, DeKlyen, & Jones, 1999; Thomas & Guskin, 2001). This may reflect the fact that oppositional and disruptive behaviors can function as one of the first manifestations of anxiety and mood-related processes. Examples include a young child's resistance to adult interference with inflexibly held beliefs or routines, or adult efforts to expose the child to novel, uncomfortable situations. Research findings pertaining to patterns of externalizing–internalizing comorbidity have been strongly affected by ascertainment criteria. For example, Speltz, McClellan, et al. (1999) found relatively low rates of internalizing symptoms in preschool boys ascertained for ODD (about 10%), whereas Luby, Heffelfinger, et al. (2003) found relatively high rates of ODD (about 60%) in a preschool sample ascertained for depression. In elementary school, children who display both depression and aggression have been found to have more severe social problems than children who have depression or aggression alone (Quiggle, Garber, Panak, & Dodge, 1993; Rudolph, Hammen, & Burge, 1993).

To some extent, these comorbidities may reflect problems with symptom definition and the lack of age-specific DSM criteria. Among studies using similar ascertainment methods and structured parent interviews to diagnose clinic-referred preschoolers, rates of certain disorders have varied tremendously and seem to reflect investigators' own age-related adaptations of DSM symptom definitions. For example, Wilens et al. (2002) found that over half of their preschoolers selected for ADHD also met criteria for ODD (using the Schedule of Affective Disorders and Schizophrenia for School-Age Children [K-SADS]), about a quarter also met criteria for CD, and slightly over a quarter (26%) were found to have bipolar disorder. Using the parent version of the Diagnostic Interview Schedule for Children (DISC) to assess a sample of preschool boys selected for ODD, Speltz, McClellan, et al. (1999) reported equivalent levels of ODD–ADHD comorbidity, but only 3% met criteria for CD and 10% for any type of mood disorder (no cases of bipolar disorder were found using the DISC screening questions for mania). Finally, Keenan and Wakschlag (2000), using the K-SADS, found that 60% of their referrals (unselected for a particular condition) had ODD, 42% met criteria for CD, and 60% had ADHD (mood disorders were not assessed). Of note, the average age of onset for CD in this sample was 28 months.

The nature of these findings and discrepancies among similar studies—all using well-known, structured interviews—highlight the difficulties in estimating the construct validity and clinical implications of DSM disorders in preschool children (McClellan & Speltz, 2003). All three studies acknowledged the absence of a validated diagnostic tool for preschoolers, but each handled this problem in a different way. Wilens et al. (2002) made a diagnosis only if it was "clinically meaningful" (i.e., of "clinical concern"). Speltz, McClellan, et al. (1999) and Keenan and Wakschlag (2000) developed specific decision rules that were intended to reflect the developmental differences between preschool- and school-age children; however, each used different, and in some cases, diametrically opposed rules. For example, Speltz, McClellan, et al. (1999) excluded the child's hitting of a parent or sibling during a tantrum from consideration of the CD symptom "often initiates physical fights" and retained the stealing requirement of "nontrivial" items, whereas Keenan and Wakschlag (2000) included physical aggression toward siblings as behavior meeting criteria for physical fights and dropped the "nontrivial" stealing criterion. Wilens et al. (2002) provided insufficient detail to determine how they might have handled these items, and it is equally unclear how these investigators wrestled with adult-based definitions of "mania" for preschoolers (e.g., how does a 4-year-old manifest grandiosity, "flight of ideas," or attention that is "too easily drawn to irrelevant stimuli"?). Speltz, McClellan, et al. (1999) required evidence for the functional impairment of symptoms (as is stipulated by DSM-IV) and the other two studies, using only DSM-III-R criteria, presumably did not. None of the studies provided details regarding how other diagnostic conundrums specific to young children were handled, including, for example, the distinction between noncompliance and inattention, and noncompliance and failure to comprehend. The latter distinction is a common problem given the relatively high rates of language impairment in preschool children referred for psychiatric evaluation (e.g., Benasich, Curtiss, & Tallal, 1993).

These important but seldom discussed uncertainties in diagnostic procedures likely explain much of the variation in reported diagnostic rates of CD and mood disorders (including bipolar disorder) in these studies. There is need for consensus among researchers regarding theoretically driven and developmentally appropriate modifications of DSM ODD criteria for young children. Research investigating specific, clearly delineated modifications of DSM criteria is needed as well, as has been done by Luby and colleagues in their investigations of depressed preschoolers (e.g., changes in language and time requirements for display of symptoms; see Luby, Mrakotsky, et al., 2003). Until this happens, current data regarding comorbidity in preschoolers with ODD, ADHD, and/or CD must be regarded as extremely tentative, pending replication and cross-laboratory confirmation.

Longitudinal Course of ODD

In cross-sectional samples, studies of changes in the prevalence of ODD with age have been inconsistent, with some studies showing declining symptoms with increasing age from preschool to adolescence (e.g., Lahey et al., 2000; Maughan et al., 2004) and others showing increasing prevalence with age (e.g., Simonoff et al., 1997). Maughan and colleagues (2004) point out that age trends in the diagnosis of ODD depend heavily on whether an overlap in diagnosis with CD is allowed. If an ODD diagnosis is excluded when a CD diagnosis is made, as is intended by DSM-IV-TR criteria, prevalence rates of ODD decline in late childhood and adolescence. However, this is not likely due to improving behavior, but rather to a change in the classification of continuing externalizing problems among some children, from ODD to CD.

The results of several longitudinal studies indicate continuity of symptoms or progression to CD for a sizable portion of young children identified with behavior problems. In her influential program of research, Campbell (1995, 2002) found that roughly 50% of the children described by their parents as "difficult to manage" as toddlers continue to show significant behavior problems up to 7 years later. Similarly, Lavigne and colleagues (1998) found that over 50% of 2- to 5-year-old pediatric clinic patients with a disruptive behavior disorder (ODD, ADHD, or CD) continued to meet criteria for a diagnosis 1 to 3 years later. When reaching elementary school, about a quarter to a half of the children from this sample initially diagnosed with ODD continued to have this diagnosis, with or without comorbid disorders (Lavigne et al., 2001). In one clinic sample, persistence was even higher, with 76% of children meeting criteria for ODD as preschoolers continuing to meet diagnostic criteria for ODD and/or ADHD 2 years later (Speltz, McClellan, et al., 1999).

Few studies have examined factors predicting persistence along diagnosed cases, an issue of vital importance to clinicians. Speltz, McClellan, et al. (1999), in their sample of preschool boys selected for ODD, found three factors that predicted the persistence of diagnosis 2 years after initial referral: (1) greater severity of externalizing behaviors, as reported by parents on a child behavior checklist; (2) comorbid ADHD; and (3) the presence of certain ODD symptoms, especially those describing heightened affective reactivity (e.g., touchy/easily annoyed, angry/resentful, spiteful/vindictive).

Most longitudinal studies of preschool children with externalizing behavior problems and/or diagnoses of ODD have focused on homotypical outcomes (i.e., later externalizing problems and diagnoses of ODD, CD, or antisocial personality disorder [ASPD]). However, there is some evidence that early-starting externalizing problems can precede a diversity of later adjustment problems and diagnoses, including "internalizing" behavior problems and related mood and emotional disorders (Fischer, Rolf, Hasazi, & Cummings, 1984; Lavigne et al., 1998). Cicchetti and Schneider-Rosen (1984) and Lavigne et al. (1998) have theorized that internalizing and externalizing disorders coexist in preschool and become more differentiated as children become more articulate about their feelings. Even adult cases of schizophrenia have been shown in retrospective "follow-back" studies to be associated with significant externalizing problems during the preschool or early elementary school years (Jones, 1997). Thus, it is possible that the early childhood externalizing pattern—commonly leading to the diagnosis of ODD—may function as a "gateway" for diverse psychopathologies in later life, although antisocial outcomes are expected to be the most prevalent. Longitudinal studies are needed to examine factors potentially associated with this distinction in the predictive specificity of early externalizing symptoms (e.g., gender, family history, comorbidity).

ETIOLOGY

There have been many studies linking specific etiological factors to one or more aspects of the externalizing–antisocial "spectrum" (e.g., Ackerman, Schoff, Levinson, Youngstrom, & Izard, 1999; Shaw, Gilliom, Ingoldsby, & Nagin, 2003). These have included both the disruptive behaviors associated with ODD and physical aggression, which is more often associated with CD and juvenile delinquency. Nearly all of the etiological factors examined in this regard can be grouped into one of three broad categories, or domains, of potential vulnerability: (1) child biological factors, including temperament; (2) parent–child relationship factors (including both attachment processes and parenting practices); and (3) family and social-contextual factors. These categories of risk have been studied in both preschool-age and older ODD samples, with demonstrated relevance across age groups (Wakschlag & Keenan, 2001). We briefly summarize research in each category, followed by a discussion of studies in which various combinations of risk factors have been examined from a multifactorial perspective.

Biological Factors

Several biological factors have been studied in relation to aggression and criminality. In a recent review of the literature on autonomic nervous system (ANS) correlates of aggressive behavior, Raine (2002) concluded that low resting heart rate is the best-replicated biological correlate of antisocial and aggressive behavior in child and adolescent populations, and is thought to reflect reduced noradrenergic functioning and a fearless, stimulation-seeking temperament.

Low levels of a serotonin metabolite in the cerebrospinal fluid have been linked to both concurrent (Kruesi et al., 1992) and future aggression (Clarke, Murphy, & Constantino, 1999; Kruesi et al., 1992). A recent review of the link between serotonin and aggression concluded that this is not a simple, direct association, but rather reflects complex processes involving neuroanatomical and neurochemical interconnectivity, executive brain function, and behavioral dysregulation (Burke, Loeber, & Birmaher, 2002).

The hypothalamic–pituitary–adrenal (HPA) axis has been the focus on several recent studies. School-age children with ODD have been found to have higher levels of dehydroepiandrosterone sulfate (DHEAS) than psychiatric and nonpsychiatric controls (van Goozen et al., 2000), indicating that adrenal androgen functioning may be higher in children with ODD, reflecting a shift in the HPA axis. Changes in the HPA axis can be related to both genetic and environmental differences, and are amenable to change with intervention. For example, Kariyawasam, Zaw, and Handley (2002) used salivary cortisol as a measure of HPA axis function in children with combined ODD and ADHD, and found that stimulant medication moderated the relation between diagnosis and cortisol. As predicted, nonmedicated children with ODD–ADHD showed relatively low levels of salivary cortisol compared to controls. However, children medicated for ODD–ADD did not differ from controls in their cortisol levels.

Although correlational studies show significant associations between externalizing psychopathology and/or criminality and a particular biological variable (Burke et al., 2002), with few exceptions, the extent to which certain biological processes are the cause or effect of various externalizing behaviors is unclear. For example, in chronically aggressive children, elevated neuroendocrine or neurotransmitter perturbations might be the cause or consequence of this behavior (or both). Furthermore, some factors may have direct influence through structural brain alterations or injury, whereas others may indirectly lead to problem behavior by altering gene products or influencing the intrauterine environment; still others may work through a learning pathway via exposure to chaotic or abusive environments (Hendren & Mullen, 2004).

Genetic Processes

Several studies have shown that the offspring of criminal or alcoholic parents raised by adoptive parents (without these problems) have higher than expected rates of criminality themselves (e.g., Cadoret, Troughton, Bagford, & Woodworth, 1990). In a well-designed longitudinal study of a large-community twin sample, Zahn-Waxler, Schmitz, Fulker, Robinson, and Emde (1996) found evidence for genetic linkage in the externalizing behavior problems of 5-year-olds who were rated by multiple informants across several assessment contexts. Slutske et al. (1998) in a large-community sample of Australian twins, reported finding substantial genetic influence on the risk of CD. Reviews of this literature (e.g., Simonoff, 2001; Comings et al., 2000) have concluded that specific genes (e.g., the dopamine, serotonin and norepinephrine genes) are significantly associated with disruptive behavior disorders, but with strong evidence for gene–environment interactions in the determination of these disorders (e.g., Burt, Krueger, McGue, & Iacono, 2001). For example, in a recent twin study of conduct problems in children and adolescents ages 5–17 years, Scourfield, Van den Bree, Martin, and McGuffin (2004) showed that both parent and teacher reports of conduct problems were predicted by the combination of genetic influence and nonshared environmental factors, such as relationships between the child and each parent.

Child Temperament

"Temperament" is regarded as the direct behavioral product of the genetic and neurobiological factors just discussed. The validity of this assumption varies with how and when temperament is measured; for example, infant Brazelton exams more closely assess "pure" temperament than did parent checklists at preschool age (which are confounded with experience and parents' report biases). Nevertheless, most early childhood measures of "difficult" temperament (e.g., "infant irritability") have shown good consistency across time (Thomas & Chess, 1977) and predict subsequent behavior problems (Rutter, Birch, Thomas, & Chess, 1964), including aggression in the early school years (Rothbart & Bates, 1998). Eisenberg et al. (1996, Eisenberg, Fabes, Nyman, Bernzweig, & Pinuelas, 1994) found that children who have difficulty focusing and shifting attention—a key indicator of emotion regulation—are more likely to exhibit externalizing behaviors than children who show more flexible deployment of attention. Temperamental adaptability has also been shown to moderate the effects of family instability on externalizing behavior problems in preschool children (Ackerman et al., 1999).

Neuropsychological Functions

At present, neuropsychological testing is not a routine part of the diagnosis of ODD in children. Most of what is known about the relation between externalizing problems and neuropsychological functioning is based on studies of school-age children with CD and adolescents. On IQ tests, juvenile delinquents have been consistently shown to score between one-half and a full standard deviation below their nondelinquent peers. Greater discrepancies are associated with problems that begin in early childhood and meet criteria for ODD, CD, or ADHD (Moffitt, 1990). Performance IQ in the adolescent delinquent population is usually higher than Verbal IQ, and antisocial children generally perform more poorly than their peers on just about any task that is administered orally, requires language mediation, and calls for a verbal response (Moffitt & Lynham, 1995).

Older children and adolescents with externalizing problems also score relatively poorly on tasks associated with frontal lobe integrity (Pennington & Ozonoff, 1996; Seguin, Pihl, Harden, Tremblay, & Boulerice, 1995), as do many other psychiatrically impaired groups (Sergeant, Geurts, & Oosterlaan, 2002). The most frequently used tasks are those associated with the "executive functions," which include the ability to monitor and control attention, to "hold" information in working memory, to make plans and set goals, to formulate mental models, and to modify these models on the basis of experience. Deficits in executive functions are most consistently found in children with ODD or CD who also have ADHD (Clark, Prior, & Kinsella, 2002; van Goozen et al., 2004), and most researchers today believe that executive function deficits are more specifically related to ADHD than to ODD or CD (Clark et al., 2002). This observation, together with the fact that children with early-onset conduct problems are more likely to have attention deficits than those with later onset (Loeber, Green, Keenan, & Lahey, 1995), suggests that deficits in executive functions may be more strongly associated with children who show an early, rather than late, onset of externalizing psychopathology.

Research on the neuropsychological characteristics of preschool children with ODD and ADHD has been limited by the lack of developmentally appropriate and psychometrically sound measures of certain functions (e.g., executive functions). Despite this deficiency, however, the study of neurodevelopment in preschoolers with ODD has certain advantages. There is the opportunity to examine the child's cognitive and language abilities before the onset of formal schooling, with its transactional effects on subsequent development (Hinshaw, 1992), and to identify neuropsychological processes closely related in time to the onset of symptoms. Early research on preschool neuropsychological functions focused on IQ and language skills (e.g., Campbell, Szumowski, Ewing, Gluck, & Breaux, 1982), with most studies finding that children clinically referred for "hyperactive" or "hard to manage" characteristics had lower scores than matched comparison groups on standardized measures. In a large nonclinic sample of 2- to 5-year-olds, Dietz, Lavigne, Arend, and Rosenbaum (1997) found that both Verbal and Performance IQ contributed to the prediction of externalizing and internalizing Child Behavior Checklist (CBCL) scales and to the presence of a diagnosis.

In one of the only studies to assess broadly a clinic-referred preschool group, Speltz, DeKlyen, and Greenberg (1999) administered IQ, language, and motor and executive function measures (motor planning and verbal fluency) to boys with ODD, with and without comorbid ADHD. In comparison with a sample of normally developing boys of similar social and family background, clinic-referred boys had (1) lower Full Scale IQ equivalent scores, (2) a higher probability of Performance IQ scores exceeding Verbal IQ scores, (3) lower performance on a latent factor of verbal ability, and (4) lower performance on a factor representing the two executive function measures. Among clinic-referred boys, those with comorbid diagnoses of ODD and ADHD were more likely to score poorly on measures of verbal ability than were those with only ODD, and they showed poorer performance on the executive function tasks. These findings are remarkably similar to those obtained with older children and adolescents with ODD and/or CD. It appears that the ODD–CD neuropsychological deficit profile begins well before the onset of formal schooling, casting doubt on the hypotheses that the deficits observed in adolescents are primarily the consequence of poor motivation and lack of participation in formal schooling.

Parent–Child Relationship Factors

Attachment Relationships

Studies of observed separation–reunion behaviors (using age-appropriate modifications of the Ainsworth Strange Situation) have shown that clinic-referred preschoolers are more likely to show insecure (ineffective) attachment patterns than matched comparison groups (for a recent review of attachment theory and research, see Carlson, Sampson, & Sroufe, 2003). This is relevant given the predominance of the ODD diagnosis among clinic-referred preschoolers. Speltz et al. (1999) found that over half (54%) of clinic-referred preschool boys with ODD exhibited an insecure attachment strategy during reunions with their mothers, as opposed to 17% of comparison boys. Father–child interactions during separations–reunions in the same sample of boys indicated a similar pattern (DeKlyen et al., 1998). Boys insecurely attached with both parents were extremely unlikely to belong to the comparison group. This pattern of attachment classification was similar for single- and two-parent families.

Although an association between a clinical diagnosis of ODD and insecure attachment seems clear, the specific factors accounting for this relationship are less certain. Greenberg, DeKlyen, Speltz, and Endriga (1997) proposed several ways in which attachment processes might be related to the development of externalizing behaviors. First, infants and young children who experience an insecure relationship with insensitive or unpredictable parents are likely to develop cognitive representations of relationships that bias subsequent social perceptions and cognitions (Sroufe & Fleeson, 1986). For example, older children with CD are more likely than typical children to attribute hostile intentions to others (Dodge, 1991), which may be due in part to a negative expectation of the availability and responsiveness of others ("felt security"; Fisher, Kramer, Hoven, King, & Bowlby, 1982). Second, insecure attachment quality may lead to a resistant motivational set for social interaction, adversely affecting readiness to identify and comply with parents and other caregivers (Waters, Kondo-Ikemura, Posada, & Richters, 1990). Third, externalizing behaviors (e.g., tantrums or noncompliance) may serve an "attachment function" for some children by regulating parent proximity and availability when caregiving is difficult to obtain (Greenberg & Speltz, 1988). Fourth, effective parent–infant interactions during times of stress may help infants to regulate their emotions. Over repeated experiences of this nature, such interactions may promote structural changes in corticolimbic structures, enabling children to regulate their own affect effectively (Greenberg & Snell, 1997). Disorders associated with emotion dysregulation (such as ODD) may be due in part to this impaired ability to tolerate and manage strong affect (Greenberg & Snell, 1997; Schore, 1996).

These hypothesized mediators of insecure attachment and behavior problems have yet to be thoroughly investigated, although two of them—biased social perceptions and poor self-regulation—have received tentative empirical support. Several studies have shown that insecurely attached infants and preschoolers are more likely than their secure counterparts to enter new relationships with distrust and negative expectations (e.g., Carslon, Sroufe, & Egeland, 2004; Ziv, Oppenheim, & Sagi-Schwartz, 2004). In the clinic-referred ODD sample followed by Speltz and colleagues (showing high rates of insecure attachment), clinic-referred boys were significantly more likely than boys in the comparison group to show hostile attributions in their response to a peer-oriented social problem-solving task (Coy, Speltz, & Jones, 2002). Studies have also shown that effective emotional self-regulation in the toddler or preschool years is predicted by secure attachment, and that assessed emotion regulation at this age predicts subsequent emotional control, social competence, and behavior problems in the early school years (Denham, Blair, Schmidt, & DeMulder, 2002; Gilliom & Shaw, 2004).

Parenting Practices

Most studies of parenting practices have focused on parents' reactions to their children's misbehavior; for example, the consistency of parents' disciplinary behavior or the severity of punishments they administer (e.g., McMahon & Forehand, 1988). The timing and contingency of parent's and children's behavior in conflicted interactions have also been examined. Patterson (2002) found that in the families of aggressive boys, one partner's aversive behavior (e.g., a child whining or a parent nagging) is commonly reinforced by the termination of the other's aversive behavior, leading to repetitive cycles of negative coercive interaction. Conflict in situations not involving child transgressions also has been examined (e.g., parental controlling behavior during play interactions with their child; Bates, Bayles, Bennett, Ridge, & Brown, 1991). In a number of investigations involving preschool children, strong associations between these dimensions of ineffective or punitive parenting practices and child problem behavior have been found (e.g., Campbell, 1991), including the types of disruptive behaviors leading to clinical referral (Gadow et al., 2001; Greenberg, Speltz, DeKlyen, & Jones, 2001). However, the extent to which such parental behaviors are the cause or result of difficult child behavior remains unclear (Anderson, Lytton, & Romney, 1986).

In addition to disciplinary action, "positive parenting practices" are also important (e.g., positive social exchanges, anticipatory guidance, monitoring of child activities, and affective expressiveness of parents). Positive parenting processes are often are more complex, longer in duration, and more distant in time from child negative behavior than parental discipline; thus, they are more difficult to measure. However, the results of some studies indicate that the absence of positive parenting practices may be as important as the presence of coercive cycles in the etiology of externalizing behavior (DeKlyen et al., 1998). For example, Pettit and Bates (1989) found that parents who initiated more positive verbal communication and physical proximity had children with lower aggression. Disruptive behavior was unrelated to the number of overt disciplinary encounters but closely associated with the proportion of ignored child initiations. Similarly, Gardner (1987) observed the families of normal preschoolers and preschoolers with behavior disorders and found that families of the problem preschoolers spent half as much time in joint play and positive conversation at home.

Family and Social Context

Family and social context can affect parents' capacity to provide optimal care to the developing child. Several researchers have used family adversity indices to summarize the total number of negative factors that have occurred or are presently active in the life of the family (e.g., Sameroff, Seifer, Barocas, Zax, & Greenspan, 1987). Such indices typically include parental characteristics (low parent education, psychiatric illness, substance abuse, criminality), family functioning (marital distress, family violence), and environmental provisions (poverty, crowded living conditions, violent neighborhoods). Ingoldsby and Shaw (2002) reviewed evidence showing that neighborhood context contributes significantly to the onset and persistence of early-onset externalizing problems. Other ecological factors of potential importance are the family's stress reactions to life events, such as divorce or job loss (Barkley, Fischer, Edelbrock, & Smallish, 1991) and the social support resources available to and utilized by the family (Jenkins & Smith, 1990). Nearly all of these aspects of family ecology have been related to externalizing behavior problems in early childhood (e.g., Erel & Kissil, 2003; Shaw et al., 2003). Although the findings in these studies were that these aspects of family ecology are specifically related to externalizing behavior, similar factors have been related to other psychiatric diagnoses, such as depression, anxiety, and withdrawal (e.g., Xue, Leventhal, Brooks-Gunn, & Earls, 2005), suggesting that family factors may be a more general risk factor for multiple forms of psychiatric illness.

Multifactorial Risk Models

The previous listing of potential etiological or risk factors for externalizing–antisocial behavior is long and remarkably heterogeneous, ranging from genetic processes to neighborhood characteristics. Most studies have examined these factors in isolation from one another, limiting our knowledge of the interrelationships among them. Yet it is unlikely that any single risk factor—or domain of similar risk factors (e.g., child biological factors)—is either necessary or sufficient to cause ODD or other forms of antisocial behavior. Rather, various combinations of risk factor domains probably lead to ODD, which is likely the end point of multiple pathways (Greenberg, Speltz, DeKlyen, & Endriga, 1991; Campbell, 1991; Loeber, 1990). Although several multifactorial models of externalizing problems have been proposed (e.g., Hill, 2002), very few studies have actually tested the concurrent or predictive significance of these models. The Rochester Longitudinal Study found that a multiple-risk index including 10 risk factors (reflecting the psychological functioning of the mother, family socioeconomic and minority status, family support, life events and family size) significantly predicted children's social–emotional competence better than any single risk factor alone. The effects could not be explained by any particular subset of the risk factors (Sameroff et al., 1987), and no particular risk patterns were uncovered across subgroups of individual (Sameroff, Seifer, Baldwin, & Baldwin, 1993). Liaw and Brooks-Gunn (1994) tested the effects of 13 risk factors on young children's behavior problems and found that as the number of risk factors increased, so did the incidence of behavior problems.

Greenberg et al. (2001) developed and tested a risk model specifically for early-onset ODD that extended previous studies of cumulative risk (e.g., Sameroff et al., 1987) by using methods that considered the relative contribution or overlap among the variables in the model. The Greenberg et al. (2001) model contained four domains of risk quite similar to those reviewed earlier: (1) child characteristics (e.g., prematurity, birth complications, teratogenic exposure, timing of developmental milestones, and IQ); (2) parenting practices (behavior management style, harsh or abusive discipline, warmth, involvement); (3) child–parent attachment; and (4) family ecology (family conflict, parental mental status and personal functioning, life stress, family structure, socioeconomic status, and the quality of family social supports). Results indicated that the combination of these factors provided relatively high sensitivity (81%) and specificity (85%) in differentiating clinic-seeking families with boys meeting criteria for ODD from demographically matched comparison boys. A dramatic increase in the probability of clinic status occurred when three or more factors were present, and specific combinations of factors were differentially predictive of conduct problems. For example, families with "high-risk" status in three domains in which *parenting practices* was one of the domains had much higher rates of disorder than did the other three combination patterns.

CLINICAL INTERVENTION

Assessment of ODD Symptoms in Preschoolers

Symptoms of ODD can vary considerably across settings and contexts. For example, children may show more significant behavior problems with one caregiver versus another, may have problems at home but not in their day care or preschool classroom, or might have particular difficulty with certain routines or activities (e.g., in public places). Thus, evaluations should be tailored to assess the "topography" of the child's behavior. As discussed below, this might include obtaining information from multiple caregivers through behavior rating scales or clinical interviews; clinic observations of caregiver–child interactions in analogue situations (e.g., play, teaching task, separation–reunion, cleanup), and (ideally) direct behavioral observations of the home and day care or preschool. In addition to contributing to a more thorough evaluation, such data are invaluable in developing an intervention to address the child's needs successfully.

Rating Scales

Caregiver-completed rating scales are a particularly efficient method for assessing symptoms of ODD. Rating scales are ideally completed by two or more caregivers who interact with the child in different settings (e.g., a parent and a teacher or day care provider). As noted earlier, this multi-informant approach helps to assess variability in a child's symptoms across settings or contexts, which can be very important in diagnostic decision making and in determining appropriate treatment modalities.

Several of the commonly used rating scales are appropriate for preschoolers and/or have age-appropriate versions. The Child Behavior Checklist for Ages 1 to 5 (CBCL 1–5; Achenbach & Rescorla, 2000) and companion Caregiver–Teacher Report Form (C-TRF; Achenbach & Rescorla, 2000) are the most popular. These broadband scales assess internalizing and externalizing problems. The current version includes a language development scale to screen for communication problems, and scores can be derived for several DSM-IV-TR categories. As with the Achenbach scales for older children, the normative data and psychometric properties of these scales are excellent (Myers & Collett, 2005). Another broadband scale developed specifically for children ages 1–3 years is the Infant and Toddler Social–Emotional Assessment (ITSEA; Carter & Briggs-Gowan, 2000). An abbreviated screening version (the Brief Infant Toddler Social–Emotional Assessment; Briggs-Gowan & Carter, 2002) is also available. The ITSEA includes Internalizing, Externalizing, Dysregulation, and Competency composite scales, as well as Maladaptive, Atypical Behavior, and Social Relatedness scales to assess more serious pathology (e.g., pervasive developmental disorders, posttraumatic stress disorder, sexualized behavior). Normative data are available for a large sample of young children; preliminary psychometric and validity data are promising (e.g., Briggs-Gowan, Carter, Irwin, Wachtel, & Cicchetti, 2004; Carter, Briggs-Gowan, Jones, & Little, 2003), and the scale is beginning to be used in other research applications with young children (e.g., Bracha et al., 2004; Briggs-Gowan et al., 2004; Ellingson, Briggs-Gowan, Carter, & Horwitz, 2004). Finally, the Eyberg Child Behavior Inventory (ECBI; Eyberg & Pincus, 1999) is a narrowband scale used to assess disruptive behaviors in young children. Although the ECBI is not disorder-specific, items correspond roughly to the DSM-IV-TR disruptive behavior disorders. The ECBI includes separate Problem and Intensity scales, allowing the caregiver to rate whether each behavior is considered problematic (yes–no) and how frequently the behavior occurs. This unique feature allows clinicians to assess parents' threshold or tolerance for disruptive behavior. For example, if a caregiver were to rate several items as problematic but low frequency, it may suggest a low tolerance level and/or developmentally inappropriate expectations for behavior (Eyberg & Pincus, 1999). Normative data are available, and the ECBI has good psychometric characteristics and well-established validity (Collett, Ohan, & Myers, 2003). The scale is commonly used as an outcome measure in treatment and other studies of children with ODD and related conduct problems.

Structured Clinical Interviews

Structured interviews can be used to obtain a more precise clinical diagnosis, assessment of severity, and description of clinical course. Unfortunately, until very recently, there were no such interviews developed specifically for toddlers or preschoolers. Researchers have tended to use interviews developed for older youth (e.g., DISC-IV, K-SADS) or to create modified versions. As noted earlier, developmental modifications have varied among research groups, making it difficult to compare across studies. Of course, this also makes it difficult for practicing clinicians to know how their diagnostic practices compare to those of their colleagues.

A recent and exciting advancement is the development of the Preschool Age Psychiatric Assessment (PAPA; Egger, Ascher, & Angold, 1999). The PAPA, a structured parent interview for children ages 2 through 5 years, can be completed by clinicians or laypersons (e.g., as in large-scale epidemiological research). A glossary is included, with objective definitions of target symptoms. The interview is a downward extension and substantially modified version of the Child and Adolescent Psychiatric Assessment (CAPA; Angold et al., 1995). The PAPA includes modified DSM-IV and International Classification of Diseases (ICD-10; World Health Organization, 1992) symptoms, symptoms from the Diagnostic Classification: 0–3 (DC:0–3; Zero to Three, 1999), and items from the CBCL for Ages 1½–5 and ITSEA. Items were also taken from the research literature on early childhood psychopathology and symptoms related to functional impairment and developmental progression (e.g., sleep behaviors, toileting). Consistent with Axis II of the DC:0–3, the PAPA can also be used to assess the relationship context. The collection of normative, psychometric, and validity data is underway (Egger & Angold, 2004). The PAPA has a great deal of potential for advancing both clinical and research practice.

Observational Methods

As in other aspects of early childhood mental health, assessment and treatment planning for preschoolers with ODD rely heavily on clinical observation. *In vivo* observations in the home, day care, or preschool setting are ideal in many respects. Though the presence of an unfamiliar observer in these settings clearly has an effect on the behavior of those observed, child and caregiver behaviors are likely to resemble day-to-day interactions more closely, and subtle factors that would not be apparent in the clinic (e.g., peer/sibling influence) may be noted. Furthermore, there is no substitute for experiencing firsthand the child's environment, including variables that caregivers themselves might fail to notice or be reticent to discuss (e.g., hygiene/safety concerns).

More commonly, observations are conducted in the clinic setting, using analogue tasks to simulate daily activities and interactions between children and their parents. For example, several observation systems (e.g., Dyadic Parent–Child Interaction Coding System–II [Eyberg, Bessmer, Newcomb, Edwards, & Robinson, 1994]; Behavioral Coding System [Forehand & McMahon, 1981]) include three stages: free play or child-directed play, parent-directed play, and cleanup. A variety of parent and child behaviors are coded. For children, target behaviors include things like compliance, "talking back," destructive behavior, yelling, and whining. Observed parent behaviors include giving commands, critical comments, and praise statements. Another popular parent–child observation system is the Clinical Problem-Solving Procedure (Crowell, Feldman, & Ginsburg, 1988). In addition to free play and cleanup activities, this system includes an activity with bubbles (to assess mutual enjoyment, turn taking, etc.), teaching during tasks that range from the child's skill level to well-above skill level (to assess the child's reliance on the parent for "scaffolding" and parent's skills), and a separation–reunion task (to assess the attachment relationship). Finally, Benham (2000) has described a mental status exam to guide observations of young children. The Infant–Toddler

Mental Status Exam can be completed based on informal observation and focuses on qualities of the child's appearance, reaction to the clinical situation, capacity for self-regulation, motor behavior, speech and language, thought, affect and mood, play, cognition, and relatedness.

Though the commonly used parent–child interaction observations have been criticized for lacking psychometric support (e.g., test–retest reliability) and normative data, they have become standard in behavioral parent training outcome studies and have proven very sensitive to treatment effects (Roberts, 2001). Clinically, these observations are easy to incorporate in the assessment process and tend to provide rich information. Videotaping interactions and later reviewing them with parents can lend insight into parent attributions and cognitions that might contribute to conflict (e.g., developmentally inappropriate expectations, attributing misbehavior to stable rather than contextual or otherwise unstable causes). Furthermore, they provide an excellent starting point for intervention with emphasis on the parent–child relationship and a way of documenting for families their improvement over the course of treatment (McDonough, 2000).

Treatment Interventions and Their Effectiveness

Child-Focused Interventions

A variety of individual therapies have been developed and are used in clinical practice with disruptive youngsters, including play therapy, psychodynamic therapy, and cognitive-behavioral therapy (CBT; see Chapters 15, and 16, this volume, for a general review of these treatment modalities). However, evidence for the efficacy of these treatments with preschoolers with ODD is limited, and some authors (e.g., Harter, 1983) have questioned whether young children are developmentally able to benefit from these traditional therapies. Furthermore, there is increasing appreciation for the need to address behavior problems on a systemic level to bring about sustained change. Research has therefore focused largely on interventions that target the parent–child relationship and the contingencies that maintain behavior problems in the home, day care, or preschool settings.

There is some evidence to support group social skills interventions with preschoolers, and such programs have been incorporated into several multimodal early intervention/prevention studies (e.g., the Montreal Longitudinal Experimental Study [Tremblay, Masse, Perrron, LeBlanc, Schwartzman, & Ledingham, 1992]; the Fast Track project [Conduct Problems Prevention Research Group, 1992]). Many of these programs are downward extensions of CBT treatments that have been validated with school-age children and adolescents (e.g., Kazdin, Esveldt-Dawson, French, & Unis, 1987; Lochman, Burch, Curry, & Lampron, 1984). Based on the social information process research discussed earlier, treatments focus on helping children to identify accurately social cues and to generate and enact prosocial solutions. CBT approaches may also include anger management strategies that "coach" children to use adaptive strategies to regulate and manage arousal. Therapists model the various skills and provide opportunities for behavioral rehearsal with therapist feedback (e.g., Webster-Stratton & Reid, 2003).

Parent Training and Consultation

Parent training and behavioral consultation is the psychosocial intervention that has received the most empirical support for the treatment of ODD (Brestan & Eyberg, 1998), and is particularly well-suited for young children. These programs are based on operant behavioral and social learning theories, with the objective of changing the environmental contingencies (e.g., parents' responses) that perpetuate disruptive child behaviors, regardless of whether such factors are truly causative (i.e., predisposing or precipitating disruptive child behavior). Several models are used, with the most well-known being Eyberg's parent–child interaction therapy (PCIT; Eyberg, Boggs, & Algina, 1995), Webster-Stratton's Incredible Years program (1994), Barkley's Defiant Children program (1997), Patterson's Living with Children program (1976; Patterson & Gullion, 1968), and Forehand and McMahon's Helping the Noncompliant Child program (2003).

These programs have all been greatly influenced by the work of Patterson and colleagues (Patterson, 1982; Patterson & Gullion, 1968) and the unpublished work of Hanf (1969). Hanf introduced the notion of coaching parents in nondirective, child-directed play (i.e., the "child's game"). In addition to facilitating relationship development, these activities were intended to increase parents' responsiveness to desirable behavior. The second stage of the Hanf model involved parent-directed activities (i.e., the "parent's game"), intended to set limits and increase child compliance. Most current models continue to use this two-stage approach. Patterson's work (1982) has been important in terms of developing a conceptual understanding of the coercive parent–child exchanges often seen in these families, and the Living with Children program (Patterson & Gullion, 1968) was among the first to be empirically validated.

Parent training has been offered in a variety of treatment formats. Programs intended for individual families (e.g., PCIT) offer the advantage of being able to focus on a particular family's needs and to incorporate sufficient guided practice, whereas group interventions (e.g., Incredible Years program) are an efficient way to reach a broader audience and can offer parents a source of social support. Several authors have studied the addition of adjunctive treatments for pretreatment motivational enhancement (e.g., Chaffin et al., 2004), to help parents manage stress and cope with depression (e.g., Webster-Stratton, 1994), and to address parental substance abuse and issues related to domestic violence (e.g., Chaffin et al., 2004). Parent training has also been used along with other treatment modalities, such as child social skills training and classroom interventions, in prevention programs for high-risk youth (e.g., Conduct Problems Prevention Research Group, 1999a, 1999b; Tremblay et al., 1992; Webster-Stratton, Reid, & Hammond, 2001).

There is a substantial body of research supporting the efficacy of behavioral parent training for the treatment of conduct problems in clinically referred children and as a preventive intervention for those considered "at-risk" (Serketitch & Dumas, 1996). In recent research, the Incredible Years program and PCIT have been especially popular. In a series of randomized, controlled trials Webster-Stratton and colleagues have shown that their intervention results in significant and clinically meaningful improvements in parents' use of effective behavior management and child behavior strategies (e.g., Webster-Stratton, Reid, & Hammond, 2001, 2004), and improvements are maintained over time (Reid, Webster-Stratton, & Hammond, 2003). An independent research group (Scott, Spender, Doolan, Jacobs, & Aspland, 2001) has replicated these positive outcomes. Randomized, controlled studies have shown that PCIT is effective in reducing disruptive child behaviors and improving parental competencies (Chaffin et al., 2004; Nixon, Sweeney, Erickson, & Touyz, 2004; Schumann, Foote, Eyberg, Boggs, & Algina, 1998), and improvements appear to be maintained at follow-up periods of up to 6 years (Nixon et al., 2004; Hood & Eyberg, 2003). Additionally, PCIT has recently been used effectively with families with a history of domestic violence (e.g., Chaffin et al., 2004; Timmer, Sedlar, & Urquiza, 2004). There is some evidence that improvement in child behavior generalizes to other settings (e.g., the classroom; McNeil, Eyberg, Eisenstadt, Newcomb, & Funderburk, 1991), though overall this appears to be the exception rather than the rule with parent training (Serketich & Dumas, 1996). It does appear that when parents' skills improve, they are able to generalize those skills to interactions with untreated siblings (Brestan, Eyberg, Boggs, & Algina, 1997).

An emerging treatment developed specifically for children with ODD is Ross Greene and colleagues' Collaborative Problem Solving approach (CPS; Greene, Ablon, & Goring, 2003). The CPS model incorporates several elements of behavioral consultation, such as psychoeducation for parents and instruction in behavioral strategies for managing child misbehavior. This portion of the program focuses largely on antecedents of behavior problems, teaching parents to think proactively to avoid behavior problems before they occur. Parents and children also learn strategies for resolving disagreements and diffusing conflict through negotiation. Parents are coached to prioritize their expectations as (1) those that are non-negotiable, (2) those that can be negotiated, and (3) those that they are willing to give up for the time being. Greene (2001) described the use of this approach in a book for parents entitled *The Explosive Child: A New Approach for Understanding and Helping Easily Frustrated, "Chronically Inflexible" Children* (second edition). Preliminary data support the efficacy of the CPS approach (Greene et al., 2004) with children as young as age 4, though some of the skills targeted appear more appropriate for older children.

A variety of factors have been found to influence outcomes in parent

training, with adjunctive treatment components developed in an effort to enhance outcomes. There is some indication that outcomes are better for two-
parent families and when both mother and father are involved in treatment
(Bagner & Eyberg, 2003; Webster-Stratton, 1985). Adjunctive treatments to
enhance parents' communication skills and address marital conflict have been
shown to improve child outcomes (Dadds, Schwartz, & Sanders, 1987; Greist
et al., 1982; Webster-Stratton, 1994). More generally, several researchers
have focused on maternal social isolation and have shown enhanced outcomes when treatments to improve interpersonal skills are added to traditional parent training (Dadds & McHugh, 1992; Wahler, Cartor, Fleischman,
& Lambert, 1993; Webster-Stratton, 1994).

Infant–Parent and Toddler–Parent Programs

There is a rich clinical literature on infant–parent and toddler–parent psychotherapies that may also be applicable for disruptive preschoolers. In general,
the theoretical underpinnings for these treatments come from psychodynamic,
object relations, and attachment theories (Lieberman, Silverman, & Pawl,
2000; see Chapter 16, this volume). Clinicians working in this tradition tend
to identify the parent–child (most often the mother–child) relationship as
their "patient," rather than the disruptive child him- or herself (Lieberman et
al., 2000). These treatments tend to be less directive than other approaches
and emphasize the role of parents' earlier life experiences (e.g., with their own
caregivers) in shaping how they relate to their child. In addition to insight and
increased awareness of these past–present relationships, the experience of being in a therapeutic relationship is thought to bring about positive change in
the parent–child relationship (Emde, Everhart, & Wise, 2004). Much of the
literature on infant– and toddler–parent psychotherapy has focused on families facing multiple stressors, particularly low socioeconomic status families,
adolescent mothers, and those involved in the child protective system (Lieberman et al., 2000). Speltz (1990) outlined an approach that combines several
aspects of these programs—particularly attachment-focused interventions—
with the social learning, parent-training models described previously.

   Relative to the behavioral parent training approaches described earlier,
rigorous empirical research (e.g., using randomized, controlled trials) on these
treatments is limited. However, there is evidence that these treatment approaches lead to improvements in parents' sensitivity and responsiveness
(Bakermans-Kranenburg, van IJzendoorn, & Juffer, 2003). For example, Cohen, Lojkask, Muir, Muir, and Parker (2002) have published outcomes data
from their Watch, Wait, and Wonder program. This intervention involves
guiding parents to observe their child's activity and foster adaptive interpretations of their child's cues. In some respects, this resembles much of what occurs during the child-directed play portion of most parent training programs.
Preliminary data suggest that the intervention results in decreased parenting
stress and increased comfort in dealing with infant behaviors for mothers,

and improvements in attachment and emotion regulation for children (Cohen et al., 2002). In the Netherlands, van den Boom (1994) has evaluated the effectiveness of a home visiting program in which clinicians worked with mothers to increase their sensitivity and responsiveness to child cues. In a sample of infants identified as highly irritable, the authors found that those whose mothers received treatment showed less irritability, greater exploration of their surroundings, and higher frequency of secure attachments than controls.

Classroom-Based Interventions

There is a great deal of research on the beneficial effects of comprehensive preschool programs, such as Head Start, for at-risk children. Although many of these projects were initially intended to enhance children's cognitive and academic development, some of the most important benefits relate to decreased behavior problems and longer-term reductions in juvenile delinquency (Yoshikawa, 1994). The more recent multimodal early intervention/prevention studies (e.g., Conduct Problems Prevention Research Group, 1992; Tremblay et al., 1992; Walker, Stiller, Severson, Feil, & Golly, 1998) continue to include classroom-based interventions along with other modalities. Most of these are downward extensions of programs developed for school-age children. Overall, there has been relatively little research on classroom-based programs specifically for preschoolers (e.g., Bryant, Vizzard, Willoughby, & Kupersmidt, 1999). This is unfortunate given that (1) preschools have the potential to be a very important resource for children whose families are not able or willing to access mental health care; (2) the setting tends to differ substantially from K–12 classrooms, with less structure and a greater emphasis on socialization versus academics; and (3) training for the early childhood educators and paraprofessionals working in these settings is highly variable, and may not include adequate training in behavior management.

The interventions with the best support involve behavioral training and consultation with teachers. For example, previous studies have supported the use of token reinforcement and response–cost interventions (McGoey & DuPaul, 2000; Reynolds & Kelley, 1997). These involve giving students the opportunity to earn tokens (e.g., stickers) that can later be redeemed for special privileges or rewards, contingent upon desired social behaviors. Tokens may be removed in response to targeted misbehaviors. There is also some evidence supporting the use of group contingencies with preschoolers. The most popular example is the Good Behavior Game developed by Barrish, Saunders, and Wolfe (1969). This involves dividing the classroom into two or more teams that compete to determine which group receives the fewest marks for undesirable behavior. Members of the winning team earn rewards or special privileges. The Good Behavior Game has been examined primarily with school-age children (e.g., Ialongo et al., 1999), though it has been shown effective with preschoolers in at least one small study (Swiezy, Matson, & Box, 1992). Recently, Filcheck, McNeil, Greco, and Bernard (2004) described the use of a classroom-wide token economy system and teacher coaching based on PCIT, with results suggesting that both strategies resulted in decreased child behavior problems. The use of compatible parent and teacher trainings appears to be a very promising approach, because it may facilitate generalization of treatment gains and promote parent–teacher collaboration.

Psychopharmacological Treatments

The prescribing of psychotropic medications to preschool-age children has increased dramatically in recent years (Zito et al., 2000), despite the lack of efficacy and safety data (Greenhill, 1998). These issues are addressed in greater detail by Luby (Chapter 14, this volume). Although there are no approved pharmacological interventions specifically for ODD, aggression and severe tantrums are a common focus of treatment. Developmental issues, and the unknown potential for long-term effects, raise caution. In comparison to older children, preschool children tend to respond less clearly to psychotropic agents and to show higher probability of side effects (Greenhill, 1998; Wilens & Spenser, 2000). Research is needed to better define valid symptom constructs as targets for treatment (Greenhill et al., 2003).

Stimulant medications have been found to be helpful for ADHD in preschoolers in placebo-controlled trials (American Academy of Child and Adolescent Psychiatry, 2002). In school-age children, stimulant medications have been shown to be effective for core ADHD symptoms as well as comorbid aggression (American Academy of Child and Adolescent Psychiatry, 2002).

Other classes of medications used to treat aggression in children include alpha-2 adrenoreceptor agonists, mood stabilizers, and antipsychotic agents (see Steiner, Saxena, & Chang, 2003). None of these agents have been well studied in preschool children. Moreover, the potential long-term developmental and neurophysiological implications of exposing very young children to psychotropic agents are unknown. Thus, although psychopharmacological intervention may be warranted for preschoolers with serious behavioral dysregulation, evidenced-based psychosocial interventions should be implemented first, if possible. Furthermore, when used, the need for ongoing medication use should be systematically reviewed over time, with careful monitoring of side effects.

FUTURE DIRECTIONS

Several trends can be anticipated in the future of research and clinical practice with disruptive preschoolers. Future research is likely to develop models of diagnostic classification based on specific etiological mechanisms such as temperament, genetic vulnerability, gene–environment interactions, and typologies of parent–child relationships (e.g., secure vs. insecure attachment). We expect to see further refinements of DSM diagnostic criteria as well, primarily in relation to developmental context (e.g., decision rules for defining "aggression" and "mania" in children under age 5). We also expect to see continued development of alternatives to DSM criteria, such as DC: 0–3 (Zero to Three, 1994).

Returning to two of the questions we posed at the beginning of this chapter, there has been little study of the many factors potentially distinguishing between referred preschoolers who outgrow their disruptive problems and those whose problems persist. And it is only suspected—but not confirmed—that ODD functions as a "gateway" to more diverse psychopathology in later life. From both a theoretical and clinical perspective, these are probably the two most important unresolved issues regarding ODD in the preschool years. Prospective longitudinal studies of large clinical samples are needed to examine predictors of continuity of ODD, including sex differences in developmental trajectories.

With respect to clinical applications, we envision increasing efforts in three areas: (1) parent–child interventions that integrate "behavior management" strategies with interventions that focus more on the quality of the parent–child relationship (e.g., attachment processes); (2) early screening and educational interventions for disruptive preschoolers that address their well-established verbal deficits, particularly in phonological processing and other early reading skills; and (3) psychopharmacology, particularly medications that might attenuate emotional reactivity. As etiological mechanisms are unraveled, biological interventions may be developed that target disrupted neurodevelopmental processes rather than symptomatic presentation. Caution will be needed in applying new treatments and technologies to young children given the potential vulnerability of developing brains, and the potential for adverse events and unexpected outcomes not predicted by studies in older individuals.

REFERENCES

Achenbach, T. W., & Rescorla, L. A. (2000). *Manual for the ASEBA Preschool Forms and Profiles*. Burlington: University of Vermont, Research Center for Children, Youth, and Families.

Ackerman, B. P., Schoff, K., Levinson, K., Youngstrom, E., & Izard, C. E. (1999). The relations between cluster indexes of risk and promotion and the problem behaviors of 6- and 7-year-old children from economically disadvantaged families. *Developmental Psychology, 35*, 1355–1366.

American Academy of Child and Adolescent Psychiatry. (2002). Practice parameter for the use of stimulant medications in the treatment of children, adolescents, and adults. *Journal of the American Academy of Child and Adolescent Psychiatry, 41*(Suppl.), 26S–49S.

American Psychiatric Association. (1980). *Diagnostic and statistical manual of mental disorders* (3rd ed.). Washington, DC: Author.

American Psychiatric Association. (1987). *Diagnostic and statistical manual of mental disorders* (3rd ed., rev.). Washington, DC: Author.

American Psychiatric Association. (1994). *Diagnostic and Statistical Manual of Mental Disorders* (4th ed.). Washington, DC: Author.

American Psychiatric Association. (2000). *Diagnostic and statistical manual of mental disorders* (4th ed., text rev.). Washington, DC: Author.

Anderson, K. E., Lytton, H., & Romney, D. M. (1986). Mothers' interactions with normal and conduct-disordered boys: Who affects whom? *Developmental Psychology, 22,* 604–609.

Angold, A., & Costello, E. J. (1996). Toward establishing an empirical basis for the diagnosis of oppositional defiant disorder. *Journal of the American Academy of Child and Adolescent Psychiatry, 35,* 1205–1212.

Angold, A., Prendergast, M., Cox, A., Harrington, R., Simonoff, E., & Rutter, M. (1995). The Child and Adolescent Psychiatric Assessment (CAPA). *Psychology and Medicine, 25,* 739–753.

Bagner, D. M., & Eyberg, S. M. (2003). Father involvement in parent training: When does it matter? *Journal of Clinical Child Adolescent Psychology, 32,* 599–605.

Bakermans-Kranenburg, M. J., van IJzendoorn, M. H., & Juffer, F. (2003). Less is more: Meta-analyses of sensitivity and attachment interventions in early childhood. *Psychological Bulletin, 129,* 195–215.

Barkley, R. A. (1997). *Defiant children: A clinician's manual for parent training* (2nd ed.). New York: Guilford Press.

Barkley, R. A., Fischer, M., Edelbrock, C., & Smallish, L. (1991). The adolescent outcome of hyperactive children diagnosed by research criteria—III: Mother–child interactions, family conflicts and maternal psychopathology. *Journal of Child Psychology and Psychiatry, 32,* 233–255.

Barrish, H., Saunders, M., & Wolfe, W. M. (1969). Good behavior game: Effects of contingencies for group consequences on disruptive behavior in a classroom. *Journal of Applied Behavior Analysis, 2,* 119–124.

Bates, J. E., Bayles, K., Bennett, D. S., Ridge, B., & Brown, M. M. (1991). Origins of externalizing problems at eight years of age. In D. J. Pepler & K. H. Rubin (Eds.), *The development and treatment of childhood aggression* (pp. 93–120). Hillsdale, NJ: Erlbaum.

Benasich, A. A., Curtiss, S., & Tallal, P. (1993). Language, learning, and behavioral disturbances in childhood: A longitudinal perspective. *Journal of the American Academy of Child and Adolescent Psychiatry, 32,* 585–594.

Benham, A. (2000). The observation and assessment of young children including use of the Infant–Toddler Mental Status Exam. In C. Zeanah (Ed.), *Handbook of infant mental health* (2nd ed., pp. 249–266). New York: Guilford Press.

Biederman, J., Faraone, S., Milberger, S., Jetton, J., Chen, L., Mick, E., et al. (1996). Is childhood oppositional defiant disorder a precursor to adolescent conduct disorder?: Findings from a four-year follow-up study of children with ADHD. *Journal of the American Academy of Child and Adolescent Psychiatry, 35,* 1193–1204.

Bird, H. R., Canino, G. J., Davies, M., Zhang, H., Ramirez, R., & Lahey, B. B. (2001). Prevalence and correlates of antisocial behaviors among three ethnic groups. *Journal of Abnormal Child Psychology, 29,* 465–478.

Bracha, Z., Perez-Diaz, F., Gerardin, P., Perriot, Y., De La Rocque, F., Flament, M., et al. (2004). A French adaptation of the Infant–Toddler Social and Emotional Assessment. *Infant Mental Health Journal, 25,* 117–129.

Brestan, E. V., & Eyberg, S. M. (1998). Effective psychosocial treatment of conduct-disordered children and adolescents: 29 years, 82 studies, and 5,272 kids. *Journal of Clinical Child Psychology, 27,* 180–189.

Brestan, E. V., Eyberg, S. M., Boggs, S. R., & Algina, J. (1997). Parent–child interaction therapy: Parents' perceptions of untreated siblings. *Child and Family Behavior Therapy, 19,* 13–28.

Briggs-Gowan, M. J., & Carter, A. S. (2002). *The Brief Infant–Toddler Social and Emotional Assessment (BITSEA).* Unpublished manual, Yale University, New Haven, CT, and University of Massachusetts, Boston.

Briggs-Gowan, M. J., Carter, A. S., Irwin, J. R., Wachtel, K., & Cicchetti, D. V. (2004). The Brief Infant–Toddler Social and Emotional Assessment: Screening for social–emotional problems and delays in competence. *Journal of Pediatric Psychology, 29,* 143–155.

Bryant, D., Vizzard, L. H., Willoughby, M., & Kupersmidt, J. (1999). A review of interventions for preschoolers with aggressive and disruptive behavior. *Early Education and Development, 10,* 47–68.

Burke, J. D., Loeber, R., & Birmaher, B. (2002). Oppositional defiant disorder and conduct disorder: A review of the past 10 years, part II. *Journal of the American Academy of Child and Adolescent Psychiatry, 41,* 1275–1293.

Burt, S. A., Krueger, R. F., McGue, M., & Iacono, W. G. (2001). Sources of covariation among attention-deficit/hyperactivity disorder, oppositional defiant disorder, and conduct disorder: The importance of shared environment. *Journal of Abnormal Psychology, 110,* 516–525.

Cadoret, R. J., Troughton, E., Bagford, J., & Woodworth, G. (1990). Genetic and environmental factors in adoptee antisocial personality. *European Archives of Psychiatry and Neurological Science, 239,* 231–240.

Campbell, S. B. (1991). Longitudinal studies of active and aggressive preschoolers: Individual differences in early behavior and outcome. In D. Cicchetti & S. Toth (Eds.), *The Rochester Symposium on Developmental Psychopathology: Vol. 1. Internalizing and externalizing expressions of dysfunction.* Hillsdale, NJ: Erlbaum.

Campbell, S. B. (1995). Behavior problems in preschool children: A review of recent research. *Journal of Child Psychology and Psychiatry, 36,* 113–149.

Campbell, S. B. (2002). *Behavior problems in preschool children: Clinical and developmental issues* (2nd ed.). New York: Guilford Press.

Campbell, S. B., Szumowski, E. K., Ewing, L. J., Gluck, D. S., & Breaux, A. M. (1982). A multidimensional assessment of parent-identified behavior problem toddlers. *Journal of Abnormal Child Psychology, 10,* 569–592.

Canino, G., Shrout, P. E., Rubio-Stipec, M., Bird, H. R., Bravo, M., Ramirez, R., et al. (2004). The DSM-IV rates of child and adolescent disorders in Puerto Rico. *Archives of General Psychiatry, 61,* 85–93.

Carlson, E. A., Sampson, M. C., & Sroufe, L. A. (2003). Implications of attachment theory and research for developmental–behavioral pediatrics. *Journal of Developmental and Behavioral Pediatrics, 24,* 364–379.

Carlson, E. A., Sroufe, L. A., & Egeland, B. (2004). The construction of experience: A longitudinal study of representation and behavior. *Child Development, 75,* 66–83.

Carter, A. S., & Briggs-Gowan. M. (2000). *The Infant–Toddler Social and Emotional Assessment (ITSEA).* Unpublished manual, University of Massachusetts, Boston and Yale University, New Haven, CT.

Carter, A. S., Briggs-Gowan, M. J., Jones, S. M., & Little, T. D. (2003). The Infant–Toddler Social and Emotional Assessment (ITSEA): Factor structure, reliability, and validity. *Journal of Abnormal Child Psychology, 31,* 495–514.

Chaffin, M., Silovsky, J. F., Funderburk, B., Valle, L. A., Brestan, E. V., Balachov, T., et al. (2004). Parent–child interaction therapy with physically abusive parents efficacy for reducing future abuse reports. *Journal of Consulting and Clinical Psychology, 72,* 500–510.

Cicchetti, D., & Schneider-Rosen, K. (1984). Theoretical and empirical considerations in the investigation of the relationship between affect and cognition. In C. Izard, J. Kagan, & R. Zajonc (Eds.), *Emotions, cognitions, and behavior* (pp. 366–406). New York: Cambridge University Press.

Clark, C. I., Prior, M., & Kinsella, G. (2002). The relationship between executive function abilities, adaptive behaviour, and academic achievement in children with externalising behaviour problems. *Journal of Child Psychology and Psychiatry, 43,* 785–796.

Clarke, R. A., Murphy, D. L., & Constantino, J. N. (1999). Serotonin and externalizing behavior in young children. *Psychiatry Research, 86,* 29–40.

Cohen, N. J., Lojkask, M., Muir, E., Muir, R., & Parker, C. J. (2002). Six month follow-up of two mother–infant psychotherapies: Convergence of therapeutic outcomes. *Infant Mental Health Journal, 23*, 361–380.

Collett, B. R., Ohan, J., & Myers, K. (2003). Ten year review of rating scales: VI. General disruptive behavior and aggression scales. *Journal of the American Academy of Child and Adolescent Psychiatry, 42*, 1143–1170.

Comings, D. E., Gade-Andavolu, R., Gonzalez, N., Wu, S., Muhleman, D., Blake, H., et al. (2000). Multivariate analysis of associations of 42 genes in ADHD, ODD, and conduct disorder. *Clinical Genetics, 58*, 31–40.

Conduct Problems Prevention Research Group. (1992). A developmental and clinical model for the prevention of conduct disorders: The FAST Track program. *Development and Psychopathology, 4*, 509–527.

Conduct Problems Prevention Research Group. (1999a). Initial impact of the Fast Track prevention trial for conduct problems: I. The high-risk sample. *Journal of Consulting and Clinical Psychology, 67*, 631–647.

Conduct Problems Prevention Research Group. (1999b). Initial impact of the Fast Track prevention trial for conduct problems: II. Classroom effects. *Journal of Consulting and Clinical Psychology, 67*, 648–657.

Costello, E. J., Mustillo, S., Erkanli, A., Keeler, G., & Angold, A. (2003). Prevalence and development of psychiatric disorders in childhood and adolescence. *Archives of General Psychiatry, 60*, 837–844.

Coy, K., Speltz, M. L., & Jones, K. (2002). Facial appearance and attachment in infants with orofacial clefts: A replication. *Cleft Palate–Craniofacial Journal, 3*, 66–72.

Crowell, J. A., Feldman, S. S., & Ginsburg, N. (1988). Assessment of mother–child interaction in preschoolers with behavior problems. *Journal of the American Academy of Child and Adolescent Psychiatry, 27*, 303–311.

Dadds, M. R., & McHugh, T. A. (1992). Social support and treatment outcome in behavioral family therapy for child conduct problems. *Journal of Consulting and Clinical Psychology, 60*, 252–259.

Dadds, M. R., Schwartz, S., & Sanders, M. R. (1987). Marital discord and treatment outcome in behavioral treatment of child conduct disorders. *Journal of Consulting and Clinical Psychology, 55*, 396–403.

DeKlyen, M., Biernbaum, M. A., Speltz, M. L., & Greenberg, M. T. (1998). Fathers and preschool behavior problems. *Developmental Psychology, 34*, 264–275.

Denham, S. A., Blair, M. A., Schmidt, M., & DeMulder, E. (2002). Compromised emotional competence: Seeds of violence sown early? *American Journal of Orthopsychiatry, 72*, 70–82.

Dietz, K. R., Lavigne, J. V., Arend, R., & Rosenbaum, D. (1997). Relation between intelligence and psychopathology among preschoolers. *Journal of Clinical Child Psychology, 26*, 99–107.

Dodge, K. A. (1991). The structure and function of reactive and proactive aggression. In D. J. Pepler & H. K. Rubin (Eds.), *The development and treatment of childhood aggression*. Hillsdale, NJ: Erlbaum.

Eaves, L., Rutter, M., Silberg, J. L., Shillady, L., Maes, H., & Pickles, A. (2000). Genetic and environmental causes of covariation in interview assessments of disruptive behavior in child and adolescent twins. *Behavior and Genetics, 30*, 321–334.

Egger, H. L., & Angold, A. (2004). The Preschool Age Psychiatric Assessment (PAPA): A structured parent interview for diagnosing psychiatric disorders in preschool children. In R. Del Carmen & A. S. Carter (Eds.), *Handbook of infant, toddler, and preschool mental health assessment* (pp. 123–140). New York: Oxford University Press.

Egger, H. L., Ascher, B. H., & Angold, A. (1999). *The Preschool Age Psychiatric Assessment: Version 1.1*. Unpublished interview schedule, Center for Developmental Epidemiology, Department of Psychiatry and Behavioral Sciences, Duke University Medical Center, Durham, NC.

Eisenberg, N., Fabes, R. A., Karbon, M., Murphy, B. C., Wosinski, M., Polazzi, L., et al. (1996). The relations of children's dispositional prosocial behavior to emotionality, regulation, and social functioning. *Child Development, 67,* 974–992.

Eisenberg, N., Fabes, R. A., Nyman, M., Bernzweig, J., & Pinuelas, A. (1994). The relations of emotionality and regulation to children's anger-related reactions. *Child Development, 65,* 109–128.

Ellingson, K. D., Briggs-Gowan, M. J., Carter, A. S., & Horwitz, S. M. (2004). Parent identification of early emerging child behavior problems: Predictors of sharing parental concern with health providers. *Archives of Pediatrics and Adolescent Medicine, 158,* 766–772.

Emde, R. N., Everhart, K. D., & Wise, B. K. (2004). Therapeutic relationships in infant mental health and the concept of leverage. In A. J. Sameroff, S. C. McDonough, & K. L. Rosenblum (Eds.), *Treating parent–infant relationship problems: Strategies for intervention* (pp. 267–292). New York: Guilford Press.

Erel, O., & Kissil, K. (2003). The linkage between multiple perspectives of the marital relationship and preschoolers' adjustment. *Journal of Child and Family Studies, 12,* 411–423.

Eyberg, S. M., Bessmer, J., Newcomb, K., Edwards, D., & Robinson, E. (1994). *Dyadic Parent–Child Interaction Coding System–II: A manual.* Retrieved May 20, 2005, from www.hp.ufl.edu/~seyberg/measures.htm.

Eyberg, S. M., Boggs, S. R., & Algina, J. (1995). Parent–child interaction therapy: A psychosocial model for the treatment of young children with conduct problem behavior and their families. *Psychopharmacology Bulletin, 31,* 83–91.

Eyberg, S. M., & Pincus, D. (1999). *Professional manual for the Eyberg Child Behavior Inventory and Sutter–Eyberg Student Behavior Inventory, Revised.* Odessa, FL: Psychological Assessment Resources.

Filcheck, H. A., McNeil, C. B., Greco, L. A., & Bernard, R. S. (2004). Using a whole-class token economy and coaching of teacher skills in a preschool classroom to manage disruptive behavior. *Psychology in the Schools, 41,* 351–361.

Fischer, M., Rolf, J. E., Hasazi, J. E., & Cummings, L. (1984). Follow-up of a preschool epidemiological sample: Cross-age continuities and predictions of later adjustment with internalizing and externalizing dimensions of behavior. *Child Development, 55,* 137–150.

Fisher, A. J., Kramer, R. A., Hoven, C. W., King, R. A., & Bowlby, J. (1982). *Attachment and loss* (Vol. 1). New York: Basic Books.

Forehand, R. L., & McMahon, R. J. (1981). *Helping the noncompliant child: A clinician's guide to parent training.* New York: Guilford Press.

Forehand, R. L., & McMahon, R. J. (2003). *Helping the noncompliant child: A clinician's guide to parent training* (2nd ed.). New York: Guilford Press.

Gadow, K. D., & Nolan, E. E. (2002). Differences between preschool children with ODD, ADHD, and ODD + ADHD symptoms. *Journal of Child Psychology and Psychiatry, 43,* 1919–1921.

Gadow, K. D., Sprafkin, J., & Nolan, E. E. (2001). DSM-IV symptoms in community and clinic preschool children. *Journal of the American Academy of Child and Adolescent Psychiatry, 40,* 1383–1392.

Gardner, F. E. M. (1987). Positive interaction between mothers and conduct-problem children: Is there training for harmony as well as fighting? *Journal of Abnormal Child Psychology, 15,* 283–293.

Gilliom, M., & Shaw, D. S. (2004). Co-development of externalizing and internalizing problems in early childhood. *Development and Psychopathology, 16,* 313–333.

Greenberg, M. T., DeKlyen, M., Speltz, M. L., & Endriga, M. C. (1997). The role of attachment processes in externalizing psychopathology in young children. In L. Atkinson & K. Zucker (Eds.), *Attachment and psychopathology* (pp. 196–222). New York: Guilford Press.

Greenberg, M. T., & Snell, J. (1997). The neurological basis of emotional development. In P.

Salovey (Ed.), *Emotional development and emotional literacy* (pp. 93–119). New York: Basic Books.

Greenberg, M. T., & Speltz, M. L. (1988). Contributions of attachment theory to the understanding of conduct problems during the preschool years. In J. Belsky & T. Nezworski (Eds.), *Clinical implications of attachment* (pp. 177–218). Hillsdale, NJ: Erlbaum.

Greenberg, M. T., Speltz, M. L., DeKlyen, M., & Endriga, M. (1991). Attachment security in preschoolers with and without externalizing behavior problems: A replication. *Development and Psychopathology, 3,* 413–430.

Greenberg, M. T., Speltz, M. L., DeKlyen, M., & Jones, K. (2001). Correlates of clinic referral for early conduct problems: Variable- and person-oriented approaches. *Development and Psychopathology, 13,* 255–276.

Greene, R. W. (2001). *The explosive child: A new approach for understanding and helping easily frustrated "chronically inflexible" children* (2nd ed.). New York: HarperCollins.

Greene, R. W., Ablon, J. S., & Goring, J. C. (2003). A transactional model of oppositional behavior: Underpinnings of the Collaborative Problem Solving approach. *Journal of Psychometric Research, 55,* 67–75.

Greene, R. W., Ablon, J. S., Monteaux, M., Goring, J., Henin, A., Raezer, L., et al. (2004). Effectiveness of collaborative problem solving in affectively dysregulated youth with oppositional defiant disorder: Initial findings. *Journal of Consulting and Clinical Psychology, 72,* 1157–1164.

Greenhill, L. (1998). The use of psychoactive medications in preschoolers: Indications, safety and efficacy. *Canadian Journal of Psychiatry, 43,* 576–581.

Greenhill, L. L., Jensen, P. S., Abikoff, H., Blumer, J. L., DeVeaugh-Gleiss, J., Fisher, C., et al. (2003). Developing strategies for psychopharmacological studies in preschool children. *Journal of the American Academy of Child and Adolescent Psychiatry, 42,* 406–414.

Greist, D. L., Forehand, R., Rogers, T., Breiner, J. L., Furey, W., & Williams, C. A. (1982). Effects of parent enhancement therapy on the treatment outcome and generalization of a parent training program. *Behaviour Research and Therapy, 20,* 429–436.

Hanf, C. (1969). *A two-stage program for modifying maternal controlling during mother–child interaction.* Paper presented at the 49th annual meeting of the Western Psychological Association, Vancouver, BC.

Harter, S. (1983). Developmental perspectives on the self-system. In P. H. Mussen (Ed.), *Handbook of child psychology* (Vol. 4, pp. 275–385). New York: Wiley.

Hendren, R. L., & Mullen, D. (2004). Conduct disorder and oppositional defiant disorder. In J. Wiener & M. Dulcan (Eds.), *Textbook of child and adolescent psychiatry* (pp. 509–528). Washington, DC: American Psychological Association.

Hill, J. (2002). Biological, psychological and social processes in the conduct disorders. *Journal of Child Psychology and Psychiatry, 43,* 133–164.

Hinshaw, S. P. (1992). Externalizing behavior problems and academic underachievement in childhood and adolescence: Causal relationships and underlying mechanisms. *Psychological Bulletin, 111,* 127–155.

Hood, K. K., & Eyberg, S. M. (2003). Outcomes of parent–child interaction therapy: Mothers' reports of maintenance three to six years after treatment. *Journal of Clinical Child and Adolescent Psychology, 32,* 419–429.

Ialongo, N. S., Werthamer, L., Kellam, S. G., Brown, C. H., Wang, S., & Lin, Y. (1999). Proximal impact of two first-grade preventive interventions on the early risk behaviors for later substance abuse, depression, and antisocial behavior. *American Journal of Community Psychology, 27,* 599–641.

Ingoldsby, E. M., & Shaw, D. S. (2002). Neighborhood contextual factors and early-starting antisocial pathways. *Clinical Child and Family Psychology Review, 5,* 21–55.

Jenkins, J. M., & Smith, M. A. (1990). Factors protecting children living in disharmonious homes: Maternal reports. *Journal of the American Academy of Child and Adolescent Psychiatry, 29,* 60–69.

Jones, P. (1997). The early origins of schizophrenia. *British Medical Bulletin, 53,* 135–155.

Kadesjo, C., Hagglof, B., Kadesjo, B., & Gillberg, C. (2003). Attention-deficit-hyperactivity disorder with and without oppositional defiant disorder in 3- to 7-year-old children. *Developmental Medicine and Child Neurology, 45,* 693–699.

Kariyawasam, S. H., Zaw, F., & Handley, S. L. (2002). Reduced salivary cortisol in children with comorbid attention deficit hyperactivity disorder and oppositional defiant disorder. *Neuroendocrinology Letters, 23,* 45–48.

Kazdin, A. E., Esveldt-Dawson, K., French, N. H., & Unis, A. S. (1987). Problem-solving skills training and relationship therapy in the treatment of antisocial child behavior. *Journal of Consulting and Clinical Psychology, 55,* 76–85.

Keenan, K., Shaw, D. S., Walsh, B., Delliquadri, E., & Giovannelli, J. (1997). DSM-III-R disorders in preschool children from low-income families. *Journal of the American Academy of Child and Adolescent Psychiatry, 36,* 620–627.

Keenan, K., & Wakschlag, L. S. (2000). More than the terrible twos: The nature and severity of behavior problems in clinic-referred preschool children. *Journal of Abnormal Child Psychology, 28,* 33–46.

Keenan, K., & Wakschlag, L. S. (2004). Are oppositional defiant and conduct disorder symptoms normative behaviors in preschoolers?: A comparison of referred and nonreferred children. *American Journal of Psychiatry, 161,* 356–358.

Kruesi, M. J., Hibbs, E. D., Zahn, T. P., Keysor, C. S., Hamburger, S. D., Bartko, J. J., et al. (1992). A 2-year prospective follow-up study of children and adolescents with disruptive behavior disorders: Prediction by cerebrospinal fluid 5–hydroxyindoleacetic acid, homovanillic acid, and autonomic measures? *Archives of General Psychiatry, 49,* 429–435.

Lahey, B. B., Applegate, B., Barkley, R. A., Garfinkel, B., McBurnett, K., Kerdyk, L., et al. (1994). DSM-IV field trials for oppositional defiant disorder and conduct disorder in children and adolescents. *American Journal of Psychiatry, 151,* 1163–1171.

Lahey, B. B., Schwab-Stone, M., Goodman, S. H., Waldman, I. D., Canino, G., Rathouz, P. J., et al. (2000). Age and gender differences in oppositional behavior and conduct problems: A cross-sectional household study of middle childhood and adolescence. *Journal of Abnormal Psychology, 109,* 488–503.

Lavigne, J. V., Arend, R., Rosenbaum, D., Binns, H. J., Christoffel, K. K., & Gibbons, R. D. (1998). Psychiatric disorders with onset in the preschool years: I. Stability of diagnoses. *Journal of the American Academy of Child and Adolescent Psychiatry, 37,* 1246–1254.

Lavigne, J. V., Cicchetti, C., Gibbons, R. D., Binns, H. J., Larsen, L., & DeVito, C. (2001). Oppositional defiant disorder with onset in preschool years: Longitudinal stability and pathways to other disorders. *Journal of the American Academy of Child and Adolescent Psychiatry, 40,* 1393–1400.

Lavigne, J. V., Gibbons, R. D., Christoffel, K. K., Arend, R., Rosenbaum, D., Binns, H., et al. (1996). Prevalence rates and correlates of psychiatric disorders among preschool children. *Journal of the American Academy of Child and Adolescent Psychiatry, 35,* 204–214.

Liaw, F., & Brooks-Gunn, J. (1994). Cumulative familial risks and low birth weight children's cognitive and behavioral development. *Journal of Clinical Child Psychology, 23,* 360–372.

Lieberman, A. F., Silverman, R., & Pawl, J. H. (2000). Infant–parent psychotherapy: Core concepts and current approaches. In C. H. Zeanah, Jr. (Ed.), *Handbook of infant mental health* (2nd ed., pp. 472–484). New York: Guilford Press.

Lochman, J. E., Burch, P. R., Curry, J. F., & Lampron, L. B. (1984). Treatment and generalization effects of cognitive-behavioral and goal-setting interventions with aggressive boys. *Journal of Consulting and Clinical Psychology, 52,* 915–916.

Loeber, R. (1990). Development and risk factors of juvenile antisocial behavior and delinquency. *Clinical Psychology Review, 10,* 1–41.

Loeber, R., Green, S. M., Keenan, K., & Lahey, B. B. (1995). Which boys will fare worse?:

Early predictors of the onset of conduct disorder in a six-year longitudinal study. *Journal of the American Academy of Child and Adolescent Psychiatry, 34*, 499–509.

Loeber, R., Green, S. M., Lahey, B. B., Frick, P. J., & McBurnett, K. (2000). Findings on disruptive behavior disorders from the first decade of the Developmental Trends Study. *Clinical Child and Family Psychology Review, 3*, 37–60.

Loeber, R., Lahey, B. B., & Thomas, C. (1991). Diagnostic conundrum of oppositional defiant disorder and conduct disorder. *Journal of Abnormal Psychology, 100*, 379–390.

Luby, J. L., Heffelfinger, A. K., Mrakotsky, C., Brown, K. M., Hessler, M. J., Wallis, J. M., et al. (2003). The clinical picture of depression in preschool children. *Journal of the American Academy of Child and Adolescent Psychiatry, 42*, 340–348.

Luby, J. L., Mrakotsky, C., Heffelfinger, A., Brown, K., Hessler, M., & Spitznagel, E. (2003). Modification of DSM-IV criteria for depressed preschool children. *American Journal of Psychiatry, 160*, 1169–1172.

Maughan, B., Rowe, R., Messer, J., Goodman, R., & Meltzer, H. (2004). Conduct disorder and oppositional defiant disorder in a national sample: Developmental epidemiology. *Journal of Child Psychology and Psychiatry, 45*, 609–621.

McClellan, J. M., & Speltz, M. L. (2003). Psychiatric diagnosis in preschool children. *Journal of the American Academy of Child and Adolescent Psychiatry, 42*, 27–28 (author reply 128–130).

McDonough, S. C. (2000). Interaction guidance: An approach for difficult-to-engage families. In C. H. Zeanah, Jr. (Ed.), *Handbook of infant mental health* (2nd ed., pp. 485–493). New York: Guilford Press.

McGoey, K. E., & DuPaul, G. J. (2000). Token reinforcement and response cost procedures: Reducing the disruptive behavior of preschool children with attention-deficit/hyperactivity disorder. *School Psychology Quarterly, 15*, 330–343.

McMahon, R. J., & Forehand, R. (1988). Conduct disorders. In E. J. Mash & L. G. Terdal (Eds.), *Behavioral assessment in childhood disorders* (2nd ed., pp. 105–153). New York: Guilford Press.

McNeil, C. B., Eyberg, S. M., Eisenstadt, T. H., Newcomb, K., & Funderburk, B. (1991). Parent–child interaction therapy with behavior problem children: Generalization of treatment effects to the school setting. *Journal of Clinical Child Psychology, 20*, 140–151.

Moffitt, T. E. (1990). Juvenile delinquency and attention deficit disorder: Boys' developmental trajectories from age 3 to age 15. *Child Development, 61*, 893–910.

Moffitt, T. E., & Caspi, A. (2001). Childhood predictors differentiate life-course persistent and adolescence-limited antisocial pathways among males and females. *Development and Psychopathology, 13*, 355–375.

Moffitt, T. E., & Lynam, D. (1995). The neuropsychology of conduct disorder and delinquency: Implications for understanding antisocial behavior. In D. Fowles, P. Sutker, & S. Goodman (Eds.), *Psychopathology and antisocial behavior: A developmental perspective* (pp. 233–262). New York: Springer.

Myers, K. M., & Collett, B. R. (2005). Psychiatric rating scales: Theory and practice. In K. Meyers & K. Cheng (Eds.), *Child and adolescent psychiatry: The essentials* (pp. 17–40). New York: Lippincott/Williams & Wilkins.

Nixon, R. D. V., Sweeney, L., Erickson, D. B., & Touyz, S. W. (2004). Parent–child interaction therapy: One and two-year follow-up of standard and abbreviated treatments for oppositional preschoolers. *Journal of Abnormal Child Psychology, 32*, 263–271.

Patterson, G. R. (1976). *Living with children: New methods for parents and teachers* (rev. ed.). Champaign, IL: Research Press.

Patterson, G. R. (1982). *Coercive family process.* Eugene, OR: Castalia.

Patterson, G. R. (2002). The early development of coercive family process. In J. B. Reid, G. R. Patterson, & J. Snyder (Eds.), *Antisocial behavior in children and adolescents: Developmental theories and models for intervention* (pp. 25–44). Washington, DC: American Psychological Association.

Patterson, G. R., & Gullion, M. E. (1968). *Living with children: New methods for parents and teachers*. Champaign, IL: Research Press.

Pennington, B. F., & Ozonoff, S. (1996). Executive functions and developmental psychopathology. *Journal of Child Psychology and Psychiatry and Allied Disciplines, 37*, 51–87.

Pettit, G. S., & Bates, J. E. (1989). Family interaction patterns and children's behavior problems from infancy to four years. *Developmental Psychology, 25*, 413–420.

Quiggle, N. L., Garber, J., Panak, W. F., & Dodge, K. A. (1993). Social information processing in aggressive and depressed children. *Child Development, 63*, 1305–1320.

Raine, A. (2002). Biosocial studies of antisocial and violent behavior in children and adults: A review. *Journal of Abnormal Child Psychology, 30*, 311–326.

Reid, M. J., Webster-Stratton, C., & Hammond, M. (2003). Follow-up of children who received the Incredible Years intervention for oppositional defiant disorder: Maintenance and prediction of 2–year outcome. *Behavior Therapy, 34*, 471–491.

Rey, J. M. (1995). Oppositional defiant disorder. *American Journal of Psychiatry, 150*, 1769–1778.

Reynolds, L. K., & Kelley, M. L. (1997). The efficacy of a response cost-based treatment package for managing aggressive behavior in preschoolers. *Behavior Modification, 21*, 216–230.

Roberts, M. W. (2001). Clinic observations of structured parent–child interactions designed to evaluate externalizing disorders. *Psychological Assessment, 13*, 46–58.

Rothbart, M. K., & Bates, J. E. (1998). Temperament. In N. Eisenberg (Ed.), *Handbook of child psychology: Vol. 3. Social, emotional, and personality development* (5th ed., pp. 105–176). New York: Wiley.

Rowe, R., Maughan, B., Pickles, A., Costello, E. J., & Angold, A. (2002). The relationship between DSM-IV oppositional defiant disorder and conduct disorder: Findings from the Great Smoky Mountains Study. *Journal of Child Psychology and Psychiatry, 43*, 365–373.

Rudolph, K. D., Hammen, C., & Burge, D. (1993). Interpersonal functioning and depressive symptoms in childhood addressing the issues of specificity and comorbidity. *Journal of Abnormal Child Psychology, 22*, 355–371.

Rutter, M., Birch, H. G., Thomas, A., & Chess, S. (1964). Temperamental characteristics in infancy and the later development of behavioural disorders. *British Journal of Psychiatry, 110*, 651–661.

Sameroff, A. J., Seifer, R., Baldwin, A., & Baldwin, C. (1993). Stability of intelligence from preschool to adolescence: The influence of social and family risk factors. *Child Development, 64*, 80–97.

Sameroff, A. J., Seifer, R., Barocas, R., Zax, M., & Greenspan, S. (1987). Intelligence quotient scores of 4 year-old children: Social–environmental risk factors. *Pediatrics, 79*, 343–350.

Schore, A. N. (1996). The experience-dependent maturation of a regulatory system in the orbital prefrontal cortex and the origin of developmental psychopathology. *Development and Psychopathology, 8*, 59–87.

Schumann, E. M., Foote, R. C., Eyberg, S. M., Boggs, S. R., & Algina, J. (1998). Efficacy of parent–child interaction therapy: Interim report of a randomized trial with short-term maintenance. *Journal of Clinical Child Psychology, 27*, 34–45.

Schwab-Stone, M. E., & Hart, E. L. (1996). Systems of psychiatric classification: DSM-IV and ICD-10. In M. Lewis (Ed.), *Child and adolescent psychiatry: A comprehensive textbook* (2nd ed., pp. 423–430). Baltimore: Williams & Wilkins.

Scott, S., Spender, Q., Doolan, M., Jacobs, B., & Aspland, H. (2001). Multi-centre controlled trial of parenting groups for childhood antisocial behaviour in clinical practice. *British Medical Journal, 323*, 194–198.

Scourfield, J., VandenBree, M., Martic, N., & McGuffin, P. (2004). Conduct problems in children and adolescents: A twin study. *Archives of General Psychiatry, 61*, 489–496.

Seguin, J. R., Pihl, R. O., Harden, P. W., Tremblay, R. E., & Boulerice, B. (1995). Cognitive and neuropsychological characteristics of physically aggressive boys. *Journal of Abnormal Psychology, 104,* 614–624.

Sergeant, J. A., Geurts, H., & Oosterlaan, J. (2002). How specific is a deficit of executive functioning for attention-deficit/hyperactivity disorder? *Behavior and Brain Research, 130,* 3–28.

Serketich, W. J., & Dumas, J. E. (1996). The effectiveness of behavioral parent training to modify antisocial behavior in children: A meta-analysis. *Behavior Therapy, 27,* 171–186.

Shaw, D. S., Gilliom, M., Ingoldsby, E. M., & Nagin, D. (2003). Trajectories leading to school-age conduct problems. *Developmental Psychology, 39,* 189–200.

Shaw, D. S., Keenan, K., Vondra, J. I., Delliquadri, E., & Giovannelli, J. (1997). Antecedents of preschool children's internalizing problems: A longitudinal study of low-income families. *Journal of the American Academy of Child and Adolescent Psychiatry, 36,* 1760–1767.

Simonoff, E. (2001). Gene–environment interplay in oppositional defiant and conduct disorder. *Child and Adolescent Psychiatry Clinics of North America, 10,* 351–374.

Simonoff, E., Pickles, A., Meyer, J. M., Silberg, J. L., Maes, H. H., Loeber, R., et al. (1997). The Virginia Twin Study of Adolescent Behavioural Development—Influences of age, sex, and impairment on rates of disorder. *Archives of General Psychiatry, 54,* 801–808.

Slutske, W. S., Heath, A. C., Dinwiddie, S. H., Madden, P. A., Bucholz, K. K., Dunne, M. P., et al. (1998). Common genetic risk factors for conduct disorder and alcohol dependence. *Journal of Abnormal Psychology, 107,* 363–374.

Sonuga-Barke, E. J., Thompson, M., Stevenson, J., & Viney, D. (1997). Patterns of behaviour problems among pre-school children. *Psychological Medicine, 27,* 909–918.

Speltz, M. L. (1990). The treatment of preschool conduct problems: An integration of behavioral and attachments constructs. In M. Greenberg, D. Cicchetti, & M. Cummings (Eds.), *Attachment in the preschool years: Theory, research, and treatment* (pp. 399–426). Chicago: University of Chicago Press.

Speltz, M. L., DeKlyen, M., Calderon, R., Greenberg, M. T., & Fisher, P. A. (1999). Neuropsychological characteristics and test behaviors of boys with early onset conduct problems. *Journal of Abnormal Psychology, 108,* 315–325.

Speltz, M. L., DeKlyen, M., & Greenberg, M. T. (1999). Attachment in boys with early onset conduct problems. *Development and Psychopathology, 11,* 269–285.

Speltz, M. L., McClellan, J., DeKlyen, M., & Jones, K. (1999). Preschool boys with oppositional defiant disorder: Clinical presentation and diagnostic change. *Journal of the American Academy of Child and Adolescent Psychiatry, 38,* 838–845.

Sroufe, L. A., & Fleeson, J. (1986). Attachment and the construction of relationships. In W. Hartup & Z. Rubin (Eds.), *Relationships and development* (pp. 51–71). Hillsdale, NJ: Erlbaum.

Steiner, H., Saxena, K., & Chang, K. (2003). Psychopharmacologic strategies for the treatment of aggression in juveniles. *CNS Spectrum, 8,* 298–308.

Stormschak, E., Speltz, M. L., DeKlyen, M., & Greenberg, M. (1997). Family interactions during clinical intake: A comparison of families containing normal or disruptive boys. *Journal of Abnormal Child Psychology, 25,* 345–357.

Swiezy, N. B., Matson, J. L., & Box, P. (1992). The good behavior game: A token reinforcement system for preschoolers. *Child and Family Behavior Therapy, 14,* 21–32.

Thomas, A., & Chess, S. (1977). *Temperament and development.* Oxford, UK: Brunner/Mazel.

Thomas, J., & Guskin, K. A. (2001). Disruptive behavior in young children: What does it mean? *Journal of the American Academy of Child and Adolescent Psychiatry, 40,* 44–51.

Thomas, J. M., & Clark, R. (1998). Disruptive behavior in the very young child: Diagnostic Classification: 0–3 guides identification of risk factors and relational interventions. *Infant Mental Health Journal, 19,* 229–244.

Timmer, S. G., Sedlar, G., & Urquiza, A. J. (2004). Challenging children in kin versus nonkin foster care: Perceived costs and benefits to caregivers. *Child Maltreatment, 9,* 251–262.

Tremblay, R. E., Masse, B., Perron, D., LeBlanc, M., Schwartzman, A. E., & Ledingham, J. E. (1992). Early disruptive behavior, poor school achievement, delinquent behavior, and delinquent personality: Longitudinal analysis. *Journal of Consulting and Clinical Psychology, 60,* 64–72.

van den Boom, D. C. (1994). The influence of temperament and mothering on attachment and exploration: An experimental manipulation of sensitive responsiveness among lower-class mothers with irritable infants. *Child Development, 65,* 1457–1477.

van Goozen, S. H., Cohen-Kettenis, P. T., Snoek, H., Matthys, W., Swaab-Barneveld, H., & van Engeland, H. (2004). Executive functioning in children: A comparison of hospitalized ODD and ODD/ADHD children and normal controls. *Journal of Child Psychology and Psychiatry, 45,* 284–292.

van Goozen, S. H., van den Ban, E., Matthys, W., Chen-Kettenis, P. T., Thijsse, J. H., & van Engeland, H. (2000). Increased adrenal androgen functioning in children with oppositional defiant disorder: A comparison with psychiatric and normal controls. *Journal of American Academy of Child and Adolescent Psychiatry, 39,* 1446–1451.

Wahler, R. G., Cartor, P. G., Fleischman, J., & Lambert, W. (1993). The impact of synthesis teaching and parent training with mothers of conduct disordered children. *Journal of Abnormal Child Psychology, 21,* 425–440.

Wakschlag, L. S., & Keenan, K. (2001). Clinical significance and correlates of disruptive behavior in environmentally at-risk preschoolers. *Journal of Clinical Child Psychology, 30,* 262–275.

Walker, H. M., Stiller, B., Severson, H. H., Feil, E. G., & Golly, A. (1998). First step to success: Intervening at the point of school entry to prevent antisocial behavior patterns. *Psychology in the Schools, 35,* 259–269.

Waters, E., Kondo-Ikemura, K., Posada, G., & Richters, J. E. (1990). Learning to love: Mechanisms and milestones. In M. Gunnar & L. A. Sroufe (Eds.), *Minnesota Symposium on Child Psychology* (Vol. 23, pp. 217–255). Hillsdale, NJ: Erlbaum.

Webster-Stratton, C. (1985). Predictors of treatment outcome in parent training for conduct disordered children. *Behavior Therapy, 16,* 223–243.

Webster-Stratton, C. (1994). Advancing videotape parent training: A comparison study. *Journal of Consulting and Clinical Psychology, 62,* 583–593.

Webster-Stratton, C., & Reid, M. (2003). Treating conduct problems and strengthening social and emotional competence in young children: The Dina Dinosaur treatment program. *Journal of Emotional and Behavioral Disorders, 11,* 130–143.

Webster-Stratton, C., Reid, M. J., & Hammond, M. (2001). Preventing conduct problems, promoting social competence: A parent and teacher training partnership in Head Start. *Journal of Clinical Child Psychology, 30,* 283–302.

Webster-Stratton, C., Reid, M. J., & Hammond, M. (2004). Treating children with early-onset conduct problems: Intervention outcomes for parent, child, and teacher training. *Journal of Clinical Child and Adolescent Psychology, 33,* 105–124.

Wilens, T. E., Biederman, J., Brown, S., Tanguay, S., Monuteaux, M. C., Blake, C., et al. (2002). Psychiatric comorbidity and functioning in clinically referred preschool children and school-age youths with ADHD. *Journal of the American Academy of Child and Adolescent Psychiatry, 41,* 262–268.

Wilens, T., & Spenser, T. (2000). The stimulants revisited. *Child and Adolescent Clinics of North America, 9,* 573–603.

Xue, Y., Leventhal, T., Brooks-Gunn, J., & Earls, F. J. (2005). Neighborhood residence and mental health problems of 5- to 11-year-olds. *Archives of General Psychiatry, 62,* 554–563.

Yoshikawa, H. (1994). Prevention as cumulative protection: Effects of early family support and education on chronic delinquency and its risks. *Psychological Bulletin, 115,* 28–54.

World Health Organization. (1992). *International Classification of Diseases, Tenth Revision*. Arlington, VA: American Psychiatric Publishing.

Zahn-Waxler, C., Schmitz, S., Fulker, D. W., Robinson, J., & Emde, R. (1996). Behavior problems in 5–year-old monozygotic and dizygotic twins: Genetic and environmental influences, patterns of regulation and internalization of control. *Development and Psychopathology, 8*, 103–122.

Zero to Three. (1994). Diagnostic Classification: 0–3. *Diagnostic classification of mental health and developmental disorders of infancy and early childhood*. Washington, DC: Zero to Three, National Center for Infant, Toddlers, and Families.

Zito, J., Safer, D., dosReis, S., Gardiner, J., Boles, M., & Lynch, F. (2000). Trends in the prescribing of psychotropic medications to preschoolers. *Journal of the American Medical Association, 283*, 1025–1030.

Ziv, Y., Oppenheim, D., & Sagi-Schwartz, A. (2004). Social-information processing in middle childhood: Relations to infant–mother attachment. *Attachment in Human Development, 6*, 327–348.

6

Eating Disorders

IRENE CHATOOR and DEEPA KHUSHLANI

PREVALENCE AND COURSE OF FEEDING AND EATING DISORDERS

During the first few years of life, when infants and young children cannot eat independently and when their food intake depends on the dyadic relationship between the infant or toddler and the caretaker, we speak of feeding disorders. However, later, as children learn to eat independently, we describe eating difficulties as eating disorders. Whereas feeding disorders are frequently seen in infants and toddlers, and eating disorders have been primarily described in adolescents and young adults, not much attention has been given to eating disorders in preschool children. However, as some longitudinal studies indicate, feeding difficulties that start during the early years may continue into childhood and be associated with behavioral problems (Galler, Ramsey, Solimano, Lowell, & Mason, 1988), cognitive delays (Drotar & Sturm, 1988; Reif, Beler, Villa, & Spirer, 1995), and anxiety disorders (Timimi, Douglas, & Tsiftsopoulou, 1997). In addition, early feeding difficulties have been correlated with eating disorders during adolescence (Marchi & Cohen, 1990) and young adulthood (Kotler, Cohen, Davies, Pine, & Walsh, 2001).

For example, Forsyth and Canny (1991) found that at 4 months of age, 36% of the infants were reported to have feeding and crying problems, and in 17% the formula had been changed. During follow-up, when the children were 3½ years of age, those who had had early feeding and crying problems, especially those with formula changes, were more often perceived as vulnerable and more often had behavioral problems. A New Zealand study by Beautrais, Fergusson, and Shannon (1982) followed children yearly from ages 2 to 4 years and found that feeding problems declined annually from 22% at 2 years to 15% at 3 years, and to 10% at 4 years of age. Feeding problems were the next common problem after temper tantrums and breath holding, which declined with age in a similar way. A small number of mothers (3% per annum) were sufficiently disturbed by the problems to seek professional help.

The only longitudinal study that has defined severe feeding problems and differentiated them from more common feeding problems is from Sweden (Dahl & Sundelin, 1986). The severe feeding problems had been present in infants without interruption for at least 1 month, and the primary help in the form of medical and psychological advice and treatment had not eliminated the problem. These severe feeding difficulties occurred in 1.4% of a large cohort of infants in an urban district of Uppsala, Sweden. Longitudinal research showed that at 2 years of age, 50% of the children's feeding problems persisted. Whereas most of the problems in the colic and vomiting groups improved and eventually disappeared, most of the children in the refusal to eat group still had feeding problems at 2 years of age. In addition, in comparison to a control group, these children had significantly higher frequencies of infections and behavioral problems (Dahl, 1987). At 4 years of age, 17 of the 24 children with early refusal to eat (71%) were reported by their parents as still having feeding problems and 10 children (42%) were reported to be hyperactive (Dahl & Sundelin, 1992). The next follow-up, when the children were in primary school, showed that in comparison to their classmates, the children who refused to eat at an early age presented more eating problems both at home and at school.

In summary, these studies demonstrate that most feeding problems are seen in the first few years of life, and some are resolved by 2 years of age. However, in a subgroup, severe feeding problems, especially those characterized by refusal to eat, persist into the preschool and school years, and may predispose the children to eating disorders during adolescence or young adulthood.

CLASSIFICATION OF FEEDING DISORDERS

One of the problems in the field has been the lack of a nationally accepted classification of feeding disorders. This has led to the use of different diagnostic labels to describe overlapping symptomatology and often the same label to describe different feeding problems. For example, Marchi and Cohen (1990) described picky eaters as "not eating enough" and as "being choosy about food," whereas Rydell, Dahl, and Sundelin (1995) called these children "choosy eaters"; Timimi et al. (1997) described them as "selective eaters." Singer, Ambuel, Wade, and Jaffe (1992) described children who refused to eat as a result of traumatic eating-related experiences as experiencing "food phobias," and Pliner and Lowen (1997) use the term "phobia" to describe children who were afraid to try new foods. In other cases, researchers and clinicians who have not distinguished between different types of feeding difficulties refer to "food refusal" as a diagnosis (Dahl, Rydell, & Sundelin, 1994; Lindberg, Bohlin, Hagekull, & Thunstroem, 1994).

The fourth edition of the *Diagnostic and Statistical Manual of Mental*

Disorders (DSM-IV; American Psychiatric Association, 1994) introduced feeding disorder of infancy and early childhood as a diagnostic category and provided a national definition of feeding disorders. Diagnostic criteria for this disorder include persistent failure to eat adequately, with significant failure to gain weight or significant loss of weight over at least 1 month; a disturbance not caused by an associated gastrointestinal or other medical condition; a condition not accounted for by another mental disorder or by lack of available food; and onset before the age of 6 years. Although this was a first step, this definition of feeding disorder is broad and does not differentiate among the various feeding disorders that can present with these symptoms. On the other hand, this definition excludes feeding disorders that do not present with general growth failure but may be associated with specific nutritional deficiencies (vitamins, iron, zinc, or protein deficiencies) and those associated with medical conditions.

To address these issues, Chatoor (2002) developed a classification scheme that differentiates between feeding disorder subtypes with different markers of inadequate nutrition. This classification scheme provides operational diagnostic criteria for six feeding disorders that arise during infancy and early childhood. It is based on previous clinical work and on empirical studies (Chatoor, Egan, Getson, Menvielle, & O'Donnell, 1988; Chatoor, Getson, et al., 1997; Chatoor, Hirsch, Ganiban, Persinger, & Hamburger, 1998; Chatoor, Ganiban, Hirsch, Borman-Spurrell, & Mrazek, 2000). The diagnostic criteria for these six feeding disorders were further refined with the help of the Task Force on Research Diagnostic Criteria: Infancy and Preschool (2003).

This chapter focuses on two eating disorders, often described as "picky eating," defined by Chatoor (2002) as infantile anorexia and sensory food aversions. Both eating disorders usually start during the transition to spoon- and self-feeding, and the introduction of baby food and table food. Both start during the time when infants learn to eat independently. However, the feeding difficulties tend to continue into childhood unless treated during the early years. In addition, we describe the posttraumatic eating disorder (Chatoor, Conley, & Dickson, 1988; Chatoor, Ganiban, Harrison, & Hirsch, 2001; Chatoor, 2002), which can occur at any age from infancy to adulthood, and address pica as it manifests in this age group. We do not address the various feeding difficulties associated with medical or neurological illnesses.

INFANTILE ANOREXIA

Diagnostic Criteria

Diagnostic criteria for infantile anorexia are as follows:

1. Refusal to eat adequate amounts of food for at least 1 month.
2. Onset of the food refusal occurs before age 3, most commonly be-

tween 9 and 18 months of age, during the transition to spoon- and self-feeding.

3. Lack of communication of hunger signals and lack of interest in food, but strong interest in exploration and/or interaction with caregivers.
4. Acute and/or chronic growth deficiency (Waterlow et al., 1977).
5. Onset of food refusal did not follow a traumatic event.
6. Food refusal is not due to an underlying medical illness or developmental disorder.

Clinical Picture and Research Findings

Chatoor and Egan (1983) first described this feeding disorder as a separation disorder, because it usually becomes apparent during the first 3 years of life, during the developmental phase of separation and individuation (Mahler, Pine, & Bergman, 1975). However, later it was referred to as "infantile anorexia" to emphasize the onset during infancy and the lack of appetite that is the cardinal symptom of this feeding disorder (Chatoor et al., 1992). This eating disorder is characterized by the child's food refusal and intense parent–child conflict over the child's poor food intake and failure to gain adequate weight. The onset of the eating disorder is most commonly between 9 and 18 months of age, during the transition to spoon- and self-feeding. During this developmental period, both motoric and cognitive maturation enable the infant to function with increasing physical and emotional independence; consequently, issues of autonomy and dependency are played out daily in the feeding situation. During the transition to self-feeding, mother and infant have to negotiate during every meal who is going to place the spoon in the infant's mouth. In addition, the infant's increasing understanding of cause and effect allows him or her to know the difference between hunger and fullness, and emotional feelings (anger, frustration, and the wish for attention). This requires that the infant signal effectively and that the caregiver read the infant's signals accurately and respond appropriately by offering food when the infant appears hungry, withdraw food when the infant is satiated, and deal with the emotional needs of the infant without using food. These developmental processes are critical in the development of internal versus external regulation of eating in general, and they take on special importance in the development of infantile anorexia in particular.

Some parents report that even during the first few months of life, infants who are later diagnosed with infantile anorexia do not signal well when they are hungry or full. They are easily distracted by external stimuli: They stop feeding when somebody enters the room, when the telephone rings, or when something else draws their attention. As they grow a little older, usually between 9 and 18 months of age, when they learn to crawl or walk and begin to talk, and their world gets more and more interesting, these infants resist staying in the high chair. After a few bites, they throw food and feeding utensils, try to climb out of the high chair, and want to get back to playing. Most parents complain that these infants do not signal when they are hungry, that they play rather than eat; moreover, the parents have to keep after these infants to get them to eat. Usually, the parents become increasingly worried about their infant's poor eating and growth. Consequently, they try to increase their infant's food intake by distracting him or her with toys or television, by coaxing or bribing, by allowing the infant to "graze," and by nursing the infant or encouraging him or her to drink from the bottle during the day and at night. Some parents get so desperate that they threaten their infants and resort to force-feeding.

The special temperament of toddlers with infantile anorexia and their disinterest in eating have been explored by Chatoor and colleagues in a series of studies. In the first study, Chatoor et al. (2000) reported that mothers of toddlers with infantile anorexia describe their children as more difficult, more irregular in their feeding and sleeping patterns, more dependent on their parents, and at the same time more unstoppable, in contrast to the way mothers of healthy eaters describe their children. An additional study of toddlers' reactions to separation from their mothers (Ganiban, Chatoor, & Gelven, 1999), revealed that toddlers with infantile anorexia showed a significantly higher level of distress and required significantly longer than the control children to recover from distress.

The emotional intensity of toddlers with infantile anorexia was further confirmed in a physiological study by Chatoor, Ganiban, Surles, and Doussard-Roosevelt (2004). When measuring heart periods and vagal tone in three situations with different levels of social and cognitive engagement, toddlers with infantile anorexia showed consistently higher levels of physiological arousal and were less adaptive than controls in their physiological regulation. In the third situation, when no social or cognitive demands were made, and the toddlers were allowed to play on their own, the control children demonstrated significantly greater vagal activation, which serves internal homeostatic needs (e.g., digestion), whereas vagal activation remained low for the toddlers with infantile anorexia (Chatoor et al., 2004). This pilot study supports the hypothesis that toddlers with infantile anorexia may operate on a higher level of physiological arousal, which supports exploration and cognitive development, but they have difficulty turning off the excitement, relaxing, experiencing hunger, and being able to transition to sleep. Such physiological dysregulation may constitute a tendency toward less optimal homeostatic regulation of feeding and growth, and may be a risk factor for infantile anorexia.

In further support of this hypothesis, in a recent study, Chatoor et al. (2004) demonstrated that, on average, toddlers with infantile anorexia perform in the normal range of cognitive development in spite of their poor nutritional state. The study demonstrated that the cognitive development of toddlers with infantile anorexia did not show a significant correlation with their nutritional state, but it correlated significantly with socioeconomic status, maternal education, and mother–toddler interactions during feeding and play. High mother–toddler reciprocity during feeding correlated positively with the mental developmental index of the toddlers, whereas mother–toddler conflict, struggle for control during feeding, and maternal intrusiveness during play correlated negatively with the cognitive development of the toddlers.

In summary, these studies indicate that toddlers with infantile anorexia demonstrate a special temperament constellation characterized by intense interest in play and interaction with their caretakers, and higher physiological arousal facilitating good cognitive development, but difficulty in calming themselves in order to eat or sleep. These special temperamental characteristics of toddlers with infantile anorexia pose a challenge to any parent; consequently, the mother–infant/toddler feeding relationship and the contribution of mothers and toddlers to the conflict in the relationship were explored. In the first study, Chatoor, Egan, et al. (1988) observed that toddlers with infantile anorexia and their mothers demonstrated less dyadic reciprocity, more dyadic conflict, more struggle for control, and more talk and distraction, with mothers exhibiting more noncontingency, than toddlers who were healthy eaters and their mothers. These findings were replicated later with a different sample (Chatoor, Egan, et al., 1998b).

With regard to parent characteristics associated with infantile anorexia, mothers of toddlers with infantile anorexia were more likely than mothers of healthy eaters to describe insecure attachment relationships to their own parents. However, they did not differ from the control mothers in marital satisfaction and attitudes toward disordered eating (Chatoor et al., 2000). Relative to the contribution of parent and child characteristics to the dyadic feeding relationship, mothers' insecure attachments, as well as their own drive for thinness, and toddlers' difficult temperament and irregular feeding and sleeping patterns correlated significantly with mother–toddler conflict during feeding; this mother–toddler conflict during feeding correlated strongly with toddlers' weight: The more mother–toddler conflict observed during feeding, the lower the toddlers' weight.

These findings support a transactional model for infantile anorexia in that both infant and parent characteristics are associated with high conflict during feeding interactions, and conflict during feeding is associated with the infant's poor growth. Reconstruction of the feeding histories, as reported by the parents, suggests that the infants' food refusal and poor weight gain trigger severe anxiety in parents, especially in first-time mothers, in mothers who have insecure attachment relationships with their own parents, or mothers who have conflicts about their own eating. However, even mothers with none of these risk factors are often so challenged by the infant's food refusal, that they fall into maladaptive feeding patterns (e.g., coaxing, distracting, bargaining, or threatening their children) in the hope of increasing their children's food intake. As time goes on, the children's food intake becomes increasingly externally regulated by their parents. Consequently, the children not only fail to develop an awareness of hunger or fullness, but they also do not learn to differentiate their physiological needs for food from their emotional feeling states in relationship to their parents. Their eating becomes totally controlled by their emotional interactions with their caretakers, and the children become stunted not only in their physical growth but also in their emotional development.

Course

No research data are available on the natural course of this feeding disorder. Clinical data and the follow-up of a treatment study by Chatoor, Hirsch, and Persinger (1997) indicate that as these children get older, they verbalize their disinterest in eating. They state that they are not hungry, that they are bored with eating, that they do not want to stop their activities to eat, and that they want to get up from the table and play. As they enter preschool or kindergarten, they are often so distracted by watching other children eat that they forget their own food and bring most of it home. Initially, their poor food intake results in poor weight gain. However, their height gradually becomes stunted, although their heads usually continue to grow at an age-appropriate rate. Such children at ages 4 and 5 may still look like 2- or 3-year-olds, and school-age children usually look a few years younger. They are usually bright children who perform well in school. As they grow older, they become aware of their small stature and may be teased by their peers. The boys in particular start suffering socially because of their small size. They become self-conscious and anxious around their peers. Girls seem to be less bothered by their peers, and some seem quite confused about their body and may experience body image distortions, not unlike adolescents with anorexia nervosa. However, in spite of the older children's suffering because of their small stature, they seem unable to make themselves eat more, and the conflict with their parents over eating often continues into adolescence. There are no data that indicate how infantile anorexia relates to anorexia nervosa or other eating disorders during the adolescent and adult years.

Treatment

Based on the transactional model for infantile anorexia described earlier, a treatment was developed that addresses the three components of the model: (1) the child's special temperament, (2) the parents' vulnerability and difficulty in limit setting because of insecure relationship experiences or difficulty regulating their own eating, and (3) conflict in the parent–child relationship during meals (Chatoor, Hirsch, et al., 1997).

The Child's Special Temperament

The therapist helps the parents understand that their child has a special temperament that seems to interfere with the awareness of hunger and fullness. It is helpful for parents to know that children with infantile anorexia, unlike other children, seem to have a higher level of arousal that supports their curiosity and interest in play and learning but interferes with their ability to calm themselves and to recognize hunger, or to settle down for sleep. Consequently, the children require more structuring of meal and sleep times and more limit setting than do other children, who can transition from play to eating and sleep more easily. At the same time, limit setting is more difficult, because these children often are very willful and have difficulty calming themselves when they are upset.

The Parents' Vulnerability and Difficulty in Limit Setting

An empathic approach is necessary to allow parents to share with the therapist their struggles with their children and explore whether these conflicts are heightened by the parents' experiences with their own parents or other life experiences. Parents also need to be helped to share their own conflicts about eating, and how they are affected by struggling with their child over food. However, it is important to keep in mind that not all parents have preexisting, pertinent intrapsychic conflicts, and that the food refusal and poor growth of these children can make otherwise well-functioning parents worried and anxious.

Conflict in the Parent–Child Relationship during Meals

After this groundwork has been laid, the parents are provided with specific guidelines on how to set limits on the children's inappropriate behaviors that interfere with eating, and how to teach their children to recognize appropriately feelings of hunger and fullness. The parents are taught to control when, what, and where they offer their children food, but to allow their children to decide "how much" they want to eat. This requires that the parents provide a regular meal schedule for their children, with meal and snack times spaced at least 3–4 hours apart, and that they not allow any snacking or drinking of milk, juice, or soda in between these scheduled times. The children are allowed to have only water if they get thirsty. This time interval allows the children to experience hunger. However, the children often rebel against these rules, and parents need to be helped to use "time out" to teach their children to accept limits and to calm themselves when frustrated and angry.

As the pilot study by Chatoor, Hirsch, et al. (1997) indicates, some children can be taught to become more aware of their hunger within days or a few weeks. However, for many children, it takes months to develop a more consistent eating pattern. In addition, it is important for parents to understand that the underlying vulnerability of these children to become overly aroused in stimulating situations and be unable to eat continues to become apparent when they travel or have house guests, or when things just get too exciting for them to think about eating.

SENSORY FOOD AVERSIONS

Diagnostic Criteria

Diagnostic criteria for sensory food aversions are as follows:

1. Consistent refusal to eat specific foods with specific tastes, textures, and/or smells.
2. Onset of the food refusal during the introduction of new and different types of food (e.g., the child may drink one type of milk but refuse another; may eat carrots but refuse green beans; may eat crunchy foods but refuse pureed food).
3. Eats without difficulty when offered preferred foods.
4. The food refusal causes specific dietary deficiencies and/or delay of oral–motor development, and/or family conflict, and/or social anxiety in the child.

Clinical Picture and Research Findings

Sensory food aversions usually become apparent when infants or toddlers are introduced to baby food or table food with a variety of tastes and textures. When specific foods are placed in the infants' or toddlers' mouths, their aversive reactions range from grimacing and spitting out the food to gagging and vomiting. After an initial aversive reaction, toddlers usually refuse to continue eating that particular food and become distressed if forced to do so. Some toddlers generalize their food refusal to other foods that look or smell like a food they have found aversive (e.g., they may refuse all green vegetables after an aversive experience with green beans). Many parents report that the children refuse to eat new foods, without ever having tried them. In extreme cases, the children insist that one food should not touch another food on their plate, or they accept food only if it is prepared by a certain company (e.g., chicken nuggets from McDonald's or Domino's pizza). If children refuse many foods or whole food groups (e.g., vegetables, fruits, or meats), their limited diet may lead to specific nutritional deficiencies (e.g., in vitamins, zinc, iron, and protein). If toddlers reject foods that require significant chewing (e.g., meats or hard vegetables), they fall behind in their oral–motor functioning, which may affect their expressive speech development. Children's refusal to eat various foods may also create conflict within their families. Interestingly, when the children go to preschool or day care, some of them imitate their peers and try to eat foods that they never touch at home. On the other hand, some children become so anxious that they cannot eat anything when they are in a strange environment. As the children get older, they may avoid social situations because of their embarrassment that they cannot eat the various foods their peers eat. Since sensory food aversions are common and occur along a spectrum of severity, the diagnosis of a feeding or eating disorder should only be made if the food aversions result in dietary deficiencies and/or oral–motor delay, and/or family conflict, and/or social anxiety.

In addition to sensitivity to certain foods, many children experience problems in other sensory areas. Parents may recall that, as toddlers, these children did not like to walk barefoot on sand or grass or to get their hands "messy," that they objected to labels in their clothing and were reluctant to change from short sleeves to long sleeves, and that they complained about odors or were bothered by loud noises.

Other authors have referred to this eating disorder as "selective eating" (Kern & Marder, 1996; Shore, Babbitt, Williams, Coe, & Snyder, 1998; Timimi et al., 1997), as "choosy eating" (Rydell et al., 1995), as "food neophobia" (Birch, 1999; Hursti & Sjödén, 1997; Pliner & Lowen, 1997), as "picky eating or choosiness, or faddiness" (Benoit, 2000), and as "taste aversion" (Garb & Stunkard, 1974; Kalat & Rozin, 1973; Logue, Ophir, & Strauss, 1981). We chose the term "sensory food aversions" because the selective eating seems to be related not only to taste but also to the texture and/or smell of food, and, as we described earlier, the children often have difficulty in other sensory areas as well.

In trying to understand why some children and adults have such strong aversions to the taste and texture of certain foods, several studies have looked at 6-propylthiouracil (PROP) and phenylthiocarbamide (PTC) as genetic markers for taste, with implications for food preferences and dietary habits (see Tepper, 1998, for a review). Both are bitter-tasting, colorless substances that can be diluted in water. The ability to taste PROP has been found to be present in young children and to decline slowly with age (Whissell-Buechy, 1990). Several studies have attempted to demonstrate a relationship between PROP taste sensitivity and rejection of bitter vegetables and other foods. Food preference surveys have consistently shown that PROP tasters have more overall food dislikes than nontasters, and that they dislike strong-tasting foods such as anchovies, sauerkraut, dark beer and ales, black coffee, and strong cheeses (Drewnowski & Rock, 1995). Tepper (1998) found that children who were PROP tasters disliked raw broccoli, whereas PROP nontasters liked raw broccoli. Anatomical studies have provided clues as to why PROP tasters may be more sensitive to a variety of tastes. Studies by Bartoshuk, Duffy, and Miller (1994) and Tepper and Nurse (1997) demonstrated that PROP tasters have both a higher density of taste papillae on the apex of the tongue and more functional taste buds. In addition, individuals who differ in taste (PROP) sensitivity also differ in lingual tactile acuity. Tactile and taste sensitivities covary and reflect individual differences in the density and diameter of fungiform papillae on the anterior tongue (Essick, Chopra, Guest, & McGlone, 2003).

Because family histories reveal that taste and texture sensitivities can be observed across generations, several studies have explored whether taste sensitivities are heritable. Various models of genetic transmission have been suggested, such as multilocus and multiallele models by Morton, Cantor, Cory, and Nance (1981) and a two-locus model by Olson, Boehnke, Neiswanger,

Roche, and Siervogel (1989). More recently, Kim, Jorgenson, Coon, Leppert, Risch, and Drayna (2003) suggested specific changes on chromosome 7q that differentiates between tasters and nontasters. Kim et al. (2003) identified a small region on chromosome 7q that shows strong linkage disequilibrium between single-nucleotide polymorphism (SNP) markers and PTC taste sensitivity in unrelated subjects.

Other studies have demonstrated that certain aspects of the eating environment can also have a strong influence on the development of food preferences and shape selective food refusal. For example, parents with extreme taste sensitivities may prepare and offer a restricted range of foods to their children. In turn, limited exposure to various foods may further the children's food selectivity (Birch, Birch, Marlin, & Kramer, 1982). If parents are selective eaters, their children may model the parents' selectivity (Harper & Sanders, 1975). On the other hand, parents' use of contingencies (e.g., promising special foods to the child if he or she eats the food the parents consider "healthy") can further enhance the child's dislikes for the foods that the parents push (Birch et al., 1982). In summary, previous studies indicate that genetic predispositions and the eating environment affect children's food preferences.

Course

To address the question of frequency of selective food refusal, Chatoor, Hamburger, Fullard, and Rivera (1994) conducted a survey of over 1,500 parents of toddlers that ranged in age from 12 to 36 months. Twenty percent of the parents reported that their children were eating only a few types of food "often" or "always," and that they considered them to be "picky eaters." This concurs with a report by Marchi and Cohen (1990), who found up to 27% maternally reported "choosiness" in a normal sample of young children. When the sample by Chatoor et al. (1994) was followed up 5 years later through telephone interviews, of the children whose parents could be reached, one-third who were considered as "picky eaters" as toddlers continued to be very selective and had a restricted diet of less than 10 foods (unpublished data). A longitudinal study of children's food preferences by Skinner, Carruth, Bounds, and Ziegler (2002) followed 70 children from 2–3 years of age to 8 years of age. Mothers completed a Food Preference Questionnaire and a Food Neophobia Scale when the children were 2, 4, and 8 years of age. Although children liked most foods, the number of liked foods did not change significantly during the 5–5.7 years of the study. The strongest predictors of the number of foods liked at age 8 years were the number of foods liked at age 4 years and the food neophobia score. Newly tasted foods were more likely to be accepted by children between 2 and 4 years than by those between 4 and 8 years of age. These findings are in agreement with informally gathered data from parents who were selective eaters as children. Very few parents remember having expanded the variety of foods in their diet as children, but many report having started to eat "new" foods as adolescents or young adults.

Treatment

The first priority of treatment has to be directed toward the nutritional adequacy of the children's diet. If the diet is deficient in specific nutrients (e.g., protein, vitamins, zinc, or iron), then supplementation with these specific nutrients should be initiated. Because some of these children have difficulties in taking specific supplements, it may be necessary to explore different flavors or to start with small amounts to allow the child to get used to the taste or texture of the supplement. This supplementation is very important to alleviate the parents' anxiety about the child's poor diet, and to allow the behavioral program to proceed.

The research by Birch, Gunder, and Grimm-Thomas (1998) indicates that infants in the first year of life are more willing to accept new foods after a single exposure, whereas toddlers age 2 years and older require repeated exposures of new foods before they become comfortable with them. At the same time, by 2 years of age, most toddlers feed themselves independently and will not accept food they do not like. Consequently, it becomes more challenging to find ways to expose them to new foods. Often parents try to coax or bargain with children to get them to eat unfamiliar or disliked foods, but as Birch et al. (1982) demonstrated, this can have the opposite effect, and the children become more and more rigid in their food preferences. On the other hand, toddlers and young children are very receptive to modeling, and there is nothing more challenging to this age group than seeing their parents eat something that is not on their own plate, and that is not being offered to them. Consequently, our recommendation is to offer young children with strong sensory food aversions only foods with which they are comfortable, and to wait for the children to ask for a new food that they see their parents or their siblings eat. Even then, if the child asks for a food that the parents eat, it is important for the parents to offer only a small bite and to keep a neutral attitude whether the child likes the food or not. In our clinical experience, this keeps young children relaxed and willing to try new foods to find out which foods they can tolerate. However, these are clinical impressions, and further research is needed to determine how to help young children with sensory food aversions expand their limited diets.

POSTTRAUMATIC EATING DISORDER

Diagnostic Criteria

Diagnostic criteria for posttraumatic eating disorder are as follows:

1. Food refusal following a traumatic event or repeated traumatic insults to the oropharynx or gastrointestinal tract (e.g., choking, severe gagging, vomiting, witnessing another person choking*) that trigger intense distress in the child.

2. Consistent refusal to eat solid foods that need to be chewed, and restriction of food intake to liquids and soft foods, such as ice cream or pureed foods.*
3. Anticipatory fear of eating and choking.*
4. Nutritional and/or emotional states interfere with the child's functioning.*

Clinical Picture and Research Findings

The term "posttraumatic eating disorder" was first coined by Chatoor, Conley, et al. (1988) in an article on food refusal in five latency-age children who experienced episodes of choking or severe gagging and later refused to eat any solid food. These children were afraid to eat any solid food that had to be chewed out of fear that the food would get stuck in their throat and cause them to choke and die. The children would get very anxious and agitated in anticipation of mealtimes and would even become combative if asked by their parents to eat solid food. Although they maintained feelings of hunger and were willing to drink liquids or eat ice cream, the hunger did not override their fear of choking on solid food, and the liquid diet was usually not enough to maintain their weight. In addition, the children reported having frightening dreams about monsters and dying, and several of the children were afraid to go to sleep by themselves. The fear of eating and dying interfered with their concentration at school, and the children became irritable, clinging to their parents.

Interestingly, most of the children seemed to have experienced a heightened level of anxiety or some depression prior to the incident of choking or gagging. This may explain why not all children who gag severely or choke develop a posttraumatic eating disorder. Clinical observation reveals that the heightened level of emotional arousal prior to the traumatic event sets the stage for the posttraumatic eating disorder. After the gagging or vomiting experience, all the anxiety seems to become focused on the fear of choking and dying.

Although this eating disorder can occur at any age and is quite common in infants and toddlers, it is rarely seen in preschool children. However, preschoolers are particularly challenging to understand and treat because they cannot verbalize their fears of choking and dying the way that older children do; at the same time, their fantasy world may be vivid and entangled in their fears. As a result, preschool children can get so frightened that they cough and gag at just the sight of food.

Several other authors have described children who develop fears of swal-

---

*To characterize the symptoms of preschool children and older children, these criteria were modified from the diagnostic criteria for infants and young children developed by Chatoor with the help of a national task force (Task Force on Research and Diagnostic Criteria, 2003).

lowing after choking on food and have labeled this eating disorder "food phobia" (Singer et al., 1992), "functional dysphagia" (Watkins & Lask, 2002), "choking phobia" (McNally, 1994), or "dysphagia and food aversion" (Culbert, Kajander, Kohen, & Reaney, 1996). However, because this is a relatively rare eating disorder, no systematic research has been published, and only case reports are available.

Course

Again, no empirical data are available that describe the course of this eating disorder in general and in preschool children in particular. Clinical observation indicates that with treatment, children can recover completely and return to a normal eating pattern within several months to a year. Anecdotal data suggest that some children may recover with the help of their parents, without special treatment.

Treatment

Some case reports (Chatoor, Conley, et al., 1988; Singer et al., 1992) described behavioral treatments for this eating disorder, but no empirical studies are available for this age group. Considering the children's conviction that any solid food will get stuck in their throat, an initial cognitive approach of helping the child understand that food passed through the throat without difficulty before the traumatic event, and will be able to pass again, is a first and often very helpful step. The children are then be encouraged to practice chewing and swallowing by eating softer, less frightening foods first, then working their way up to harder, chewier foods (hard vegetables, fruits, and meats). They can be encouraged in this process of gradually overcoming their fears by earning stickers or points for courage when trying to eat new foods. The excitement of earning stickers or special rewards for courage can help the children to focus away from their fears. However, some children are so anxious that they seem immobilized by their fears. These children benefit from anxiolytic medication (e.g., sertraline or fluoxetine), which seems to control their excessive fears and helps them to engage in the gradual desensitization process. In some instances, the children are so trapped and disabled by their fears that they need to be hospitalized and treated with a very controlled behavioral plan of gradually introducing feared foods. In general, it may take weeks or months to overcome their fears, but eventually, the children seem to be able to resume a normal eating pattern.

PICA

Diagnostic Criteria

Diagnostic criteria for pica are as follows (American Psychiatric Association, 1994):

1. Persistent eating of non-nutritive substances for at least 1 month.
2. The eating of such substances is inappropriate to the developmental level.
3. The eating behavior is not part of a culturally sanctioned practice.
4. If such behavior occurs only during the course of another mental disorder, it is serious enough to warrant independent clinical attention.

Clinical Picture

The eating of non-nutritive substances can be seen most frequently in infants and young children. The typical substances ingested vary with children's ages, and preschool children typically eat plaster, paper, paint, cloth, hair, strings, leaves, insects, animal droppings, sand, pebbles, dirt, and colorful objects. The word "pica" is derived from the Latin word for magpie (Barnes, Monagle, & McNamara, 2003), a bird renowned for its bold attitude, voracious appetite, and indiscriminate eating of a variety of food and nonfood articles. Several types of pica have been described based on the type of material ingested: geophagia (ingestion of earth substances, including dirt, clay and soil); pagophagia (ingestion of ice); plumbophagia (eating lead); lithophagia (ingestion of stones); trichophagia (eating hair); phytophagia (eating plants); coprophagia (eating feces); amylophagia (eating laundry starch or cornstarch); acuphagia (eating sharp objects); and cautopyreiophagia (eating burnt matches).

Because mouthing of objects is still common in toddlers between ages 1 and 2 years, the diagnosis of pica should be made only if the behavior is persistent and inappropriate for the child's developmental level. However, the diagnosis of pica should be explored in children presenting with accidental poisoning, lead intoxication, worm infestation, signs of malnutrition, or iron deficiency anemia. It is also important to suspect this disorder in preschool children who present with unexplained signs and symptoms, such as early satiety, lack of weight gain, abdominal pain, nausea, vomiting, change in bowel habit (diarrhea or constipation), a painless upper abdominal mass, or acute behavioral alteration.

If the diagnosis is delayed, pica can be potentially life threatening as a result of its associated complications. Malnutrition, accidental poisoning (e.g., plumbism from paint or plaster ingestion), mercury and heavy metal poisoning, and soil-borne parasitic infections (e.g., toxoplasmosis, toxocariasis, and trichuriasis) have resulted from pica.

Pica may also result in a high incidence of surgical complications, such as intestinal obstruction (secondary to trichobezoar, geophagia, or lithophagia), intestinal perforations from sharp objects, and infestations by gastrointestinal parasites. Gonzales et al. (2000) reported 16 cases of toxocariasis with liver involvement in a 2-year period. Mean age was 2 years, 9 months. Sex distribution was 1:1. Thirteen children (81%) presented with pica, 8 (50%) had pets at home, and 10 (62.5%) presented with anemia and long-standing fever, and all had eosinophilic leukocytosis.

The assessment should include the history of the child's development, feeding history, information regarding other oral activities (e.g., thumb-sucking or nail-biting) that the child may use for self-soothing, caregiver–child interaction, and psychosocial conditions. The home environment and the parents' relationship with the child are particularly relevant to assess the parents' ability to nurture and supervise the child. It is also helpful to observe the caregiver and child during a meal and during play to gain a better understanding of the dyadic relationship, caregiver adequacy, responsivity, and involvement, and how the symptoms of pica can be understood in the context of that relationship. Once the diagnosis of pica is made or suspected, the child needs a comprehensive physical examination to rule out any of the complications associated with this disorder, such as nutritional deficiencies (especially iron deficiency), lead poisoning, intestinal infections (toxoplasmosis or intestinal parasites), or gastrointestinal bezoars (Sayetta, 1986; Glickman, Cypess, Crunrine, & Gitlin, 1979).

Epidemiology

Chatoor et al. (1994) did a survey of over 1,500 toddlers, 1–3 years of age, in a pediatric clinic with a population representing a broad spectrum of ethnic and socioeconomic backgrounds. They found that 22% of the mothers observed that their children put nonfood objects in their mouths and that this behavior generally declined with age. Most of these toddlers (88%) were good eaters, and their mothers had little concern about their growth. Robinson, Tolan, and Golding-Beecher (1990) compared the clinical profiles of 108 children, ages 1.5–10 years, with pica to that of 50 children of the same age without pica. Their findings revealed that of the patients with pica, 85% were younger than 5 years and 29% were 1.5–2 years of age. The male:female ratio was 1:1.4, with the most common form of pica being geophagia. Forty-one percent of the children had a positive family history of pica and were more susceptible to complications of malnutrition, anemia, diarrhea, or constipation, and worm infestation. Millican, Layman, Lourie, Takahashi, and Dublin (1962) studied the prevalence of pica in three groups of children ages 1–6 years. They found that pica occurred in 32% of an African American, low-income group and in 10% of a white middle- and upper-class population. The prevalence was highest (55%) in a group of children hospitalized for accidental poisoning. They also noted that 63% of mothers with children with pica had pica themselves. Gutelius, Millican, Layman, Cohen, and Dublin (1962) reported that 87% of children with pica had either mothers or siblings with pica.

Etiology

Currently, no single theory explains this disorder. Several theoretical considerations have been proposed. These include organic, nutritional, psychodynamic, socioeconomic, and cultural factors, all of which appear to play a role in the etiology of this disorder. Nutritional factors that have been linked to this disorder include deficiencies in iron, zinc, and calcium. Some authors have proposed that inadequate dietary intake of iron or calcium can lead to abnormal cravings and induce pica (Crosby, 1976; Johnson & Tenuta, 1979; Singhi & Singhi, 1982). Animal models also support the hypothesis that iron deficiency (Woods & Wessinger, 1970) and a low calcium diet (Jacobsen & Snowdon, 1976) can induce pica. A study of 213 preschool children with low zinc levels, assessed by means of hair sampling, showed pica to be a frequent presenting complaint. Subsequent zinc supplementation resulted in elimination of pica (Chen et al., 1985). To determine the trace elements in the causation of pica, with specific reference to zinc and iron, Singhi and Bakker (1984) studied plasma levels of iron, zinc, lead, calcium, and magnesium by atomic absorption spectrophotometry in 31 children with pica and in 60 controls. Their findings suggested that hypozincemia and low iron levels are associated with pica.

Blood lead levels were assessed in 293 children ages 4–6 years attending preschool centers in metropolitan Cape Town. Results of this assessment revealed a significantly higher incidence of pica in children with higher lead levels (Devereaux, Kibel, Dempster, Pocock, & Formenti, 1986). Pica appears to have an unusually high prevalence in children with sickle-cell disease and a correlation with lower hemoglobin levels (Ivascu et al., 2001).

Psychosocial, family, and cultural factors have also been implicated in this disorder and may put an individual at risk either directly or indirectly. Some authors (Lourie, 1977; Madden, Russo, & Michael, 1980; Singhi, Singhi, & Adwani, 1981) have associated family factors such as psychosocial stress, maternal deprivation, parental neglect and abuse, inadequate daily living skills, and family dysfunction with this disorder. In some Southern African American cultures, there is an association between cultural factors and pica. Clay may be fed to infants as a pacifier. (Danford, 1982; Forsyth & Benoit, 1989; Vermeer & Frate, 1979). In some African cultures, well-being is promoted by the ingestion of soil, which is believed to have magical properties (Danford, 1982).

Millican, Dublin, and Lourie (1979) have proposed a complex multifactorial etiology whereby constitutional, developmental, familial, socioeconomic, and cultural factors interact. These authors noted that the children who engaged in pica had experienced separation from one or both parents early in life, followed by frequent changes and misattuned caregivers who seemed to encourage oral gratification in response to the child's distress. These children often demonstrated a high degree of other oral activities (e.g., thumbsucking or nailbiting), and the pica behavior was interpreted as an aberrant form of seeking gratification caused by the lack of parental availability and nurture.

Course and Natural History

Pica may have its onset in infancy; in most instances, this disorder is believed to be self-limited. Most cases of pica remit spontaneously after a few months, and patient outcomes are generally favorable. The symptoms of pica are inversely related to age, with symptom onset and severity decreasing across the lifespan. Occasionally, symptoms continue into adolescence or, less frequently, into adulthood. Such cases are rare and generally occur in the context of another developmental disorder (e.g., mental retardation or developmental delays). Millican et al. (1979) pointed to the seriousness of the developmental impact of the symptoms of pica in childhood and adolescence. The younger children were somewhat retarded in their use of speech and showed conflicts centered around their dependency needs and aggressive feelings. Half of the adolescents evidenced some degree of depression; several had passive, dependent, or borderline personality disorders, engaged in other forms of disturbed oral activities (e.g., thumbsucking, nail-biting), and abused tobacco, alcohol, and drugs. Marchi and Cohen (1990) documented a strong relationship between pica in early childhood and problems with bulimia nervosa during adolescence.

Treatment

In treating pica, one must consider the multiplicity of factors that appear to contribute to its development, as well as address any complications. The initial focus should be on improving parental education, such as food safety and nutrition, and to address any medical or surgical complications (e.g., correcting anemia, nutritional deficiencies, or lead poisoning). However, in order to facilitate any long-term changes in the child's behavior, parenting practices and the psychosocial needs of the parents and child need to be addressed. Essential are home visits by paraprofessionals, with early involvement of families to heighten their awareness to the risks of pica; assistance in providing a childproof environment; support; and counseling of parents, as well as continuity of services. Interventions might include removing the preferred nonnutritive substance from accessible areas, removal of lead from paint in old housing, or antihelminthic therapy for family pets (Sayetta, 1986). Lourie (1977) proposed a psychoeducational treatment approach for pica and stressed that in addition to awareness of the potential risks of pica, mothers needed increased social support to alleviate stress, so that they become more available to their children. In culturally transmitted pica, it seems important to alter the attitudes of parents engaging in such practices by educating them about the dangers of pica.

Some authors have suggested behavioral interventions in the treatment of pica. These include aversive and nonaversive behavioral therapy (e.g., differential reinforcement of other behavior, noncontingent attention, or overcorrection; McAdam, Sherman, Sheldon, & Napolitano, 2004), physical restraints (Singhi & Bakker, 2003), environmental enrichment with group or individual play (Madden et al., 1980), and time out and overcorrection (Foxx & Martin, 1975). Education on pica prevention by increasing community awareness should be an integral component of all soil transmitted parasite control programs and prevention of plumbism.

CONCLUSION

In conclusion, a comprehensive evaluation in identifying the salient individual and family factors should determine which type of treatment is best suited for preschool children and their families. This may be behavioral intervention, family therapy, environmental enrichment and education, and/or medical treatment of the complications of pica.

REFERENCES

American Psychiatric Association. (1994). *Diagnostic and statistical manual of mental disorders* (4th ed.). Washington, DC: Author.

American Psychiatric Association. (2000). *Diagnostic and statistical manual of mental disorders* (4th ed., text rev.). Washington, DC: Author.

Barnes, C., Monagle, P., & McNamara, J. (2003). Velcroholism. *Journal of Paediatrics and Child Health, 39*(5), 392.

Bartoshuk, L. M., Duffy, V. B., & Miller, I. J. (1994). PTC/PROP tasting: Anatomy, psychophysics, and sex effects. *Physiology and Behavior, 56*, 1165–1171.

Beautrais, A. L., Fergusson, D. M., & Shannon, F. T. (1982). Family life events and behavioral problems in preschool-aged children. *Pediatrics, 70*(5), 774–779.

Benoit, D. (2000). Feeding disorders, failure to thrive, and obesity. In C. H. Zeanah (Ed.), *Handbook of infant mental health* (2nd ed., pp. 339–352). New York: Guilford Press.

Birch, L. L. (1999). Development of food preferences. *Annual Review of Nutrition, 19*, 41–62.

Birch, L. L., Birch, D., Marlin, D. W., & Kramer, L. (1982). Effects of instrumental eating on children's food preferences. *Appetite, 3*, 125–134.

Birch, L. L., Gunder, L., & Grimm-Thomas, K. (1988). Infants' consumption of a new food enhances acceptance of similar foods. *Appetite, 30*, 283–295.

Chatoor, I. (2002). Feeding disorders in infants and toddlers: Diagnosis and treatment. *Child and Adolescent Psychiatric Clinics of North America, 11*, 163–183.

Chatoor, I., Conley, C., & Dickson, L. (1988). Food refusal after an incident of choking: A posttraumatic eating disorder. *Journal of the American Academy of Child and Adolescent Psychiatry, 27*, 105–110.

Chatoor, I., & Egan, J. (1983). Nonorganic failure to thrive and dwarfism due to food refusal: A separation disorder. *Journal of the American Academy of Child and Adolescent Psychiatry, 22*, 294–301.

Chatoor, I., Egan, J., Getson, P., Menvielle, E., & O'Donnell, R. (1988). Mother–infant interactions in infantile anorexia nervosa. *Journal of the American Academy of Child and Adolescent Psychiatry, 27*, 535–540.

Chatoor, I., Ganiban, J., Colin, V., Plummer, N., & Harmon, R. J. (1998). Attachment and feeding problems: A reexamination of nonorganic failure to thrive and attachment insecurity. *Journal of the American Academy of Child and Adolescent Psychiatry, 37*, 1217–1224.

Chatoor, I., Ganiban, J., Harrison, J., & Hirsch, R. (2001). The observation of feeding in the diagnosis of posttraumatic feeding disorder of infancy. *Journal of the American Academy of Child and Adolescent Psychiatry, 40*(5), 595–602.

Chatoor, I., Ganiban, J., Hirsch, R., Borman-Spurrell, E., & Mrazek, D. (2000). Maternal characteristics and toddler temperament in infantile anorexia. *Journal of the American Academy of Child and Adolescent Psychiatry, 39*(6), 743–751.

Chatoor, I., Ganiban, J., Surles, J., & Doussard-Roosevelt, J. (2004). Physiological regulation in infantile anorexia: A pilot study. *Journal of the American Academy of Child and Adolescent Psychiatry, 43*(8), 1019–1025.

Chatoor, I., Getson, P., Menvielle, E., O'Donnell, R., Rivera, Y., Brasseaux, C., et al. (1997). A feeding scale for research and clinical practice to assess mother–infant interactions in the first three years of life. *Infant Mental Health Journal, 18*, 76–91.

Chatoor, I., Hamburger, E., Fullard, R., & Rivera, Y. (1994). *A survey of picky eating and pica behaviors in toddlers.* Paper presented at the Scientific Proceedings of the 50th annual meeting of the American Academy of Child and Adolescent Psychiatry, New York, NY.

Chatoor, I., Hirsch, R., Ganiban, J., Persinger, M., & Hamburger, E. (1998). Diagnosing infantile anorexia: The observation of mother–infant interactions. *Journal of the American Academy of Child and Adolescent Psychiatry, 37*(9), 959–967.

Chatoor, I., Hirsch, R., & Persinger, M. (1997). Facilitating the internal regulation of eating: A treatment model for infantile anorexia. *Infants and Young Children, 9*, 12–22.

Chatoor, I., Kerzner, B., Zorc, L., Persinger, M., Simenson, R., & Mrazek, D. (1992). Two-year old twins refuse to eat: A multidisciplinary approach to diagnosis and treatment. *Infant Mental Health Journal, 13*, 252–268.

Chen, X. C., Yin, T. A., He, J. S., Ma, Q. Y., Han, Z. M., & Li, L. X. (1985). Low levels of zinc in hair and blood, pica, anorexia, and poor growth in Chinese preschool children. *American Journal of Clinical Nutrition, 42*, 694–700.

Crosby, W. H. (1976). Pica: A compulsion caused by iron deficiency. *British Journal of Haematology, 34*, 341–342.

Culbert, T. P., Kajander, R. L., Kohen, D. P., & Reaney, J. B. (1996). Hypnobehavioral approaches for school-age children with dysphagia and food aversion: A case series. *Journal of Developmental and Behavioral Pediatrics, 17*, 335–341.

Dahl, M. (1987). Early feeding problems in an affluent society: III. Follow-up at two years: Natural course, health, behaviour and development. *Acta Paediatricia Scandinavia, 76*:872–880.

Dahl, M., Rydell, A. M., & Sundelin, C. (1994). Children with early refusal to eat: Follow-up during primary school. *Acta Paediatricia Scandinavica, 83*, 54–58.

Dahl, M., & Sundelin, C. (1986). Early feeding problems in an affluent society: I. Categories and clinical signs. *Acta Paediatricia Scandinavica, 75*, 370–379.

Dahl, M., & Sundelin, C. (1992). Feeding problems in an affluent society: Follow-up at four years of age in children with early refusal to eat. *Acta Paediatricia Scandinavica, 81*, 575–579.

Danford, D. E. (1982). Pica and nutrition. *Annual Review of Nutrition, 2*, 303–322.

Devereaux, P., Kibel, M. A., Dempster, W. S., Pocock, F., & Formenti, K. (1986). Blood lead levels in preschool children in Cape Town. *South African Medical Journal, 69*(7), 421–424.

Drewnowski, A., & Rock, C. L. (1995). The influence of genetic taste markers on food acceptance. *American Journal of Clinical Nutrition, 62*, 506–511.

Drotar, D., & Sturm, L. (1988). Prediction of intellectual development in young children with early histories of nonorganic failure to thrive. *Journal of Pediatric Psychology, 13*, 281–296.

Ellis, C. R., & Schnoes, J. C. (2002). eMedicine—Eating disorder: Pica.

Essick, G. K., Chopra, A., Guest, S., & McGlone, F. (2003). Lingual tactile acuity, taste perception, and the density and diameter of fungiform papillae in female subjects. *Physiology and Behavior, 80*, 289–302.

Forsyth, B. W., & Canny, P. F. (1991). Perceptions of vulnerability 3½ years after problems of feeding and crying behavior in early infancy. *Pediatrics, 88*(4), 757–763.

Forsyth, C. J., & Benoit, G. M. (1989). "Rare ole dirty snacks": Some research notes on dirt eating. *Deviant Behavior, 10*, 61–68.

Foxx, R. M., & Martin E. D. (1975). Treatment of scavenging behavior (coprophagy and pica) by overcorrection, *Behaviour Research and Therapy, 13*, 153–162.

Galler, J. R., Ramsey, R. L., Solimano, G., Lowell, W. E., & Mason, E. (1988). The influence of early malnutrition on subsequent behavioral development: I. Degree of impairment in intellectual performance. *Journal of the American Academy of Child and Adolescent Psychiatry, 22*, 8–15.

Ganiban, J., Chatoor, I., & Gelven, E. (1999). *Emotional reactivity and regulation in infantile anorexia.* Poster presented at the Biennial Meeting of the Society for Research in Child Development, Albuquerque, NM.

Garb, J. L., & Stunkard, A. J. (1974). Taste aversions in man. *American Journal of Psychology*, *131*, 1204–1207.

Glickman, L. T., Cypess, R. H., Crunrine, P. K., & Gitlin, D. A. (1979). Toxocara infection and epilepsy in children. *Journal of Pediatrics*, *94*, 75–78.

Gonzalez, M. T., Ibanez, O., Balcarce, N., Nanfito, G., Kozubsky, L., Radman, N., et al. (2000). Toxocariasis with liver involvement. *Acta Gastroenterologica Latinoamericana*, *30*(3), 187–190.

Gutelius, M. F., Millican, F. K., Layman, E. M., Cohen, G. J., & Dublin, C. C. (1962). Children with pica: Treatment of pica with iron given intramuscularly. *Pediatrics*, *29*, 1018–1023.

Harper, L. V., & Sanders, K. M. (1975). The effect of adults' eating on young children's acceptance of unfamiliar foods. *Journal of Experimental Child Psychology*, *20*, 206–214.

Hursti, U. K. K., & Sjödén, P. O. (1997). Food and general neophobia and their relationship with self-reported food choice: Familial resemblance in Swedish families with children of ages 7–17 years. *Appetite*, *29*, 89–103.

Ivascu, N. S., Sarnaik, S., McCrae, J., Whitten-Shurney, W., Thomas, R., & Bond, S. (2001). Characterization of pica prevalence among patients with sickle cell disease. *Archives of Pediatrics and Adolescent Medicine*, *155*(11), 1243–1247.

Jacobsen, J. L., & Snowdon, C. T. (1976). Increased lead ingestion in calcium deficient monkeys. *Nature*, *162*, 51–52.

Johnson, N. E., & Tenuta, K. (1979). Diets and lead blood levels of children who practice pica. *Environmental Research*, *18*, 369–376.

Kalat, J. W., & Rozin, P. (1973). "Learned safety" as a mechanism in long delay taste aversion learning in rats. *Journal of Comparative and Physiological Psychology*, *83*, 198–207.

Kern, L., & Marder, T. J. (1996). A comparison of simultaneous and delayed reinforcement as treatments for food selectivity. *Journal of Applied Behavior Analysis*, *29*(2), 243–246.

Kim, U., Jorgenson, E., Coon, H., Leppert, M., Risch, N., & Drayna, D. (2003). Positional cloning of the human quantitative trait locus underlying taste sensitivity to phenylthiocarbamide. *Science*, *299*, 1221–1225

Kotler, L. A., Cohen, P., Davies, M., Pine, D.S., & Walsh, B.T. (2001). Longitudinal relationships between childhood, adolescent, and adult eating disorders. *Journal of the American Academy of Child Adolescent Psychiatry*, *40*(12), 1434–1440.

Lindberg, L., Bohlin, G., Hagekull, B., & Thunstroem, M. (1994). Early food refusal: Infant and family characteristics. *Infant Mental Health Journal*, *15*(3), 262.

Logue, A. W., Ophir, I., & Strauss, K. (1981). The acquisition of taste aversions in humans. *Behaviour Research and Therapy*, *19*, 319–333.

Lourie, R. S. (1977). Pica and lead poisoning. *American Journal of Orthopsychiatry*, *41*, 697–699.

Madden, N. A., Russo, D. C., & Michael, F. C. (1980). Environmental influences on mouthing in children with lead intoxication. *Journal of Pediatric Psychology*, *5*, 207–216.

Mahler, M. S., Pine, F., & Bergman, A. (1975). *The psychological birth of the human infant*. New York: Basic Books.

Marchi, M., & Cohen, P. (1990). Early childhood eating behaviors and adolescent eating disorders. *Journal of the American Academy of Child and Adolescent Psychiatry*, *29*, 112–117.

McAdam, D. B., Sherman, J. A., Sheldon, J. B., & Napolitano, D. A. (2004). Behavioral interventions to reduce the pica of persons with developmental disabilities. *Behavior Modification*, *28*(1), 45–72.

McNally, R. J. (1994). Choking phobia: A review of the literature. *Comprehensive Psychiatry*, *35*, 83–89.

Mihailidou, H., Galanakis, E., Paspalaki, P., Borgia, P., & Mantzouranis, E. (2002). Pica and the elephant's ear. *Journal of Child Neurology*, *17*(11), 855–856.

Millican, F. K,, Dublin, C. C., & Lourie, R. S. (1979). Pica. In J. D. Noshpitz (Ed.), *Basic handbook of child psychiatry: Vol. II. Disturbances in development* (pp. 660–666). New York: Basic Books.

Millican, F. K., Layman, E. M., Lourie, R. S., Takahashi, L. Y., & Dublin, C. C. (1962). The prevalence of ingestion and mouthing of nonedible substances by children. *Clinical Proceedings: Children's Hospital, Washington, DC*, *18*, 207–214.

Morton, C. C., Cantor, R. M., Cory, L. A., & Nance, W. E. (1981). A genetic analysis of taste threshold for phenylthiocarbamide. *Acta Geneticae Medicae et Gemellologiae (Roma), 30,* 51–57.

Olson, J. M., Boehnke, M., Neiswanger, K., Roche, A. F., & Siervogel, R. M. (1989). Alternative genetic models for the inheritance of the phenylthiocarbamide (PTC) taste deficiency. *Genetic Epidemiology, 6*(3), 423–434.

Pliner, P., & Lowen, E. R. (1997). Temperament and food neophobia in children and their mothers. *Appetite, 28*(3), 239–254.

Reif, S., Beler, B., Villa, Y., & Spirer, Z. (1995). Long-term follow-up and outcome of infants with non-organic failure to thrive. *Israel Journal of Medical Sciences, 31*(8), 483–489.

Robinson, B. A., Tolan, W., & Golding-Beecher, O. (1990). Childhood pica. Some aspects of the clinical profile in Manchester, Jamaica. *West Indian Medical Journal, 39,* 20–26.

Rydell, A. M., Dahl, M., & Sundelin, C. (1995). Characteristics of school children who are choosy eaters. *Journal of Genetic Psychology, 156*(2), 217–229.

Sayetta, R. B. (1986). Pica: An overview. *American Family Physician, 33,* 181–185.

Shore, B. A., Babbitt, R. L., Williams, K. E., Coe, D. A., & Snyder, A. (1998). Use of texture fading in the treatment of food selectivity. *Journal of Applied Behavior Analysis, 31*(4), 621–633.

Singer, L. T., Ambuel, B., Wade, S., & Jaffe, A. C. (1992). Cognitive-behavioral treatment of health-impairing food phobias in children. *Journal of American Academy of Child and Adolescent Psychiatry, 31*(5), 847–852.

Singhi, N. N., & Bakker, L. W. (1984). Suppression of pica by overcorrection and physical restraint: A comparative analysis. *Journal of Autism and Developmental Disorders, 14,* 331–341.

Singhi, P., & Singhi, S. (1982). Pica type of "nonfood articles" eaten by Ajmer children and their significance. *Indian Journal of Pediatrics, 49,* 681–684.

Singhi, S., Ravishanker, R., Singhi, P., & Nath, R. (2003). Low plasma zinc and iron in pica. *Indian Journal of Pediatrics, 70*(2), 139–143.

Singhi, S., Singhi, P., & Adwani, G. B. (1981). Role of psychosocial stress in the case of pica. *Clinical Pediatrics, 20,* 783–785.

Skinner, J. D., Carruth, B. R., Bounds, B., & Ziegler, P. J. (2002). Children's food preferences: A longitudinal analysis. *Journal of the American Dietetic Association, 102*(11), 1638–1647.

Task Force on Research Diagnostic Criteria: Infancy and Preschool. (2003). Research diagnostic criteria for infants and preschool children: The process and empirical support. *Journal of the American Academy of Child and Adolescent Psychiatry, 42*(12), 1504–1512.

Tepper, B. J. (1998). 6-n-propylthiouracil: A genetic marker for taste, with implications for food preference and dietary habits. *American Journal of Human Genetics, 63,* 1271–1276.

Tepper, B. J., & Nurse, R. J. (1997). Fat perception is related to PROP taster status. *Physiology and Behavior, 61,* 949–954.

Timimi, S., Douglas, J., & Tsiftsopoulou, K. (1997). Selective eaters: A retrospective case note study. *Child: Care, Health and Development, 23*(3), 265–278.

Vermeer, D. E., & Frate, D. A. (1979). Geophagia in rural Mississippi: Environmental and cultural contexts and nutritional implications. *American Journal of Clinical Nutrition, 32,* 2129–2135.

Waterlow, J. C., Buzina, R., Keller, W., Lan, J. M., Nichaman, M. Z., & Tanner, J. M. (1977). The presentation and use of height and weight data for comparing the nutritional status of groups of children under the age of 10 years. *Bulletin of the World Health Organization, 55,* 489–498.

Watkins, B., & Lask, B. (2002). Eating disorders in school-aged children. *Child and Adolescent Psychiatric Clinics of North America, 11*(2), 185–199.

Whissell-Buechy, D. (1990). Effects of age and sex on taste sensitivity to phenylthiocarbamide (PTC) in the Berkeley Guidance sample. *Chemical Senses, 15,* 39–57

Woods, S. C., & Wessinger, R. S. (1970). Pagophasia in the albino rat. *Science, 169,* 1334–1336.

7

Anxiety Disorders

HELEN LINK EGGER and ADRIAN ANGOLD

Anxiety is among the most common and disabling psychiatric problems of childhood (Costello, Egger, & Angold, 2004). Effective psychopharmacological and psychotherapeutic treatments for older children have been developed (Ollendick & March, 2004), and younger children, too, could potentially be helped, if they have similar patterns of symptoms, impairment, and prognosis. However, remarkably little clinical or epidemiological research has examined the prevalence or characteristics of clinically significant anxiety symptoms and disorders in preschool children. Most of the research on anxiety and fear in young children has been conducted from the perspective of temperament and normal development, not psychiatric symptoms and disorders, and it has not been clinically focused. This chapter reviews the approaches to and the classification of anxiety symptoms and disorders in preschool children, the prevalence and associated features of preschool anxiety disorders, assessment of preschool anxiety disorders, and their treatment.

CLASSIFICATION OF ANXIETY SYMPTOMS AND DISORDERS IN PRESCHOOL CHILDREN

Fears and Anxiety in the Preschool Period

From the perspective of developmental psychology and temperament research, anxiety and fear in young children has typically been seen either as a normative phase of development or, in a subset of children, as a temperament style that increases the child's risk for developing an anxiety disorder later in childhood or adulthood.

Most infants develop a degree of a fear of strangers and express distress when separated from their primary caregivers between 6 and 12 months of

137

age, with these fears peaking between 9 and 13 months and decreasing for most children by 30 months (Marks, 1987; Warren & Sroufe, 2004). Both stranger anxiety and separation anxiety reflect evolutionary selection of an infant's adaptive response to danger posed by unfamiliar adults and by being alone. For the majority of children, these anxieties would not be classified as symptoms of a disorder because they reflect the baby's attachment to a primary caregiver and the ability to distinguish between loved ones and strangers. These anxieties and fear responses are transient and do not derail the child's cognitive, social, or emotional development.

Early developmental studies of children within the community (e.g., Macfarlane, Allen, & Honzik, 1954; Richman et al., 1974; Earls, 1980; Richman, Stevenson, & Graham, 1982) have also revealed that specific fears, including fear of animals and fear of the dark, are common in young children, with peak prevalence between ages 2 and 6 years (for reviews see Marks, 1987; Warren & Sroufe, 2004). In Macfarlane and colleagues' (1954) longitudinal study of 252 children assessed from 18 months to 14 years of age, 62% of 3-year-olds were reported to have specific fears, with these rates being the highest compared with the rates at the other ages. The two most common fears of preschoolers were fear of dogs and fear of the dark. At age 5, fears in girls were correlated with irritability, mood swings, tantrums, timidity, and overdependence, while in boys they were associated only with negativism. In two community studies of preschoolers in the 1970s, 9–14% of parents reported that their 3-year-olds "often" had fears (Richman et al., 1974; Earls, 1980). In the Richman study ($N = 705$), 2.6% of parents reported that their child often worried, compared with 7.9% in the Earls study ($N = 100$). In all three studies, girls age 3 were reported to be more fearful than boys (25.5% vs. 3.7% in the Earls study; 17.2% vs. 8.0% in the Richman et al. [1974] study; 67% vs. 56% in the Macfarlane et al. [1954] study).

For a subset of children, fear of strangers and of novel situations is more extreme. About 15% of young children display intense and persistent fear, shyness, and social withdrawal in response to unfamiliar people, situations, or objects. These children are said to be "behaviorally inhibited" (Biederman et al., 1993; Fox et al., 2001; Hirshfeld et al., 1992; Kagan & Snidman, 1991). Behaviorally inhibited infants and preschoolers display characteristic patterns of physiological reactions to novelty (high heart rate, low heart rate variability, high baseline morning cortisol, elevated startle responses; Calkins, Fox, & Marshall, 1996; Fox et al., 2001; Kagan, Reznick, & Snidman, 1987), and are more likely to develop an anxiety disorder, particularly social phobia, later in childhood or adolescence, or to have first-degree relatives with anxiety disorders (Hirshfeld et al., 1992; Schwartz, 1999; Rosenbaum, Biederman, Hirshfeld, Bolduc, & Chaloff, 1991; Rosenbaum et al., 1991, 1992; Kagan & Snidman, 1999; Biederman et al., 1993). They also show greater amygdalal functional MRI signal response to novel versus familiar faces as adults, compared to adults who had not been uninhibited as children (Schwartz, Wright, Shin, Kagan, & Rauch, 2003).

In general, temperamental characteristics, including those identifying behaviorally inhibited children, have been treated as *risk factors* for a variety of disorders across the lifespan. However, as with extreme manifestations of developmentally normative anxieties, it is also possible that these temperamental characteristics could represent the early presence of anxiety disorders themselves. Only recently have researchers and clinicians begun to explore whether it is possible to identify clinically significant anxiety in preschoolers, and to define constellations of anxiety symptoms and associated symptoms that we might identify as anxiety disorders.

Anxiety Disorders and Clinically Significant Anxiety Symptoms in Preschoolers

We review three approaches to defining and categorizing clinically significant anxiety in preschool children: (1) the use of "clinically significant" cutpoints on checklist-derived symptoms counts, (2) the fourth edition of the *Diagnostic and Statistical Manual of Mental Disorders* (DSM-IV), and (3) Diagnostic Classification 0–3 (DC:0–3). There has been a longstanding debate in the child psychiatric literature about whether psychopathology in children is "dimensional," with clinically significant problems representing the extreme end of a continuum, or "categorical," with individuals either meeting or not meeting criteria for a specific disorder (Sonuga-Barke, 1998; Pickles & Angold, 2003; Achenbach, 1991; Arend, Lavigne, Rosenbaum, Binns, & Christoffel, 1996). The first approach listed here is dimensional, whereas the following two are diagnostic classifications that define categories of anxiety disorders. Clearly, the challenge of distinguishing between developmentally normal anxiety, temperamental variation, and clinically significant anxiety in very young children arises because there seems to be a continuum of anxieties and fears during the preschool period, with gradations based on degrees of severity, persistence, and impairment. On the other hand, clinical evaluation and intervention require that the clinician decide whether to treat or not to treat a child. So whether this involves defining "caseness" based on a cutpoint on a dimensional measure or applying diagnostic criteria, it is a categorical decision. From the medical point of view, this decision is called making a diagnosis. Echoing Pickles and Angold in their article on this topic, we agree that the central question is not whether anxiety symptomatology in preschoolers is best conceptualized as scalar or categorical, but rather "under what circumstances" (Pickles & Angold, 2003, p. 529) is it useful to measure and define clinically significant anxiety from dimensional and categorical points of view.

"Clinically Significant" Cutpoints on Symptom Counts Defined by Checklists

BROAD ANXIETY DIMENSIONS

In a number of studies of emotional and behavioral problems in preschoolers, using checklists of widely varying length and content, with different informants (parents, preschool teachers), the broad distinction between emotional (internalizing) and behavioral (externalizing) syndromes has consistently emerged (Crowther, Bond, & Rolf, 1981; Behar & Stringfield, 1974; Richman et al., 1982; McGuire & Richman, 1986; Koot & Verhulst, 1991; Koot, van den Oord, Verhulst, & Boomsma, 1997; Achenbach & Rescorla, 2000; Achenbach, Edelbrock, & Howell, 1987; van den Oord, Koot, Boomsma, Verhulst, & Orlebeke, 1995). Although attempts to extract more than two factors have had much less consistent results, at least one factor representing some mixture of fear–anxiety–depression–withdrawal is typically seen. For example, in the Achenbach and colleagues (1987) study of over 500 non-referred preschoolers using the Child Behavior Checklist (CBCL 1½–5), 17% of the children were in the clinical range of the internalizing scale, 8% were in the clinical range for the anxious–depressed syndrome, and 8% were in the clinical range for anxiety problems on the DSM-oriented scales, suggesting that clinically significant anxiety symptoms are not uncommon in preschool children (Achenbach & Rescorla, 2000). In a study of the CBCL 2–3 in clinical (N = 426), community (N = 469), and twins (N = 1,306 twin pairs) samples of 2- and 3-year-olds, Koot and colleagues (1997) identified an anxious factor, distinct from a withdrawn–depressed factor. Cutpoints for clinically significant anxiety were not reported from these data.

EVIDENCE FOR SUBTYPES OF ANXIETY SYMPTOMS

There have also been a few studies using checklist measures that reflect the symptoms domains of the DSM-IV diagnostic categories to examine whether preschool anxiety can be grouped into subtypes similar to anxiety disorders found in older children, or whether preschool anxiety is better described as a single anxiety dimension, as it is in the CBCL. Spencer and colleagues (2001) assessed anxiety in 755 preschoolers attending preschool or kindergarten in Australia, based on maternal report on the 28-item Preschool Anxiety Scale (PAS). A confirmatory factor analysis found that preschool anxiety symptoms clustered into five factors similar to the DSM-IV anxiety subtypes of separation anxiety disorder (SAD), social phobia, obsessive–compulsive disorder (OCD), generalized anxiety disorder (GAD), and specific phobias (here limited to the specific fear of physical injury), suggesting differentiation of anxiety in early childhood. Although social phobia, OCD, and fear of physical injury seemed to be separate dimensions, there were suggestions that separation anxiety and generalized anxiety might be measuring the same or highly similar dimensions (Spencer, Rapee, McDonald, & Ingram, 2001). No significant differences were found between boys and girls.

A study of 4,564 4-year-old twins provides similar evidence for phenotypic and genetic differentiation between specific categories of anxious behavior in young children. A confirmatory factor analysis of a 16-item anxiety survey, which included anxiety-related items from psychiatric and temperament checklists, identified five factors: general distress, separation anxiety, fear, obsessive–compulsive behaviors, and shyness–inhibition (Eley et al., 2003). Although all of the factors were correlated, there was differentiation. Interestingly, the correlation between the general distress, separation anxiety, and fear factors and the shyness–inhibition factor ranged from about .17 to .28, suggesting that anxiety symptoms were distinct from behaviorally inhibited temperament.

In a study of a community sample of preschoolers ($N = 271$) using the Early Childhood Inventory–4 (ECI), a parent- and teacher-completed DSM-IV–referenced rating scale (Gadow & Sprafkin, 1997, 2000; Gadow, Sprafkin, & Nolan, 2001; Sparking & Gadow, 1996), rates of anxiety disorder symptom clusters were as follows: 3.7% of boys and 2.3% of girls had GAD, 4.1% of boys and 3.9% of girls had SAD, and 2.2% of boys and 1.2% of girls had social phobia. Teacher-reported rates for GAD were 5.3% for boys and 4.7% for girls (Gadow et al., 2001).

Although checklist measures like these do not include enough symptom specificity (e.g., frequency, duration, onset) to enable researchers or clinicians to make the sorts of psychiatric diagnoses that are familiar to them at every other stage of life, these data do support the hypothesis that already in the preschool period, clinically significant anxiety can be subtype into patterns similar to those identified for older children (e.g., March, Parker, Sullivan, Stalling, & Canners, 1997; Marisa, Mayer, Barbells, Tourney, & Bogie, 2001; Spencer, 1997).

DSM-IV

Because the DSM-IV was developed with essentially no attention to the emotional and behavioral problems of preschoolers, there are many questions about the validity of the anxiety disorder criteria for young children.

Table 7.1 lists the DSM-IV anxiety disorder subtypes, specifying the four domains the DSM uses to identify "clinically significant" anxiety symptoms and disorders: (1) descriptors defining the characteristics of the anxiety, (2) duration criterion for the syndrome, (3) association of the syndrome with distress and/or impairment, and (4) presentations of symptoms specific to children. Here we examine the application of these domains to preschool anxiety and assess how they can be interpreted and implemented to identify "clinically significant" anxiety and anxiety disorders in preschoolers.

Descriptors Defining Characteristics of the Anxiety

As Table 7.1 shows, the DSM-IV (American Psychiatric Association, 2000) anxiety disorders use various adjectives to describe clinically significant anxiety: developmentally inappropriate (SAD), excessive (SAD, GAD), marked (specific phobia, social phobia), persistent (SAD, specific phobia, social phobia), repeated (SAD), difficult to control (GAD), and recurrent (panic disorder, SAD). These descriptors refer to the intensity (e.g., marked), frequency

TABLE 7.1. DSM-IV Anxiety Disorders

DSM-IV disorder	Key symptoms	Duration	Impairment/distress	Child-specific criteria
Separation anxiety disorder (SAD)	Three out of eight symptoms of persistent, developmentally inappropriate behavior.	At least 4 weeks.	Causes clinically significant distress or impairment.	• In "disorders usually first diagnosed in infancy, childhood, or adolescence" section. • Must begin before age 18. • Early onset if onset occurs before age 6 years.
Selective mutism	Child does not speak to others in certain social situations, despite speaking in other situations.	At least 1 month.	Interferes with educational achievement or with social communication.	• In "disorders usually first diagnosed in infancy, childhood, or adolescence" section.
Panic disorder with and without agoraphobia	Recurrent panic attacks with and without agoraphobia.	At least 1 month of worry about or change in behavior due to panic attacks.	No impairment criteria specified. Distress inherent in the symptoms.	None
Specific phobia	• Marked, persistent fear that is unreasonable, cued by presence or anticipation of feared stimulus. • Exposure almost invariably provokes an immediate anxiety response.	If the person is under age 18, duration is at least 6 months. No duration criterion specified for adults.	Causes clinically significant distress or impairment.	• In children, anxiety may be expressed by crying, tantrums, freezing, or clinging. • Children need not recognize that the fear is excessive or unreasonable. • If the person is under age 18, duration is at least 6 months.

Social phobia	• Marked, persistent fear of one or more social or performance situations. Fear that he or she will be humiliated or embarrassed. • Exposure almost invariably provokes an immediate anxiety response.	If the person is under age 18, duration is at least 6 months. No duration criterion specified for adults.	Causes clinically significant distress or impairment.	• In children, must be evidence of capacity for age-appropriate social relationship with familiar people, and the anxiety must occur with unfamiliar peers and adults. • In children, anxiety may be expressed by crying, tantrums, freezing, or clinging. • Children need not recognize that the fear is excessive or unreasonable. • If the person is under age 18, duration is at least 6 months.
Obsessive–compulsive disorder (OCD)	Obsessions and/or compulsions.	No duration criteria specified.	Causes marked distress, is time consuming (takes more than 1 hour a day), or causes impairment.	• Children need not recognize that the obsession or compulsions are excessive or unreasonable.
Generalized anxiety disorder (GAD)	• Excessive, difficult-to-control anxiety and worry. • Three of six associated symptoms.	More days than not for at least 6 months.	Causes clinically significant distress or impairment.	• States that GAD includes the DSM-III-R diagnosis overanxious disorder of childhood. • In children only one of six associated symptoms is required.

Note. Posttraumatic stress disorder and acute stress disorder, although included in the "anxiety disorders" section, are not included here because they are covered in a separate chapter (Chapter 8 in this book). Anxiety disorder due to a general medical condition and substance-induced anxiety disorder are not reviewed here.

143

(e.g., recurrent), and duration (e.g., persistent) of the anxiety. No further guidance is provided for determining when separation distress is developmentally inappropriate, what constitutes persistent versus transient anxiety, or why the worries of GAD are specified as "difficult to control," whereas SAD symptoms are not (although, perhaps the terms "persistent" and "excessive" suggest difficulty with control). The challenge of translating these criteria into specific expressions of emotion and behaviors is not unique to young children. The inherent ambiguity of many of the DSM symptoms affects the assessment of anxiety in older children (and adults). However, older children and adults are better at reliably describing their internal experiences and emotions, whereas young children, particularly those younger than age 4, usually do not have the cognitive, verbal, or emotional capacity to describe their own anxiety. Assessment of anxiety, then, depends on descriptions of the young child's affect state that (1) are based on the child's behaviors and manifest distress, and (2) are primarily based on adult report (e.g., parent, teacher/day care provider) and/or observational assessments (e.g., structured observations in a lab or at home or school/day care). This becomes particularly problematic for identifying symptoms such as the worries of GAD or the obsessions of OCD. The few measures that directly assess young children's psychiatric symptoms and internal experiences, including anxious affect and specific fears or worries (e.g., the Berkeley Puppet Interview [Ablow & Measelle, 1993; Ablow et al., 1999; Measelle, Ablow, Cowan, & Cowan, 1998] and the MacArthur Narrative Story Stems [Warren, 2003; Robinson, Mantz-Simmons, MacFie, & MacArthur Narrative Working Group, 1996]) show promise but are not reliable for children under the age of 4.

Duration Criteria for the Anxiety Disorders

There is great variety in the duration criterion for each of the anxiety disorders. For example, SAD and selective autism require at least 1 month of symptoms, whereas GAD, specific phobia, and social phobia must persist for at least 6 months in children, although no duration criterion is specified for social or specific phobia in those over 18 years old. OCD does not include a duration criterion. Prospective longitudinal data on the course of anxiety symptoms from toddler hood through the preschool period are needed to test whether these durations are appropriate for young children.

Association of the Syndrome with Distress and/or Impairment

The DSM-IV criteria for SAD, specific phobia, social phobia, GAD, and OCD specify that the symptoms must cause clinically significant distress *or* impairment (American Psychiatric Association, 2000). Because the anxiety symptoms are by definition and description distressing, this means that impairment is not required to diagnose an anxiety disorder. Selective mutism is the only anxiety disorder with an impairment criterion (refusal to talk must lead to impairment in either educational functioning or social communication). However, because separation anxiety, stranger anxiety and specific fears peak in the toddler–preschool period, we suggest that a diagnosis of SAD, specific phobia, or social phobia in young children should be associated with impairment to be considered "clinically significant" and a disorder. Because the syndromes of GAD, OCD, and panic disorder are not developmentally normative, we do not recommend changing the current DSM-IV criteria to require impairment. Clearly, more empirical evidence is needed to determine whether these recommendations are appropriate; however, at this point, they make clinical sense and seem to have face validity.

The other difficult issue that affects all preschoolers' disorders but is particularly pertinent to anxiety disorder based on the aforementioned criteria, is how to define impairment in preschoolers. The DSM-IV specifies that impairment must occur in social, occupational, academic, or "other important areas of functioning" (American Psychiatric Association, 2000). Because not all preschoolers are in day care or preschool, impairment may only be manifest in the home setting or in relationship to the child's primary caregivers. Moreover, a parent may limit the anxious preschooler's exposure to anxiety-provoking situations, such as day care for the child with SAD or birthday parties or other social events for the child with social phobia, or significantly modify family routines to accommodate the child's anxiety (e.g., the child sleeps in parents' bed because of separation fears or fear of the dark; prolonged morning routine to accommodate the rituals of a child with OCD). Because preschoolers have much less independence from their caregivers and less control over their activities and relationships than older children, we suggest that impairment be assessed in two domains: (1) the impact of the child's anxiety on his or her functioning and cognitive, social, and emotional development; and (2) the impact of the child's anxiety on parental and family functioning (e.g., a parent is unable to work because the child is too fearful to attend preschool, or parents are unable to leave the child with a babysitter due to the child's anxious distress).

Child-Specific Symptoms

The DSM-IV does attempt to identify child-specific aspects of anxiety disorders, yet they apply to children from 0 to 18 years old, a very wide range of developmental levels! Despite the fact that anxiety disorders commonly have their onset during childhood (Costello, Egger, & Angold, 2005), only two of the anxiety disorders are included in the DSM-IV section on disorders usually first diagnosed in infancy, childhood, or adolescence, whereas the other anxiety disorders are in the anxiety disorders section. The last column of Table 7.1 lists the modifications proposed for children. Most useful for preschoolers is the caveat, found in the specific and social phobia criteria, that anxiety in children may be expressed by crying, tantrums, freezing, or clinging. It is less clear whether the increased duration criterion (6 months for children, no duration criterion for adults) for these two disorders is the right cut point for distinguishing between normative fears and stranger anxiety–social reticence and disorders, or whether the reduced symptom requirement for GAD is appropriate either for preschoolers or older children.

Responding to the need for developmentally appropriate criteria for psychiatric disorders diagnosed in young children, infant and preschool mental health researchers, sponsored by the American Academy of Child and Adolescent Psychiatry, proposed modifications of DSM diagnostic criteria for use with preschool children (Task Force on Research Diagnostic Criteria, 2003). The purpose of this effort was to define developmentally appropriate criteria so as to facilitate further research on the diagnostic validity of psychiatric disorders in preschoolers. However, the Research Diagnostic Criteria— Preschool Age (RDC-PA) anxiety disorders' recommendations reflect the lack of empirical evidence about the nosology of preschool anxiety disorders. Although significant changes were proposed for posttraumatic stress disorder (PTSD), which is covered in Scheeringa, Chapter 8, this volume, minor modifications were proposed for SAD, with the addition of descriptors detailing how SAD symptom might appear in young children with limited ability to verbalize their fears (Task Force on Research Diagnostic Criteria, 2003). No modifications were proposed for specific phobia. Criteria for social phobia, panic disorder, GAD, and OCD were not addressed, because "not enough empirical data has accumulated to justify and/or provide guidance on whether or how to modify them at this point" (Task Force on Research Diagnostic Criteria, 2003, p. 12). Criteria for a new disorder named "disorder of inhibition/avoidance" were included in the appendix as needing further study, but to date, there are not sufficient data to warrant its support as a new disorder. Thus, whereas the RDC-PA provided some preliminary guidance, the clinician (and researcher) who is attempting to evaluate preschoolers with anxiety symptoms needs more specific guidelines for understanding how to apply the DSM-IV nomenclature to preschoolers.

Diagnostic Classification: 0–3

The Diagnostic Classification: 0–3 (DC:0–3) identifies mental health problems affecting infants and toddlers (Zero to Three, 1994, 2005). The DC:0–3 includes both alternative versions of DSM-IV diagnoses (e.g., for anxiety and depressive disorders) and new diagnostic categories (e.g., regulatory disorders). Little research has been conducted with or on this diagnostic approach, although a start has been made (Boris, Zeanah, Larrien, Scheeringa, & Heller, 1998; Reams, 1999; Scheeringa, Zeanah, Drell, & Larrien, 1995; Thomas & Clark, 1998). Despite this lack of adequate validation, it is widely used in service settings; indeed, it is often mandated by public funding agencies. A revised version (DC:0–3R) that incorporates research findings from the last decade and operational the original DC:0–3 criteria was published in 2005. Although the DC:0–3 offered few specific criteria for anxiety disorders, the

DC:0–3R does define specific anxiety disorders based on the DSM-IV criteria, but modifies them for use with young children. For example, in an attempt to define the difference between developmentally expected anxiety or fear and developmentally inappropriate and excessive anxiety, the DC:0–3R identifies general criteria that must be met for a young child's anxiety or fears to be considered as a possible symptom of an anxiety disorder: They must (1) cause the child distress, or lead to avoidance of activities or settings associated with the anxiety or fear; (2) occur during two or more everyday activities, or within two or more relationships; (3) be uncontrollable, at least some of the time; (4) persist for at least 2 weeks (note that for some disorders, the duration is longer than 2 weeks); and (5) impair the child's or the family's functioning, and/or the child's expected development (Zero to Three, 2005). Although there is no research on the validity of these specifications, they certainly make clinical sense and provide guidance for the clinician assessing a young child with concerning symptoms of anxiety.

PREVALENCE OF ANXIETY DISORDERS

Clinical Studies

There have been few clinical studies of anxiety disorders in preschool children. In a 1987 article, Wolfson, Fields, and Rose (1987) compared 27 preschoolers diagnosed with a DSM-III anxiety disorder (overanxious disorder (OAD), SAD, avoidant disorder, and adjustment disorder with either anxious or mixed mood features) diagnosed using a clinical consensus approach to 20 community children without an anxiety disorder. They found that the anxious preschoolers had higher rates of both emotional and behavioral symptoms on a rating scale, had poorer social relationships with adults and peers, and on temperament measures were high on negative mood, low adaptability, and distractibility. In studies of preschoolers seen in specialty mental health clinics (Frankel, Boyum, & Harmon, 2004; Lee, 1987; Hooks, Mayes, & Volkmar, 1988; Luby & Morgan, 1997), rates of anxiety disorders, overall, ranged from 4 to 10%. In the Wilens and colleagues (2002) study of patterns of psychopathology in clinically referred preschoolers (ages 2–6; mean age 5), the rates of specific anxiety disorders reported were 34% for SAD, 3% for panic disorder, 18% for agoraphobia, 20% for overanxious disorder, 17% for specific phobia, and 7% for social phobia; 28% of children had two or more anxiety disorders. The mean age of onset was about 3.5 years old.

Community Studies

A very small group of nonclinical studies has assessed the prevalence of DSM defined anxiety disorders in young children. Until the recent Preschool Age Psychiatric Assessment (PAPA) Test–Retest Study (PTRTS; Egger, Erkanli, Keeler, Potts, Walter, & Angold, in press; Angold, Egger,

Erkanli, & Keeler, submitted for publication), only four studies could approximate community-based estimates of the prevalence of DSM disorders in preschoolers. The Earls study (1982) was far ahead of its time, and employed questionnaires followed by clinical judgment to identify DSM-III disorders on all the 3-year-old children on Martha's Vineyard. Fifteen years later, Keenan studied another small sample, this time of children in poverty assessed with the Schedule of Affective Disorders and Schizophrenia for School-Age Children (K-SADS), an interview developed for use with older children (Keenan, Shaw, Walsh, Delliquadri, & Giovannelli, 1997). Lavigne and colleagues (1996) used a combination of the CBCL, observational assessments, and measures of adaptive behaviors to make clinical consensus diagnoses of the preschoolers they studied in a pediatric primary care setting. Briggs-Gowan and colleagues assessed a representative sample of children in a primary care clinic, 516 of whom were ages 4–6 years old, using an unmodified version of the Diagnostic Interview Schedule for Children, 1999 (DISC) (Briggs-Gowan, Horwitz, Schwab-Stone, Leventhal, & Leaf, 2000). The PTRTS is the only study to use a structured diagnostic psychiatric interview (PAPA; Egger, Ascher, & Angold 1999; Egger & Angold, 2004) developed for use with parents of children ages 2–5 years old. Table 7.2 shows the prevalence rates of anxiety disorders from these five available studies of preschool psychiatric disorders in nonpsychiatric settings (providing an approximation to expected general population rates).

The Lavigne et al. (1996) study reported much lower rates of anxiety disorders than any of the other studies. Although the reasons for these low rates are not known, it is possible that the use of a nonstructured assessment led to undercounting of anxiety symptoms or that the study's 45% response rate led to recruitment biases.

The PTRTS is the only study to present data on the characteristics associated with specific anxiety disorders in preschoolers. The prevalence rates by anxiety disorder are noted in Table 7.2. There were no significant gender differences for anxiety disorders overall or for specific anxiety disorders. Four- and 5-year-olds were significantly more likely than 2- and 3-year-olds to have any anxiety disorder (11.9 vs. 7.7%; odds ratio [OR] = 1.4 [1.1, 1.9]; $p = .02$) or PTSD (1.3 vs. 0%; odds ratio [OR] = 2.5 [1.1, 5.8]; $p = .03$). African American children were less likely to meet criteria for any anxiety disorder (6.4 vs. 14.0%; OR = 0.4 [0.2, 0.9]; $p = .02$) or social phobia (0.6 vs. 4.3%; OR = 0.1 [0.0, 0.6]; $p = .005$) than non–African American children.

Table 7.3 shows the rates and patterns of comorbidity for preschoolers with specific anxiety disorders in the PTRTS (Angold, Egger, Erklani, & Keeler, unpublished). Children with one anxiety disorder were significantly more likely to have another anxiety disorder. About one-third (29%) of children with an anxiety disorder also met criteria for depression, attention-deficit/hyperactivity disorder, oppositional defiant disorder, conduct disorder, or depression.

TABLE 7.2. Prevalence of Anxiety Disorder in Community Studies of Preschoolers

Study and year	Measure/diagnostic criteria	Ages	N	Any anxiety disorder	SAD	GAD	OAD	Specific phobia	Social phobia	Selective mutism
Lavigne et al. (1996)	Clinical consensus DSM-III-R	2–5 years	510	NR	0.5%	NR	NR	0.6%	0.7%	NR
Keenan et al. (1997)	Modified K-SADS DSM-III-R	5 years	104	NR	11.5%	NR	NR	4.6%	2.3%	NR
Earls (1982)	Questionnaire and clinical interview DSM-III	3 years	100	NR	5%	NR	NR	0	2%	NR
Briggs-Gowan et al. (2000)	DISC DSM-III-R	4–6 years	516 (out of total sample of 1,060)	6.1%	3.6%	NR	0.5%	3.7%	NR	NR
Angold et al. (submitted)	PAPA DSM-IV	2–5 years	307 (data weighted back to screening population of 1,073)	9.5%	2.4%	6.5%	0	2.3%	2.2%	0.6%

Note. DISC, Diagnostic Interview Schedule for Children; GAD, generalized anxiety disorder; K-SADS, Schedule for Affective Disorders and Schizophrenia for School-Age Children; NR, not reported; OAD, overanxious disorder; PAPA, Preschool Age Psychiatric Assessment; SAD, separation anxiety disorder.

TABLE 7.3. Comorbidity of Preschool Anxiety Disorders in the PTRTS

Disorder	Pure disorder (%)	Comorbid[a] (%)	Associated with these disorders when controlling for comorbidity between all disorders
SAD	21	79	Depression, social phobia, PTSD (negative association with ADHD)
GAD	47	53	ADHD, SAD, PTSD
Social phobia	45	55	SAD, specific phobia
Specific phobia	0	100	Depression, social phobia, PTSD (negative association with ADHD)
PTSD	15	85	—
Selective mutism	41	59	Depression

[a]Comorbid with other anxiety disorder(s), depression, oppositional defiant disorder (ODD), conduct disorder (CD), or attention-deficit/hyperactivity disorder (ADHD). PTRTS, PAPA Test–Retest Study.

In the PTRTS, preschoolers with anxiety disorders were significantly more impaired than children without disorders (OR = 9.3 [4.2, 21]; $p < .0001$). On an impairment scale (range, 0–30), children with an anxiety disorder had a mean scale score of 7.6 compared to 0.9 for children without a disorder. The mean scores for each disorder were as follows: SAD, 13.6; GAD, 7.7; social phobia, 10.6; specific phobia, 12.4; selective mutism, 8.4; and PTSD, 14.3. Of the parents of preschoolers with an anxiety disorder, 61% felt that their child had problems and needed help. Despite this degree of impairment, only 9.9% of preschoolers with an anxiety disorder had been referred for a mental health evaluation.

These findings suggest that specific anxiety disorders can be diagnosed in preschool children and that these disorders show high rates of comorbidity and significant psychosocial impairment. Further research using multimodal, multi-informant assessments of anxiety symptoms and disorders and longitudinal designs are needed to further describe the prevalence, characteristics, and clinical implications of early-onset anxiety disorders.

Risk Factors Associated with Anxiety Disorders in Preschoolers

Studies of older children with anxiety disorders have identified a variety of putative risk factors or vulnerabilities associated with childhood anxiety disorders (for a review, see Merikangas, Avenevoli, Dierker, & Grillon, 1999). Putative risk factors associated with childhood anxiety disorders include age; sex; socioeconomic status; attention bias; high life stress; parenting behaviors, including emotional overinvolvement, support of children's avoidant behavior, and high levels of aversive and controlling parenting strategies (including criticism, intrusiveness, and punishment), particularly when coupled with low warmth or general negative affect; insecure or resistant infant attachment; temperament factors, including behavioral inhibition, anxiety sensitivity, and fearfulness; psychophysiological functions associated with autonomic regulation (including CO^2 sensitivity, pulse, respiration rate, and galvanic skin response); sexual abuse; physical illness; low academic achievement; family disruption and disharmony; and family history of depression and/or anxiety and/or alcoholism (Angold, Costello, & Worthman, 1999; Angold, Worthman, & Costello, 2003; Beidel & Turner, 1997; Biederman, Rosenbaum, Bolduc, Faraone, & Hirshfeld, 1991; Dadds & Roth, 2001; Eaves et al., 1997; Eley et al., 2003; Goodyer, 1990a, 1990b, 1996, 1999; Goodyer, Ashby, Altham, Vize, & Ashby, 1993; Goodyer, Herbert, Tamplin, Secher, & Pearson, 1997; Goodyer, Kolvin, & Gatzanis, 1985, 1987; Goodyer, Wright, & Altham, 1990; Hirshfeld, Biederman, Brody, Faraone, & Rosenbaum, 1997; Hirshfield et al., 2003; Last, Hersen, Kazden, Orvashel, & Perrin, 1991; Lewinsohn, Gotlib, & Seeley, 1995; Lewinsohn et al., 1994; Lewinsohn, Rohde, & Seeley, 1993, 1994, 1998; Merikangas et al., 1999; Merikangas, Dierker, & Szatmari, 1998; Monroe, Rohde, Seeley, & Lewinsohn, 1999; Nolen-Hoeksma & Girgus, 1994; Nolen-Hoeksma, Girgus, & Seligman, 1992; Silberg, Noale, Rutter, & Eaves, 2001; Thapar & McGuffin, 1995; Topolski et al., 1997, 1999; Turner et al., 1987; Warren, Huston, Egeland, & Sroufe, 1997; Warren, Schmitz, & Emde, 1999; Warren & Sroufe, 2004; Weissman, Leckman, Merikangas, Gammon, & Prusoff, 1984; Weissman, Warner, Wickramaratne, Moreau, & Olfson, 1997).

Given the lack of diagnostic measures and lack of studies examining specific preschool anxiety disorders, it is not surprising that we know little about the putative risk factors associated with preschool anxiety disorders. Heritability of specific patterns of anxiety symptoms in preschoolers was demonstrated in the Eley et al. (2003) large preschool twin study which found genetic differentiation between general distress, separation anxiety, and fear factors, with additive genetic, shared and nonshared environments contributing to these anxieties. Shared environment had the largest effect for separation anxiety. On the other hand, genetic effects accounted for more than two-thirds of the variance in obsessive–compulsive behaviors and shyness/inhibition, with the other one-third due to nonshared environmental effects (Eley et al., 2003). Studies in young children have found that behavioral inhibition is heritable, related to parental anxiety disorders, has physiological accompaniments (sympathetic, cardiovascular, and cortisol hyperreactivity), and is a risk factor for anxiety disorder later in childhood and adulthood (Hirshfeld et al., 1992, 1997, 2003; Biederman et al., 1993). Further research is needed to understand the risk factors associated with preschool anxiety disorders.

ASSESSMENT OF PRESCHOOL ANXIETY DISORDERS

In light of the recommendations of the RDC-PA, as well as the ambiguities and difficulties in applying the current DSM-IV criteria to preschoolers, we make the following recommendations for clinicians who are trying to identify "clinically significant" anxiety in preschoolers (Table 7.4). These guidelines have been adopted in the DC:0–3R (Zero to Three, 2005). At this point, we recommend that clinicians either use the DSM-IV criteria, within the context of the RDC-PA provisional recommendations, or the DC:0–3R criteria. While these parameters and the DSM-IV/DC:0–3 nosology reflect the current state of our knowledge, they are derived from a relatively underdeveloped research base. Clinicians evaluating, diagnosing, and treating preschoolers with anxiety disorders are encouraged to keep abreast of emerging knowledge, because we can expect greater understanding of preschool anxiety disorders in the next decade.

Table 7.5 provides an overview of the domains to be assessed in a comprehensive evaluation of a preschool child. Use of structured measures with psychometric validity are recommended both to assess child domains (e.g., child symptomatology) and parental domains (e.g., parental anxiety). These measures can be administered over the course of treatment to evaluate the efficacy of treatment. Producing empirical data on the effectiveness of treatments is essential, particularly because there are no empirically validated treatments for anxiety disorders in preschoolers at the present time. The *Handbook of Infant, Toddler, and Preschool Mental Health Assessment* (DelCarmen-Wiggins & Carter, 2004) is an excellent resource about measures to be used to assess preschool mental health symptoms and disorders, including anxiety. A 2004 article by Carter, Briggs-Gowan, and Davis also provides a useful overview of measures. The American Psychiatric Association's *Handbook of Psychiatric Measures* is good resource for measures of parental psychopathology, functioning, and parental stress (Task Force for the Handbook of Psychiatric Measures, 2000).

The CBCL, which has parent and teacher versions for children ages 18

TABLE 7.4. Features Associated with Potentially Clinically Significant Anxiety in Preschoolers

Anxiety or fear should be . . .

- *Distressing*: Causes the child distress or leads to avoidance of activities or settings associated with the anxiety or fear to avoid distress.

- *Pervasive*: Occurs during two or more everyday activities or within two or more relationships. In the case of specific fears, including social fears and separation fears, the feared stimulus or situation must almost always provoke an immediate anxiety response.

- *Uncontrollable*: Is uncontrollable by the child or by adult admonition, at least some of the time.

- *Persistent*: Persists for at least 2 weeks (duration may be longer for specific disorders—e.g., GAD, 6-month duration).

- *Impairing*: Impairs the child's or the family's functioning and/or the child's expected development.

TABLE 7.5. Comprehensive Psychiatric Assessment of a Preschool Child

- Current and past history of emotional and behavioral symptoms, including frequency, duration, content, onset, relationship context, and triggers for positive symptoms.
- Developmental history, including history of pregnancy, maternal prenatal care (e.g., use of alcohol, tobacco, or drugs during pregnancy), neonatal history, and developmental milestones and delays (e.g., motor, language).
- Sleep, feeding and eating, and toileting history.
- Child's play (e.g., content, enjoyment of, variety of).
- Parent–child relationship (e.g., affect of parent and child during interaction, child's reactions to separation and reunion, level of conflict/coercion/instrusiveness).
- Current cognitive and developmental assessment of expressive and receptive language ability, gross and fine motor capacities, and adaptive functioning.
- Medical history, including history of strep infections, ear infections, hospitalizations, and traumatic medical experiences.
- Medication history, including psychotropic medications and other medications such as antibiotics and asthma medication (name, dosage, length of treatment, adverse side effects).
- Laboratory test, if indicated (e.g., strep antibodies to assess the child for PANDAS; thyroid function).
- History of potentially stressful life events, including both major traumas (e.g., death in the family, abuse, witness to violence), "minor" stressors (e.g., birth of sibling, changing day care/school), and ongoing stressors (e.g., economic hardship, parental illness).
- Family structure and functioning, including discipline practices involving the use of corporal punishment and marital/adult relationship functioning.
- Daycare/school experiences, including type of setting, teacher/child ratios, length of time in setting, relationships with teachers/child care providers, and relationship with peers, number of daycare/school changes.
- Three-generation family psychiatric/substance abuse/criminal history (ideally collected as a genogram) with record of symptoms/diagnoses/events; age of onset; treatments, including inpatient and outpatient interventions; and psychotherapy and medications (name, dosage, any adverse side effects), including details about anxiety disorders and depression.
- Current history of parental psychiatric symptoms, including symptoms of depression, anxiety, and substance use/abuse. Obtain histories about both biological parents (if possible) and parent figures living in the child's home (e.g., stepfather, grandmother).
- Current and past history of domestic violence between adults and between adult and child in the child's home.
- Assessment of the child's impairment in activities and relationships as a result of symptoms.
- Impact of the child's symptoms on the family's functioning (e.g., parents unable to leave the child with a babysitter due to the child's anxious distress).
- Degree of parental stress, both overall and in relationship to the child who is being evaluated.

months to 5 years old, can help to identify problematic anxiety in preschoolers, primarily from separation or generalized anxieties, but does not provide enough symptom coverage or specificity to make a diagnosis (Achenbach & Rescorla, 2000). Checklist measures specifically developed to assess preschool anxiety such as the PAS (Spence et al., 2001), the Fear Survey Schedule for Infants and Preschoolers (Warren, 2004), and the Infant–Preschool Scale for Inhibited Behaviors (Warren, 2004) have been developed, but no psychometric data are yet available on their reliability or validity in relationship to anxiety disorders in preschoolers. The ECI, a checklist reflecting the symptom domains of the DSM, assesses symptoms of SAD, social phobia, GAD, and OCD, and is useful in screening for specific anxiety domains in young children (Gadow & Sprafkin, 1997, 2000; Gadow et al., 2001). The ECI is used for children ages 3–6 and has both parent and teacher versions. Future research is needed to see whether anxiety measures such as the Multidimensional Anxiety Scale for Children (MASC), developed for use with older children, can be reliably used with preschool children (March et al., 1997).

In the future, structured diagnostic interviews for assessing preschool psychiatric symptoms and disorders will be the best way to obtain a comprehensive mental health assessments of preschoolers, but these measures are not yet "user-friendly" enough for use in clinical settings. The PAPA is currently the only comprehensive parent psychiatric interview for assessing psychiatric symptoms and disorders (including all of the anxiety disorders) in children ages 2–5 with demonstrated test–retest reliability and validity (Egger, Erklani, Keeler, Potts, Walter, et al., in press). The ePAPA, a Web-based version of the PAPA that is administered on a tablet PC, has recently been developed and will facilitate the use of the PAPA in clinical settings. Direct interviews with the young child about his or her feelings and experiences is also an essential component of a comprehensive assessment, particularly for the emotional disorders. In most clinical practices, unstructured play is the method used to learn about the child's emotions. Two structured child interviews show significant promise in assessing depressive mood and anxieties in preschoolers. The Berkeley Puppet Interview (BPI) is an interactive interview for children 4–8 years old (Ablow et al., 1999; Measelle et al., 1998). Children are interviewed with two identical puppets that present opposing statement about themselves (i.e., "I am a sad kid" or "I am not a sad kid"), then ask the child, "How about you?" The symptomatology scales of the BPI provide a child's report of emotional and behavioral symptoms. The MacArthur Story-Stem Battery (MSSB; Toth, Cicchetti, Macfie, & Emde, 1997; Macfie et al., 1999; Oppenheim, Emde, & Wamboldt, 1996; Oppenheim, Emde, & Warren, 1997; Oppenheim, Nir, Warren, & Emde, 1997; Petrill et al., 1998; Warren, Oppenheim, & Emde, 1996; Warren et al., 1999, 2000), which has been used with children as young as 3 years old, consists of a systematic group of story beginnings, enacted in play with Lego figurines. The child is asked to complete the story by showing "what happens next," using the Lego toys. Warren's Narrative Emotional Coding (NEC; Warren et al., 2000) system can be used to assess the child's emotion regulation, anxiety, and depression.

TREATMENT

When a comprehensive psychiatric evaluation has been conducted with an anxious preschool child and his or her family and the DSM or DC:0–3 axes have been completed, a treatment plan addressing each problem area should be developed. Clearly defined symptoms within the child must be identified and targeted interventions planned. Of course, a comprehensive assessment also identifies targets for treatment beyond the child's mental health symptomatology. For example, a treatment plan might include referral of the child for speech or occupational therapy; recommendations that the parents seek an individualized education plan (IEP) from the school system; referral of a parent for evaluation and treatment of psychopathology, particularly anxiety and depression; referral to marital therapy to address conflict in the parents' relationship; and/or recommendations for reducing parental stress, including respite care provided by a grandparent or sitter, or regular exercise or other opportunities for self-care for the primary caregiver.

There are no treatment studies specifically addressing preschoolers with anxiety disorders. In older children, psychosocial treatments including cognitive behavioral therapy (CBT), family management training and medications, particularly selective serotonin reuptake inhibitors (SSRIs) such as Prozac, have been shown to be effective in treating specific anxiety disorders in prepubertal children, as well as adolescents (for detailed reviews of the evidence base for psychosocial and pharmacological treatment of pediatric anxiety disorders, see Compton, Burns, Egger, & Robertson, 2002; Hibbs & Jensen, 2005; Ollendick & March, 2004) A few of these studies have included small groups of 4- or 5-year-olds but not enough to demonstrate specific effectiveness and/or tolerability in young children. However, the lack of empirically supported or validated treatments for preschool disorders overall, or preschool anxiety disorders in particular, is not unique to this age group. Despite the lack of data to guide treatment, clinicians caring for preschoolers will need to make decisions about how to treat preschoolers with anxiety disorders. Because we expect the treatment literature on preschool psychiatric disorders to expand over the next decade, it is imperative that clinicians have methods for evaluating new research findings and implementing them into their practice. One useful approach is that of evidence-based medicine (EBM). Outlining an EBM approach and the parameters of an evidence-based psychiatric practice is beyond the scope of this article but excellent and practical reviews and didactic materials can be found in Gray (2004), Burns, Hoagwood, and Lewis (2005), and Sackett, Straus, Richardson, Rosenberg, and Haynes (2000).

In implementing an intervention with a preschool child, we recommend a structured, empirically based approach to determine whether the treatments, psychosocial and/or pharmacological, are effective. Commonly, when there is a lack of treatment evidence, clinicians treat the patient and deem the treatment a success if the symptoms remit. Although it may appear that a reduction in symptoms with treatment is due to the intervention, it may well be that remission is due to placebo effect, regression to the mean, or lack of precision in the measurement of problems in the first place. The history of child psychiatric interventions is rife with application of costly, long-term therapies with no demonstrated efficacy. Data showing a 2.2-fold increase in the use of antidepressants in children ages 2–4 years old from 1990–1995 (Zito, Daniel, DosReis, Gardner, Boles, & Lynch, 2000), despite the lack of studies showing their efficacy in this age group or the long-term impact of these medications on the developing brain (and the developing child), are deeply concerning, particularly because children prescribed psychotropic medications tend to be treated for extended periods of time (often more than a year). Although common wisdom is that psychosocial treatments have fewer "side effects" or associated morbidity than psychotropic medications, one can certainly argue that treatment of a preschool child who presents with pediatric autoimmune neuropsychiatric disorders associated with streptococcal infections (PANDAS)-induced OCD with play therapy, rather than antibiotics and developmentally modified CBT, is harmful because potentially effective treatment has been withheld.

Because of the lack of treatment studies, as well as the potential risks of treatment, we believe that it is medically and ethically imperative that physicians who treat anxious preschoolers use a single-case experimental design in planning, implementing, and determining the efficacy of treatment of anxiety in young children. The key to this approach is establishing an adequate baseline describing the patient, his or her symptoms, functioning, and biological and social context. Establishing a baseline (A) is accomplished during the assessment process. In the second phase, treatment, the first type of treatment is B, with subsequent treatments labeled C, D, and so forth. In a simple A/B design, an assessment is conducted, a treatment is implemented, and the clinician determines whether change (improvement, no change, or deterioration) in the target(s) of treatment was seen from time point A to time point B. In an A/B/A design, the treatment is withdrawn to see whether the symptoms return to baseline (i.e., deteriorate), stay the same, or continue to improve. If there is deterioration, then the clinician may decide to restart treatment; if there is continued improvement but at a slower rate, then the clinician may still decide to restart treatment. If no change is noted, then the clinician may decide to extend the no-treatment period to see whether this improvement is stable or transitory. Details about the design, implementation, and interpretation of single-case experimental designs can be found in *The Scientist Practitioner* by Hayes, Barlow, and Nelson-Gray (1999).

The *n*-of-1 trial is a specific type of single-case experimental design that uses the methodology of clinical trials to address the efficacy of pharmacological treatment for an individual patient. In the classic *n*-of-1 trial, the clinician (1) assesses the patient and determines the symptoms, signs, or other manifestations (e.g., impairment) that will be the target(s) of treatment; (2) defines an active treatment dose and a nonactive placebo (pharmacists can help with this), duration, and rules for stopping a period of treatment; (3) implements a series of treatment periods in which the order of active and placebo treatments is randomized and the patient (and caregivers) and the clinician are blind to the order of treatment; and (4) repeats active and placebo pairs of treatment, and follows the effect on the target symptoms evaluated, until the clinician and family decide to unblind the results and decide whether the evidence is convincing that the active treatment is effective and should be continued (Sackett et al., 2000).

Although these approaches are quite different than those used in many mental health practices, they provide an empirically based, structured way to evaluate whether treatment is effective in the absence of appropriate treatment studies to guide clinical practice. They also require that the clinician and family work together, really as co-investigators, to determine whether the child is responding to treatment. This cooperation between clinician and family can strengthen the clinical alliance and support treatment compliance.

CONCLUSION

We have a far distance to travel to define, assess, and treat anxiety disorders in young children. Because we expect that clinically significant preschool anxiety, like extreme behavioral inhibition, increases the child's risk for later anxiety disorders, as well as depression and other types of psychopathology, we hope that this chapter demonstrates that anxiety disorders themselves start during the preschool period. Young children experience highly distressing anxiety symptoms and anxiety disorders that already impair their functioning within and outside the home, and adversely impact their relationships with caregivers, siblings, peers, and other adults. Identification and treatment of these children are critical and, we believe, will contribute to ameliorating or even preventing the onset or progression of these disorders into later childhood and adulthood.

ACKNOWLEDGMENTS

Dr. Egger and Dr. Angold's work described in this chapter was supported by grants from the National Institute of Mental Heath (RO1 MH-63670 and K23 MH-02016) and from a NARSAD Young Investigator Award and Pfizer Scholar Grant for Faculty Development in Clinical Epidemiology awarded to Helen Link Egger.

REFERENCES

Ablow, J. C., & Measelle, J. R. (1993). *The Berkeley Puppet Interview (BPI): Interviewing and coding system manuals.* Berkeley: University of California, Berkeley.

Ablow, J. C., Measelle, J. R., Kraemer, H. C., Harrington, R., Luby, J., Smider, N., et al. (1999). The MacArthur Three-City Outcome Study: Evaluating multi-informant measures of young children's symptomatology. *Journal of the American Academy of Child and Adolescent Psychiatry, 38,* 1580–1590.

Achenbach, T. M. (1991). The derivation of taxonomic constructs: A necessary stage in the development of developmental psychopathology. In D. Cicchetti & S. Toth (Ed.), *Roch-*

ester Symposium on Developmental Psychopathology: Vol. 3. Models and integrations (pp. 43–74). Rochester, NY: University of Rochester Press,

Achenbach, T. M., Edelbrock, C., & Howell, C. T. (1987). Empirically based assessment of the behavioral/emotional problems of 2- and 3-year-old children. *Journal of Abnormal Child Psychology, 15,* 629–650.

Achenbach, T. M., & Rescorla, L. A. (2000). *Manual for the ASEBA Preschool Forms and Profiles: An integrated system of multi-informant assessment.* Burlington: University of Vermont, Department of Psychiatry.

American Psychiatric Association. (2000). *Diagnostic and statistical manual of mental disorders* (4th ed., text rev.). Washington, DC: Author.

Angold, A., Costello, E. J., & Worthman, C. M. (1998). Puberty and depression: The roles of age, pubertal status, and pubertal timing. *Psychological Medicine, 28,* 51–61.

Angold, A., Costello, E. J., & Worthman, C. M. (1999). Pubertal changes in hormone levels and depression in girls. *Psychological Medicine, 29,* 1043–1053.

Angold, A., Egger, H. L., Erkanli, A., & Keeler, G. (2006). *Prevalence and comorbidity of psychiatric disorders in preschoolers attending a large pediatric service.* Manuscript under review.

Angold, A., Worthman, C. M., & Costello, E. J. (2003). Puberty and depression. In C. Hayward (Ed.), *Gender differences at puberty* (pp. 137–164). New York: Cambridge University Press.

Arend, R., Lavigne, J. V., Rosenbaum, D., Binns, H. J., & Christoffel, K. K. (1996). Relation between taxonomic and quantitative diagnostic systems in preschool children: Emphasis on disruptive disorders. *Journal of Clinical Child Psychology, 25,* 388–387.

Behar, L., & Stringfield, S. (1974). A behavior rating scale for the preschool child. *Developmental Psychology, 10,* 601–610.

Beidel, D., & Turner, S. M. (1997). At risk for anxiety: I. Psychopathology in the offspring of anxious parents. *Journal of the American Academy of Child and Adolescent Psychiatry, 36,* 918–924.

Biederman, J., Rosenbaum, J. F., Bolduc, E. A., Faraone, S. V., & Hirshfeld, D. R. (1991). A high risk study of young children of parents with panic disorder and agoraphobia with and without comorbid major depression. *Psychiatry Research, 37,* 333–348.

Biederman, J., Rosenbaum, J. F., Bolduc-Murphy, E. A., Faraone, S. V., Chaloff, J., Hirshfeld, D. R., et al. (1993). A 3-year follow-up of children with and without behavioral inhibition. *Journal of the American Academy of Child and Adolescent Psychiatry, 32,* 814–821.

Biederman, J., Rosenbaum, J. F., Hirshfeld, D. R., Faraone, S. V., Bolduc, E. A., Gersten, M., et al. (1990). Psychiatric correlates of behavioral inhibition in young children of parents with and without psychiatric disorders. *Archives of General Psychiatry, 47,* 21–26.

Boris, N. W., Zeanah, C. H., Larrieu, J. A., Scheeringa, M. S., & Heller, S. S. (1998). Attachment disorders in infancy and early childhood: A preliminary investigation of diagnostic criteria. *American Journal of Psychiatry, 155,* 295–297.

Briggs-Gowan, M. J., Horwitz, S. M., Schwab-Stone, M. E., Leventhal, J. M., & Leaf, P. J. (2000). Mental health in pediatric settings: Distribution of disorders and factors related to service use. *Journal of the American Academy of Child and Adolescent Psychiatry, 39,* 841–849.

Burns, B. J., Hoagwood, K. E., & Lewis, M. (Eds.). (2005). Evidence-based practice, part II: Effecting change. *Child and Adolescent Psychiatric Clinics of North America, 14.*

Calkins, S. D., Fox, N., & Marshall, T. R. (1996). Behavioral and physiological antecedents of inhibited and uninhibited behavior. *Child Development, 67,* 523–540.

Carter, A. S., Briggs-Gowan, M. J., & Davis, N. O. (2004). Assessment of young children's social-emotional development and psychopathology: Recent advances and recommendations for practice. *Journal of Child Psychology and Psychiatry, 45,* 109–134.

Compton, S. N., Burns, B. J., Egger, H. L., & Robertson, E. (2002). Review of the evidence base for treatment of childhood psychopathology: Internalizing disorders. *Journal of Consulting and Clinical Psychology, 70*, 1240–1266.

Costello, E. J., Egger, H. L., & Angold, A. (2004). The developmental epidemiology of anxiety disorders. In T. Ollendick & J. March (Eds.), *Phobic and anxiety disorders in children and adolescents: A clinician's guide to effective psychosocial and pharmacological interventions* (pp. 61–91). New York: Oxford University Press.

Costello, E. J., Egger, H. L., & Angold, A. (2005). The developmental epidemiology of anxiety disorders: Phenomenology, prevalence, and comorbidity. In S. Swedo & D. Pine (Eds.), *Anxiety disorders* (pp. 631–648). New York: Elsevier Saunders.

Crowther, J. H., Bond, L. A., & Rolf, J. E. (1981). The incidence, prevalence, and severity of behavior disorders among preschool-age children in day care. *Journal of Abnormal Child Psychology, 9*, 23–42.

Dadds, M., & Roth, J. H. (2001). Family processes in the development of anxiety problems. In M. W. Vasey & M. Dadds (Eds.), *The developmental psychopathology of anxiety* (pp. 278–303). New York: Oxford University Press.

DelCarmen-Wiggins, R., & Carter, A. (2004). *Handbook of infant, toddler, and preschool mental health assessment*. New York: Oxford University Press.

Earls, F. (1980). Prevalence of behavior problems in 3-year-old children: A cross-national replication. *Archives of General Psychiatry, 37*, 1153–1157.

Earls, F. (1982). Application of DSM-III in an epidemiological study of preschool children. *American Journal of Psychiatry, 139*, 242–243.

Eaves, L. J., Silberg, J. L., Maes, H. H., Simonoff, E., Pickles, A., Rutter, M., et al. (1997). Genetics and developmental psychopathology: 2. The main effects of genes and environment on behavioral problems in the Virginia Twin Study of adolescent behavior development. *Journal of Child Psychology and Psychiatry and Allied Disciplines, 38*, 965–980.

Egger, H. L., & Angold, A. (2004). The Preschool Age Psychiatric Assessment (PAPA): A structured parent interview for diagnosing psychiatric disorders in preschool children. In R. DelCarmen-Wiggins & A. Carter (Eds.), *Handbook of infant, toddler, and preschool mental assessment* (pp. 223–243). New York: Oxford University Press.

Egger, H. L., Ascher, B. H., & Angold, A. (1999). *The Preschool Age Psychiatric Assessment: Version 1.1*. Durham, NC: Center for Developmental Epidemiology, Department of Psychiatry and Behavioral Sciences, Duke University Medical Center.

Egger, H. L., Erkanli, A., Keeler, G., Potts, E., Walter, B., & Angold, A. (in press). The test–retest reliability of the Preschool Age Psychiatric Assessment. *Journal of the American Academy of Child and Adolescent Psychiatry*.

Eley, T. C., Bolton, D., O'Connor, T. G., Perrin, S., Smith, P., & Plomin, R. (2003). A twin study of anxiety-related behaviours in pre-school children. *Journal of Child Psychology and Psychiatry, 44*, 945–960.

Fox, N., Henderson, H., Rubin, K., Calkins, S., & Schmidt, L. (2001). Continuity and discontinuity of behavioral inhibition and exuberance: Psychophysiological and behavioral influences across the first four years of life. *Child Development, 72*, 1–21.

Frankel, K. A., Boyum, L. A., & Harmon, R. J. (2004). Diagnoses and presenting symptoms in an infant psychiatry clinic: Comparison of two diagnostic systems. *Journal of the American Academy of Child and Adolescent Psychiatry, 43*, 578–587.

Gadow, K. D., & Sprafkin, J. (1997). *Early Childhood Symptom Inventory–4 norms manual*. Stony Brook, NY: Checkmate Plus.

Gadow, K. D., & Sprafkin, J. (2000). *Early Childhood Symptom Inventory–4 screening manual*. Stony Brook, NY: Checkmate Plus.

Gadow, K. D., Sprafkin, J., & Nolan, E. E. (2001). DSM-IV symptoms in community and clinic preschool children. *Journal of the American Academy of Child and Adolescent Psychiatry, 40*, 1383–1392.

Goodyer, I. (1990a). Annotation: Recent life events and psychiatric disorder in school age children. *Journal of Child Psychology and Psychiatry, 31*, 839–848.

Goodyer, I. (1990b). Family relationships, life events and childhood psychopathology. *Journal of Child Psychology and Psychiatry and Allied Disciplines, 31*, 161–192.

Goodyer, I. (1996). Recent undesireable life events: Their influence on subsequent psychopathology. *European Child and Adolescent Psychiatry, 5*(1), 33–37.

Goodyer, I. (1999). The influence of recent life events on the onset and outcome of major depression in young people. In C. A. Essau & F. Petermann (Eds.), *Depressive disorders in children and adolescents: Epidemiology, risk factors, and treatment* (pp. 237–260). Northvale, NJ: Jason Aronson.

Goodyer, I., Ashby, L., Altham, P., Vize, C., & Cooper, P. (1993). Temperament and major depression in 11 to 16 year olds. *Journal of Child Psychology and Psychiatry and Allies Disciplines, 34*, 1409–1423.

Goodyer, I., Cooper, P., Vize, C., & Ashby, L. (1993). Depression in 11–16 year-old girls: The role of past parental psychopathology and exposure to recent life events. *Journal of Child Psychology and Psychiatry and Allied Disciplines, 34*, 1103–1115.

Goodyer, I., Herbert, J., Tamplin, A., Secher, S., & Pearson, J. (1997). Short-term outcome of major depression: II. Life events, family dysfunction, and friendship difficulties as predictors or persistent disorder. *Journal of American Academy of Child and Adolescent Psychiatry, 36*, 474–480.

Goodyer, I., Kolvin, I., & Gatzanis, S. (1985). Recent undesirable life events and psychiatric disorder in childhood and adolescence. *British Journal of Psychiatry, 147*, 517–523.

Goodyer, I., Kolvin, I., & Gatzanis, S. (1987). The impact of recent undesirable life events on psychiatric disorders in childhood and adolescence. *British Journal of Psychiatry, 151*, 179–184.

Goodyer, I., Wright, C., & Altham, P. (1990). Recent achievements and adversities in anxious and depressed school age children. *Journal of Child Psychology and Psychiatry and Allied Disciplines, 31*, 1063–1077.

Gray, G. E. (2004). *Concise guide to evidence-based psychiatry.* Arlington, VA: American Psychiatric Press.

Hayes, S. C., Barlow, D. H., & Nelson-Gray, R. O. (1999). *The scientist practitioner.* Boston: Allyn & Bacon.

Hibbs, E. D., & Jensen, P. S. (2005). *Psychological treatments for child and adolescent disorders: Empirically based strategies for clinical practice.* Washington, DC: American Psychological Association.

Hirshfeld, D. R., Biederman, J., Brody, L., Faraone, S. V., & Rosenbaum, J. F. (1997). Associations between expressed emotion and child behavioral inhibition and psychopathology: A pilot study. *Journal of the American Academy of Child and Adolescent Psychiatry, 36*, 205–213.

Hirshfeld, D. R., Rosenbaum, J. F., Biederman, J., Bolduc, E. A., Faraone, S. V., Snidman, N. S., et al. (1992). Stable behavioral inhibition and its association with anxiety disorder. *Journal of the American Academy of Child and Adolescent Psychiatry, 31*, 103–111.

Hirshfeld-Becker, D. R., Biederman, J., Calltharp, S., Rosenbaum, E. D., Faraone, S. V., & Rosenbaum, J. F. (2003). Behavioral inhibition and disinhibition as hypothesized precursors to psychopathology: Implications for pediatric bipolar disorder. *Society of Biological Psychiatry, 53*, 985–999.

Hooks, M. Y., Mayes, L. C., & Volkmar, F. R. (1988). Psychiatric disorders among preschool children. *Journal of the American Academy of Child and Adolescent Psychiatry, 27*, 623–627.

Kagan, J., Reznick, J. S., & Snidman, N. (1987). The physiology and psychology of behavioral inhibition in young children. *Child Development, 58*, 1459–1473.

Kagan, J., & Snidman, N. (1991). Infant predictors of inhibited and uninhibited profiles. *Psychological Science, 2*, 40–44.

Kagan, J., & Snidman, N. (1999). Early childhood predictors of adult anxiety disorders. *Biological Psychiatry, 46*, 1536–1541.

Keenan, K., Shaw, D. S., Walsh, B., Delliquadri, E., & Giovannelli, J. (1997). DSM-III-R disorders in preschool children from low-income families. *Journal of the American Academy of Child and Adolescent Psychiatry, 36*, 620–627.

Koot, H. M., van den Oord, E. J. C. G., Verhulst, F. C., & Boomsma, D. I. (1997). Behavioral and emotional problems in young preschoolers: Cross-cultural testing of the validity of the Child Behavior Checklist/2–3. *Journal of Abnormal Child Psychology, 25*, 183–196.

Koot, H. M., & Verhulst, F. C. (1991). Prevalence of problem behavior in Dutch children aged 2–3. *Acta Psychiatrica Scandinavica, 83*, 1–37.

Last, C. G., Hersen, M., Kazden, A., Orvaschel, H., & Perrin, S. (1991). Anxiety disorders in children and their families. *Archives of General Psychiatry, 48*, 928–934.

Lavigne, J. V., Gibbons, R. D., Christoffel, K. K., Arend, R., Rosenbaum, D., Binns, H., et al. (1996). Prevalence rates and correlates of psychiatric disorders among preschool children. *Journal of the American Academy of Child and Adolescent Psychiatry, 35*, 204–214.

Lee, B. (1987). Multidisciplinary evaluation of preschool children and its demography in a military psychiatric clinic. *Journal of the American Academy Child and Adolescent Psychiatry, 26*, 313–316.

Lewinsohn, P. M., Gotlib, I. H., & Seeley, J. R. (1995). Adolescent psychopathology: IV. Specificity of psychosocial risk factors for depression and substance abuse in older adolescents. *Journal of the American Academy of Child and Adolescent Psychiatry, 34*, 1221–1229.

Lewinsohn, P. M., Roberts, R. E., Seeley, J. R., Rohde, P., Gotlib, I. H., & Hops, H. (1994). Adolescent psychopathology: II. Psychosocial risk factors for depression. *Journal of Abnormal Psychology, 103*, 302–315.

Lewinsohn, P. M., Rohde, P., & Seeley, J. R. (1993). Psychosocial characteristics of adolescents with a history of suicide attempt. *Journal of the American Academy of Child and Adolescent Psychiatry, 32*, 60–68.

Lewinsohn, P. M., Rohde, P., & Seeley, J. R. (1994). Psychosocial risk factors for future adolescent suicide attempts. *Journal of Consulting and Clinical Psychology, 62*, 297–305.

Lewinsohn, P. M., Rohde, P., & Seeley, J. R. (1998). Major depressive disorder in older adolescents: Prevalence, risk factors, and clinical implications. *Clinical Psychology Review, 18*, 765–794.

Luby, J. L., & Morgan, K. (1997). Characteristics of an infant/preschool psychiatric clinic sample: Implications for clinical assessment and nosology. *Infant Mental Health Journal, 18*, 209–220.

Macfarlane, J. W., Allen, L., & Honzik, M. P. (1954). *A developmental study of the behavior problems of normal children between twenty-one months and fourteen years*. Berkeley: University of California Press.

Macfie, J., Toth, S. L., Rogosch, F. A., Robinson, J., Emde, R. N., & Cicchetti, D. (1999). Effect of maltreatment on preschoolers' narrative representations of responses to relieve distress and of role reversal. *Developmental Psychology, 35*, 460–465.

March, J. S., Parker, J. D. A., Sullivan, K., Stallings, P., & Conners, C. K. (1997). The Multidimensional Anxiety Scale for Children (MASC): Factor structure, reliability, and validity. *Journal of the American Academy of Child and Adolescent Psychiatry, 36*, 554–565.

Marks, I. (1987). The development of normal fear: A review. *Journal of Child Psychology and Psychiatry, 28*, 667–697.

McGuire, J., & Richman, N. (1986). The prevalence of behavioral problems in three types of preschool group. *Journal of Child Psychology and Psychiatry and Allied Disciplines, 27*, 455–472.

Measelle, J. R., Ablow, J. C., Cowan, P. A., & Cowan, C. P. (1998). Assessing young children's views of their academic, social, and emotional lives: An evaluation of the self-perception scales of the Berkeley Puppet Interview. *Child Development, 69*, 1556–1576.

Merikangas, K. R., Avenevoli, S., Dierker, L., & Grillon, C. (1999). Vulnerability factors among children at risk for anxiety disorders. *Biological Psychiatry, 46*, 1523–1535.

Merikangas, K., Dierker, L., & Szatmari, P. (1998). Psychopathology among offspring of parents with substance abuse and/or anxiety disorders: A high-risk study. *Journal of Child Psychology and Psychiatry, 39,* 711–720.

Monroe, S. M., Rohde, P., Seeley, J. R., & Lewinsohn, P. M. (1999). Life events and depression in adolescence: Relationship loss as a prospective risk factor for first onset of major depressive disorder. *Journal of Abnormal Psychology, 108,* 606–614.

Muris, P., Mayer, B., Bartelds, E., Tierney, S., & Bogie, N. (2001). The revised version of the Screen for Child Anxiety Related Emotional Disorders (SCARED-R): Treatment sensitivity in an early intervention trial for childhood anxiety disorders. *British Journal of Clinical Psychology, 40,* 323–336.

Nolen-Hoeksema, S., & Girgus, J. S. (1994). The emergence of gender differences in depression during adolescence. *Psychological Bulletin, 115,* 424–441.

Nolen-Hoeksema, S., Girgus, J. S., & Seligman, M. E. P. (1992). Predictors and consequences of childhood depressive symptoms: A 5-year longitudinal study. *Journal of Abnormal Psychology, 101,* 405–422.

Ollendick, T., & March, J. S. (Eds.). (2004). *Phobic and anxiety disorders in children and adolescents: A clinician's guide to effective psychosocial and pharmacological interventions.* New York: Oxford University Press.

Oppenheim, D., Emde, R. N., & Wamboldt, F. S. (1996). Associations between 3-year-olds' narrative co-constructions with mothers and fathers and their story completions about affective themes. *Early Development and Parenting, 5,* 149–160.

Oppenheim, D., Emde, R. N., & Warren, S. (1997). Children's narrative representations of mothers: Their development and associations with child and mother adaptation. *Child Development, 68,* 127–138.

Oppenheim, D., Nir, A., Warren, S., & Emde, R. N. (1997). Emotion regulation in mother-child narrative co-construction: Associations with children's narratives and adaptation. *Developmental Psychology, 33,* 284–294.

Petrill, S. A., Saudino, K., Cherny, S. S., Emde, R. N., Fulker, D. W., Hewitt, J. K., et al. (1998). Exploring the genetic and environmental etiology of high general cognitive ability in fourteen- to thirty-six-month-old twins. *Child Development, 69,* 68–74.

Pickles, A., & Angold, A. (2003). Natural categories or fundamental dimensions: On carving nature at the joints and the rearticulation of psychopathology. *Development and Psychopathology, 15,* 529–551.

Reams, R. (1999). Children birth to three entering the state's custody. *Infant Mental Health Journal, 20,* 166–174.

Richman, N., Stevenson, J., & Graham, P. (1982). *Preschool to school: A behavioural study.* London: Academic Press.

Richman, N., Stevenson, J. E., Graham, P. J., Ridgely, M. S., Goldman, H. H., & Talbott, J. A. C. (1974). Prevalence of behaviour problems in 3-year-old children: An epidemiological study in a London borough. *Journal of Child Psychology and Psychiatry, 16,* 277–287.

Robinson, J., Mantz-Simmons, L., MacFie, J., & MacArthur Narrative Working Group. (1996). *MacArthur Narrative coding manual.* Unpublished manuscript, University of Colorado Health Sciences Center, Denver.

Rosenbaum, J. F., Biederman, J., Bolduc, E. A., Hirshfeld, D. R., Faraone, S. V., & Kagan, J. (1992). Comorbidity of parental anxiety disorders as risk for childhood-onset anxiety in inhibited children. *American Journal of Psychiatry, 149,* 475–481.

Rosenbaum, J. F., Biederman, J., Hirshfeld, D. R., Bolduc, E. A., & Chaloff, J. (1991). Behavioral inhibition in children: A possible precursor to panic disorder or social phobia. *Journal of Clinical Psychiatry, 52,* 5–9.

Rosenbaum, J. F., Biederman, J., Hirshfeld, D. R., Bolduc, E. A., Faraone, S. V., Kagan, J., et al. (1991). Further evidence of an association between behavioral inhibition and anxiety disorders: Results from a family study of children from a non-clinical sample. *Journal of Psychiatric Research, 25,* 49–65.

Sackett, D. L., Straus, S. E., Richardson, W. S., Rosenberg, W., & Haynes, R. B. (2000). *Evidence-based medicine: How to practice and teach EBM*. New York: Churchill Livingstone.

Scheeringa, M. S., Zeanah, C. H., Drell, M. J., & Larrieu, J. A. (1995). Two approaches to the diagnosis of posttraumatic stress disorder in infancy and early childhood. *Journal of the American Academy of Child and Adolescent Psychiatry, 34*, 191–200.

Schwartz, C. E. (1999). Adolescent social anxiety as an outcome of inhibited temperament in childhood. *Journal of the American Academy of Child and Adolescent Psychiatry, 38*, 1008–1015.

Schwartz, C. E., Wright, C. I., Shin, L. M., Kagan, J., & Rauch, S. L. (2003). Inhibited and uninhibited infants "grown up": Adult amygdalar response to novelty. *Science, 300*, 1952–1953.

Silberg, J., Neale, M., Rutter, M., & Eaves, L. (2001). Genetic moderation of environmental risk for depression and anxiety in adolescent girls. *British Journal of Psychiatry, 179*, 116–121.

Sonuga-Barke, E. J. S. (1998). Categorical models of childhood disorder: A conceptual and empirical analysis. *Journal of Child Psychology and Psychiatry, 39*, 115–133.

Spence, S. H. (1997). Structure of anxiety symptoms among children: A confirmatory factor-analytic study. *Journal of Abnormal Psychology, 106*, 280–297.

Spence, S. H., Rapee, R., McDonald, C., & Ingram, M. (2001). The structure of anxiety symptoms among preschoolers. *Behavior Research and Therapy, 39*, 1293–1316.

Sprafkin, J., & Gadow, K. D. (1996). *Early Childhood Inventories manual*. Stony Brook, NY: Checkmate Plus.

Task Force for the *Handbook of Psychiatric Measures*. (2000). *Handbook of psychiatric measures*. Washington, DC: American Psychiatric Association.

Task Force on Research Diagnostic Criteria: Infancy and Preschool. (2003). Research diagnostic criteria for infants and preschool children: The process and empirical support. *Journal of the American Academy of Child and Adolescent Psychiatry, 42*, 1504–1512.

Thapar, A., & McGuffin, P. (1995). Are anxiety symptoms in childhood heritable? *Journal of Child Psychology and Psychiatry, 36*, 439–447.

Thomas, J. M., & Clark, R. (1998). Disruptive behavior in the very young child: Diagnostic classification: 0–3 guides identification of risk factors and relational interventions. *Infant Mental Health Journal, 19*, 229–244.

Topolski, T., Hewitt, J., Eaves, L., Silberg, J., Meyer, J., Rutter, M., et al. (1997). Genetic and environmental influences on child reports of manifest anxiety and symptoms of separation anxiety and overanxious disorders: A community-based twin study. *Behavior Genetics, 27*, 15–28.

Topolski, T. D., Hewitt, J. K., Eaves, L., Meyer, M., Silberg, J. L., Simonoff, E., et al. (1999). Genetic and environmental influences on rating of manifest anxiety by parents and children. *Journal of Anxiety Disorders, 13*, 371–397.

Toth, S. L., Cicchetti, D., Macfie, J., & Emde, R. N. (1997). Representations of self and other in the narratives of neglected, physically abused, and sexually abused preschoolers. *Development and Psychopathology, 9*, 781–796.

Turner, S. M., Beidel, D. C., & Costello, A. (1987). Psychopathology in the offspring of anxiety disorders patients. *Journal of Consulting and Clinical Psychology, 55*, 229–235.

van den Oord, E. J. C. G., Koot, H. M., Boomsma, D. I., Verhulst, F. C., & Orlebeke, J. F. (1995). A twin-singleton comparison of problem behaviour in 2–3 year-olds. *Journal of Child Psychology and Psychiatry, 36*, 449–458.

Warren, S. L. (2003). Narratives in risk and clinical populations. In R. Emde, D. P. Wolfe, & D. Oppenheim (Eds.), *Revealing the inner worlds of young children: The MacArthur Story Stem Battery and Parent–Child Narratives* (pp. 222–239). New York: Oxford University Press.

Warren, S. L. (2004). Anxiety disorders. In R. DelCarmen-Wiggins & A. S. Carter (Eds.),

Handbook of infant, toddler, and preschool mental assessment (pp. 355–375). New York: Oxford University Press.

Warren, S. L., Emde, R. N., & Sroufe, A. (2000). Internal representations: Predicting anxiety from children's play narratives. *Journal of the American Academy of Child and Adolescent Psychiatry, 39*, 100–107.

Warren, S. L., Huston, L., Egeland, B., & Sroufe, L. A. (1997). Child and adolescent anxiety disorders and early attachment. *Journal of the American Academy of Child and Adolescent Psychiatry, 36*, 637–644.

Warren, S. L., Oppenheim, D., & Emde, R. N. (1996). Can emotions and themes in children's play predict behavior problems? *Journal of the American Academy of Child and Adolescent Psychiatry, 35*, 1331–1337.

Warren, S. L., Schmitz, S., & Emde, R. N. (1999). Behavioral genetic analyses of self-reported anxiety at 7 years of age. *Journal of the American Academy of Child and Adolescent Psychiatry, 38*, 1403–1408.

Warren, S. L., & Sroufe, L. A. (2004). Developmental issues. In H. Ollendick & J. S. March (Eds.), *Phobic and anxiety disorders in children and adolescents: A clinician's guide to effective psychosocial and pharmacological interventions* (pp. 92–115). New York: Oxford University Press.

Weissman, M., Leckman, J., Merikangas, K., Gammon, G., & Prusoff, A. (1984). Depression and anxiety disorders in parents and children: Results from the Yale family study. *Archives of General Psychiatry, 41*, 845–852.

Weissman, M. M., Warner, V., Wickramaratne, P., Moreau, D., & Olfson, M. (1997). Offspring of depressed parents. *Archives of General Psychiatry, 54*, 932–940.

Wilens, T. E., Biederman, J., Brown, S., Monuteaux, M., Prince, J., & Spencer, T. J. (2002). Patterns of psychopathology and dysfunction in clinically referred preschoolers. *Journal of Developmental and Behavioral Pediatrics, 23*, 531–537.

Wolfson, J., Fields, J. H., & Rose, S. A. (1987). Symptoms, temperament, resiliency, and control in anxiety-disordered preschool children. *Journal of the American Academy of Child and Adolescent Psychiatry, 26*, 16–22.

Zero to Three. (1994). *Diagnostic classification of mental health and development disorders of infancy and early childhood.* Washington, DC: Zero to Three: National Center for Infants, Toddlers, and Families.

Zero to Three. (2005). *Diagnostic Classification: 0–3R: Diagnostic classification of mental health and developmental disorders of infancy and early childhood: Revised edition.* Washington, DC: Zero To Three Press.

Zito, J. M., Daniel, J. S., dosReis, S., Gardner, J. F., Boles, M., & Lynch, F. (2000). Trends in the prescribing of psychotropic medications to preschoolers. *Journal of the American Medical Association, 283*, 1025–1030.

8

Posttraumatic Stress Disorder
Clinical Guidelines and Research Findings

MICHAEL S. SCHEERINGA

Current discussions in the field about posttraumatic syndromes in children include vastly different opinions and practices. Some of these represent healthy debates about competing plausible ideas, whereas others represent the unfortunately typical slowness with which evidence-based practices seep into clinical practices. One of these issues is whether posttraumatic stress disorder (PTSD) is an appropriate diagnosis for children. It is common at professional gatherings for colleagues to claim that PTSD is not a fitting diagnosis for children, because children show all sorts of non-PTSD symptomatology after traumatic events. An alternative nosology has already been proposed for a subset of children who suffer complex trauma (van der Kolk, 2005). This debate is a useful starting point for making a few introductory explanations.

First, it must be noted that no expert has ever claimed that PTSD captures every iota of posttraumatic symptomatology, and to claim that PTSD is inappropriate for children because it does not capture every facet of symptomatology misses the point of why we need diagnoses (Spitzer & Williams, 1980).

Second, it is worth framing the question clearly in terms of three options: (1) PTSD exists within an individual but there is also more symptomatology there; (2) PTSD is not there at all, and some decidedly different syndrome exists; or (3) both preceding options are correct in that PTSD is there in a subset of children, but a decidedly different syndrome develops in a different subset of children. This is not a trivial question, and it is forefront in many people's minds and ultimately determines how children are diagnosed and treated. In response, it can be stated definitively that the majority of PTSD symptomatology, as defined in the fourth edition of the *Diagnostic and Statistical Manual of Mental Disorders* (DSM-IV; American Psychiatric Association, 1994), can be detected when looked for in young children. When the effort is made to ask the relevant questions of caregivers, PTSD symptomatology is detected consistently (Ghosh-Ippen, Briscoe-Smith, & Lieberman, 2004; Scheeringa, Zeanah, Drell, & Larrieu, 1995) and reliably (Scheeringa, Peebles, Cook, & Zeanah, 2001; Scheeringa, Zeanah, Myers, & Putnam, 2003). This rules out option 2. For option 1, it is also clear that there is almost always more symptomatology present than the 17 PTSD items, which I discuss later. The relevant question is whether these additional signs and symptoms are comorbid disorders, associated symptoms, or whether they ought to be blended with PTSD symptomatology to fashion a more comprehensive syndrome. For option 3, the relevant question is whether a subset of children does not develop enough criteria for PTSD but develops some other coherent constellation of symptomatology. Although this is an intriguing issue, no known systematic group studies or even case reports yet support this option.

Restricting our focus for the remainder of this chapter to the data base, the first logical clinical and research issues are how PTSD in young children is similar to that in adults and how it is uniquely different, since there is an enormously large and useful data base on adults. The main categories to consider for how PTSD may be different in young children due to developmental considerations (Table 8.1) are the types of events that may cause PTSD, manifestation of symptomatology, longitudinal course, psychophysiology, and the influence of the caregiver–child relationship.

TRAUMATIC EVENTS

The types of events that may be perceived as traumatic to preschool-age children are similar to those that are life-threatening to older populations, such as disasters (Ohmi et al., 2002), motor vehicle accidents (Scheeringa et al., 2003), war experiences (Laor et al., 1996), and witnessing gruesome deaths (Pruett, 1979). Other types of events are perceived as relatively more life-threatening in younger compared to older children, such as dog and large animal attacks (Gaensbauer, 1994; MacLean, 1977), physical and sexual abuse (Terr, 1988), witnessing domestic violence (Levendosky, Huth-Bocks, Semel, & Shapiro, 2002; Pruett, 1979), and invasive medical procedures (Scheeringa et al., 2003).

All of the known group studies of exclusively or primarily preschool children are summarized in Table 8.2, which conveniently summarizes the age ranges, sample sizes, type of traumatic events, measures used, and key findings from this growing literature. Despite the prevalence and concern about child abuse, there is a notable absence of studies that have used a standardized instrument to assess PTSD in maltreated preschool children.

TABLE 8.1. Developmental Considerations in the Measurement, Epidemiology, and Treatment of PTSD in Preschool-Age Children

Domain	Developmental considerations
Abstract cognitive	Abstract reasoning, symbolic representation, and means–end understanding of causal relationships that aid in understanding the meaning and salience of external and internal events emerge around 36 months of age.
Language	First words emerge around 20 months of age, and grammatically correct sentences emerge around 36 months of age, which aid in encoding and self-reporting about life experiences.
Memory	Behavioral memory emerges around 9 months and declarative memory for coherent autobiographical narrative emerges around 36 months. Important for developing a temporally organized memory of life events.
Dependence on the caregiving context	Dependent on caregivers for protection from life-threatening traumatic experiences, for protection from inappropriate traumatic reexposures that may provoke recurrent fear reactions, and for reassurance and soothing to prevent excessive emotional dysregulation.
Maturity of neural networks/ affect regulation	First 3 years are the most active postnatal years for the progressive processes of brain development (neuronal cell growth, whole brain volume growth, and glial and myelin proliferation), and for the regressive processes of brain development (synapse pruning and use-dependent consolidation of neural networks). Period of vulnerability or resilience?

PTSD SYMPTOMATOLOGY AND DIAGNOSIS

As noted earlier, more than PTSD may result following trauma, but we focus on PTSD in this section. In our first study on the diagnostic validity of PTSD in young children (Scheeringa et al., 1995), we asked the simple question: Are the DSM-IV criteria developmentally sensitive enough to cover the salient posttraumatic signs and symptoms, and able to diagnose PTSD validly in infants and preschool children? The details from the programmatic series of studies that followed cannot be summarized in this space, but the answer is that DSM-IV criteria are not sensitive enough to diagnose extremely symptomatic and impaired young children. Instead, an alternative set of criteria with a different algorithm has been proposed and found to have greater diagnostic validity.

This alternative set of criteria possesses superior content validity (Scheeringa et al., 1995), discriminant and convergent validity (Scheeringa et al., 2001), criterion validity (Ghosh-Ippen et al., 2004; Ohmi et al., 2002; Scheeringa et al., 2003), and predictive validity (Scheeringa, Zeanah, Myers, & Putnam, 2005).

TABLE 8.2. Systematic Group Studies of Traumatized Preschool Children

Study	Age	Sample	Measure	Findings
Scheeringa et al. (1995)	18–48 months	N = 12 clinic patients; 50% DV, 50% other	Interview of treating clinicians that covered all PTSD items	Created alternative criteria and algorithm through an empirical process. Four investigators rated cases; 13% met DSM-IV diagnosis and 69% met alternative diagnosis.
Laor et al. (1996) (followed up in Laor et al., 1997)	3–5 years	N = 72 homes destroyed by missile attacks (displaced) N = 81 homes not destroyed N = 77 distant from missile attacks	PCASS interview. CFS checklist.	PTSD not diagnosed, but the displaced group scored higher on all PCASS scales (separation, mood, fears, sleep, regression, and tension) and the CFS.
Scheeringa et al. (2001)	13–47 months	N = 15 clinic patients; 60% DV, 67% abuse, 20% CV, 40% other	PTSD SSIORIYC interview	20% met DSM-IV diagnosis and 60% met alternative diagnosis. Mean 9.9 symptoms[a] in those with alternative diagnosis. Superior criterion validity shown for the alternative set.
Levendosky et al. (2002)	3–5 years	N = 39 response to flyers; DV	PTSD-PAC checklist	3% met DSM-IV diagnosis and 26% met an alternative diagnosis. Measure did not include all PTSD items.
Ohmi et al. (2002)	32–73 months	N = 32 gas explosion in a nursery school	Modified CPTSD-RI checklist	Zero met DSM-IV diagnosis and 25% met alternative diagnosis. Mean 5.9 symptoms[a] in those with alternative diagnosis.
Scheeringa et al. (2003)	20 months–6 years	N = 62 mostly hospital cohort and DV cohort	PTSD SSIORIYC interview	Zero met DSM-IV diagnosis and 26% met revised alternative criteria diagnosis. Mean 6.1 symptoms in those with alternative diagnosis.
Ghosh-Ippen et al. (2004)	0–6 years	N = 156 clinic referred; 95% DV	DC:0–3 interview	2% of 0- to 3-year-olds and 1% of 4- to 6-year-olds met DSM-IV diagnosis, compared to 47% of 0- to 3-year-olds and 39% of 4- to 6-year-olds who met the alternative diagnosis. Factor analysis supported a five-factor structure.

Note. DV, witnessed domestic violence; CV, witnessed community violence; abuse, physical or sexual abuse; PCASS, Preschool Children's Assessment of Stress Scale; CFS, Change of Functioning Scale; PTSD SSIORIYC, Posttraumatic Stress Disorder Semi-Structured Interview and Observational Record for Infants and Young Children; CPTSD-RI, Child Posttraumatic Stress Disorder Reaction Index; PTSD-PAC, PTSD Symptoms in Preschool Age Children.

[a]Includes four novel items: regression in skills, separation anxiety, aggression, and new fears unrelated to the traumatic event.

Recommendations for the Definition of PTSD in Preschool Children

The alternative set of criteria for PTSD for preschool children differs from the DSM-IV in two main ways. First, the wording of five of the 17 DSM-IV items need to be qualified. Three items are manifest differently in young children compared to adults due to developmental differences.

1. The symptom of intrusive and recurrent recollections is often evident in children without obvious distress; that is, young children, just like adults, appear pressured to talk about their traumatic experience but their distress is not always apparent. The reason for this is unclear. One speculation may be that young children are uninhibited about retelling their stories to family and strangers, and the distress is quickly discharged by the retelling, whereas adults do not have the "freedom" to discharge personally sensitive information to family and strangers. Another speculation is that distress is truly absent from the recollections. Young children may not be as aware as adults that intrusive recollections are "abnormal," thereby preventing a cascade of distress feelings.

2. Diminished interest in significant activities can mostly be observed in young children's play since they do not attend school or work.

3. The sign of irritability and outbursts of anger can be manifest in young children as an increase in frequency and intensity of temper tantrums. Young children are not as capable of the explosive and physically violent rage of adults associated with this item because of their limited size, strength, and capacity for violence.

Two items that were worded as highly internalized phenomena in DSM-IV ought to be modified, because young children cannot adequately verbalize such internal experiences.

4. Young children can have flashbacks, but if they are preverbal or barely verbal, then they cannot relate the content of the flashbacks. This item ought to be counted as present if only the behavioral components of a flashback or dissociation are evident, such as a sustained period of appearing disconnected from reality.

5. Young children cannot recount the internalized feeling of detachment and estrangement from others, yet this item ought to be counted if the behavioral manifestations of detachment are evident, such as a new onset or increased frequency of withdrawal from social situations.

Second, the algorithm for the avoidance/numbing criterion needs to be lowered from three items to one item. Young children cannot meet the DSM-IV threshold of three out of seven possible avoidance/numbing items, even though they may be severely symptomatic and functionally impaired. It is unclear whether this is explained by the true absence of some avoidance/numbing items (due to developmental reasons) or by the difficulty in detecting highly internalized and abstract items in children with emerging verbal and cognitive capacities.

The superior validity of this alternative set of criteria and algorithm compared to DSM-IV criteria has now been shown in six studies at four sites, which are summarized in Table 8.2. In these studies, the rates of PTSD are higher in the three studies drawn from help-seeking clinical samples— 43, 69, and 60% (Ghosh-Ippen et al., 2004; Scheeringa et al., 1995, 2001, respectively)—and lower in the three studies drawn from trauma-exposed cohorts in the community—26, 25, and 26% (Levendosky et al., 2002; Ohmi et al., 2002; Scheeringa et al., 2003, respectively), as would be expected.

Four novel items that are not in DSM-IV criteria were detected in the search for content validity (Scheeringa et al., 1995) and were common in subsequent studies (Ghosh-Ippen et al., 2004; Levendosky et al., 2002; Ohmi et al., 2002; Scheeringa et al., 2001, 2003). These four items—regression in skills, separation anxiety, aggression, and new fears—were systematically examined but were found not to be useful for increasing the sensitivity of the diagnosis criteria (Scheeringa et al., 2003); however, these items may have other utility, for example, as constituents of dimensional symptom checklists or treatment outcome measures.

The PTSD items and the four novel items are listed in Table 8.3 in decreasing order of prevalence relative to the four studies that have published prevalence rates for each item. Table 8.3 also gives overall weighted average rank prevalences from the four studies. Larger studies were given proportionately more weight in the ratings; the reverse is true for smaller studies. Notably, the three most common items are all reexperiencing items (criterion B), and five of the six least common items are numbing and avoidance items (criterion C), consistent with studies on all age groups.

COURSE

The only prospective longitudinal data on the course of PTSD in preschool children showed that, contrary to the pattern in adult populations, the number of PTSD symptoms did not significantly decrease over the course of 2 years (Scheeringa et al., 2005). The sample for this study began with 62 children, ages 20 months through 6 years, recruited mostly from a hospital and battered women shelters, plus other sources (see Scheeringa et al., 2003, for details). They were first assessed at a median duration of 7 months after their latest traumatic events, reassessed 1 year later ($N = 47$), and again 2 years later ($N = 35$). Furthermore, 19 of these participants received community treatment after their traumas, but there was no effect of treatment on their PTSD symptomatology. This unremitting course of symptom manifestation has also been demonstrated in older children (McFarlane, 1987; Stuber, Nader, & Yasuda, 1991).

Laor, Wolmer, Mayes, and Gershon (1997) conducted the only other known prospective longitudinal study of preschool children. Their measure

TABLE 8.3. Relative Ranks of PTSD Items and Four Novel Items

	Scheeringa et al. (2001); N = 15	Levendosky et al. (2002); N = 39	Ohmi et al. (2002); N = 32	Scheeringa et al. (2003); N = 62	Weighted overall rank
PTSD items					
B.1. Intrusive recollections	5 (37%)	1 (77%)	3 (28%)	5 (53%)	3
B.2. Nightmares	11 (26%)	7 (21%)	10 (3%)	5 (53%)	12
B.3. Flashbacks/dissociation	15 (6%)	10 (13%)	3 (28%)	17 (7%)	15
B.4. Psychological distress at reminders	2 (45%)	2 (44%)	1 (59%)	1 (80%)	1
B.5. Physiological distress at reminders	Not asked	Not asked	Not asked	5 (53%)	2
C.1. Avoidance of thoughts, feelings, conversations	Not asked	Combined with C.2.	Not asked	13 (33%)	10
C.2. Avoidance of people, places, activities	5 (37%)	5 (26%)	Not asked	5 (53%)	5
C.3. Inability to recall	Not asked	Not asked	Not asked	20 (0%)	20
C.4. Diminished interests	16 (2%)	16 (0%)	3 (28%)	17 (7%)	16
C.5. Detachment and estrangement	14 (13%)	16 (0%)	14 (0%)	15 (13%)	19
C.6. Restricted range of affect	17 (0%)	11 (8%)	14 (0%)	15 (13%)	18
C.7. Foreshortened future	Not asked	Not asked	Not asked	20 (0%)	20
D.1. Difficulty sleeping	10 (31%)	14 (3%)	10 (3%)	3 (67%)	11
D.2. Irritability/anger	1 (47%)	9 (15%)	10 (3%)	3 (67%)	6
D.3. Difficulty concentrating	11 (26%)	11 (8%)	14 (0%)	17 (7%)	17
D.4. Hypervigilance	8 (32%)	3 (41%)	7 (19%)	10 (40%)	8
D.5. Exaggerated startle	8 (32%)	11 (8%)	1 (59%)	10 (40%)	7
Novel items					
Regression in skills	11 (26%)	14 (3%)	9 (9%)	10 (40%)	14
New aggression	2 (45%)	8 (18%)	10 (3%)	1 (80%)	4
New separation anxiety	7 (35%)	4 (36%)	6 (22%)	14 (20%)	13
New fears unrelated to the trauma	4 (40%)	5 (26%)	7 (19%)	9 (47%)	9

Note. The table shows the relative rank of each item in relation to the other items for each study (and the percentage of participants who showed the item in parentheses).

was not confined to diagnostic items of PTSD, and was derived from questionnaires rather than interviews, so it is not clear how their findings relate strictly to interview-based PTSD symptomatology. Nevertheless, after assessing 51 3- to 5-year-old Israeli children displaced from their homes by missile attacks during the Gulf War, and 56 children exposed to the attacks but not displaced, they found that stress symptoms of the displaced group decreased after 30 months, but stress symptoms of the undisplaced group did not decrease. The reason for the discrepancy between the displaced versus the undisplaced groups is probably that the displaced group had significantly higher levels of stress at the first assessment, so they had much more room to change over time. Even though members of the displaced group improved over time, they still had a higher mean level of stress symptoms compared to the undisplaced group at the 30-month follow-up.

Overall, these early findings paint an ominous picture for PTSD in young children and lend support to theories that trauma in the preschool period may have more permanent and pernicious effects relative to older populations because of the vulnerability of the rapidly developing central nervous system (Schore, 2002).

IMPAIRMENT

The presence of either functional impairment or emotional distress is required to make a diagnosis of PTSD, in addition to signs and symptoms. Impairment and distress are quite different constructs, and it is conceivable that one could be emotionally distressed but not show functional impairment, and vice versa. However, researchers have rarely bothered to report these two constructs separately. We present preliminary data on the rates of impairment and distress from our research on traumatized young children.

In our previously mentioned study (Scheeringa et al., 2003), 62 traumatized children ages 20 months through 6 years were assessed with a diagnostic measure that did not measure symptoms separately from impairment. However, at the prospective follow-up assessments 1 and 2 years later, we used a modified version of the National Institute of Mental Health (NIMH) Diagnostic Interview Schedule for Children—Version IV (DISC-IV; Shaffer, Fisher, & Lucas, 2000) that separated the assessment of symptoms from impairment. Parents were interviewed about five child impairment items: annoying to parents, preventing activities with family, preventing activities with peers, interfering with schoolwork, and annoying to teachers.

At the 1-year follow-up, 23.4% of the sample had the full diagnosis of PTSD by the alternative criteria for preschool children, but significantly more children (48.9%) were impaired in at least one domain (binomial test $p < .0001$; Scheeringa et al., 2005). The most common domain of impairment among all subjects was annoyed parents (32%), followed by restricted participation in activities with the family (26%), restricted participation with peers (19%), annoyed teachers (17%), and schoolwork (6%). Child emotional distress was also measured, and this was more common (34%) than any single impairment domain.

At the 2-year follow-up, the discrepancy between rates of PTSD diagnosis (22.9%) and impairment in at least one domain (74.3%) was even more pronounced (binomial test $p < .0001$) than at the 1-year follow-up. The most common domain of impairment at the 2-year follow-up was parent annoyed (66%), followed by restricted activities with the family (51%), restricted participation with peers (37%), schoolwork (31%), and teacher annoyed (29%). The rates of impairment in all domains were greater compared to the 1-year follow-up, including child emotional distress (40%).

These findings suggest that even though there are fewer opportunities to observe functional impairment in young children, impairment can still be observed at high rates. This also suggests that it is appropriate to require impairment for the diagnosis in preschool children. In fact, it appears that the threshold for diagnosing PTSD is too high to capture all of the children who have impaired functioning and may need intervention. The discrepancy between children with a full diagnosis of PTSD and children in need of treatment for PTSD symptomatology would be even greater if the standard DSM-IV algorithm, which captures significantly fewer children than the proposed alternative criteria, were used.

ASSESSMENT

Interviewing caregivers about their children's PTSD symptomatology is enormously difficult. Many of the PTSD items are abstract, internalized, and complicated phenomena. It is difficult to ask adults about their own symptomatology, much less to ask caregivers to validly report about that of their children. Assessment of PTSD in preschool children is constrained to parental report, because children under the age of 6 or 7 years do not yet have the capacity to validly self-report about symptomatology. Two interview measures have been developed for this purpose. The Posttraumatic Stress Disorder Semi-Structured Interview and Observational Record for Infants and Young Children (PTSD-SSIORIYC; Scheeringa & Zeanah, 1994) has been used in three studies and has shown adequate reliability and validity (Scheeringa et al., 1995, 2001, 2003). Ghosh-Ippen and colleagues (2004) used a measure created by Scheeringa that turned Diagnostic Classification 0–3 (DC:0–3; Zero to Three, 1994) into interview questions, and the PTSD section is very similar to the PTSD-SSIORIYC. The second interview measure is the PTSD module of the Preschool Age Psychiatric Assessment (PAPA; Egger, Ascher, & Angold, 2002). Psychometric data on the PAPA PTSD module have not yet been published. These two interviews differ slightly on the coverage of life events and symptomatology, but both adequately cover DSM and alternative criteria.

Two parental checklist measures have been developed for this population. The PTSD Symptoms in Preschool Age Children (PTSD-PAC), an 18-item measure that asks parents to rate items as present or absent (Levendosky et al., 2002), does not provide coverage of all DSM items but does include several developmentally appropriate items (e.g., separation anxiety and regression in skills). The Trauma Symptom Checklist for Young Children (TSCYC; Briere et al., 2001) is an expansive 90-item checklist for assessing 3- to 12-year-old children.

The Traumatic Events Screening Inventory—Parent Report Revised (Ghosh-Ippen et al., 2002), a new 24-item measure, assesses exposure to a variety of life-threatening and stressful events.

Important tasks for the future include sophisticated assessments of the validity of parent report, such as whether there exist clinical subgroups of caregivers who under- or overreport symptomatology and impairment, and how to characterize those subgroups for easy identification in clinical settings. Also, it is well-known that parents generally are not aware of all internalizing symptoms of their children, and it would be helpful to understand how parental report underestimates PTSD symptomatology. One task will be to understand whether particular symptoms are consistently underestimated and to what extent this happens.

TREATMENT

The majority of trauma-exposed, symptomatic, and impaired young children are not brought to clinics for treatment. For example, in our longitudinal study, 74% were rated as impaired after 2 years, but only 31% of families ever sought treatment. The fact that young children cannot bring themselves to treatment is one unique barrier to treatment access for preschool children, but most other barriers are common for all age groups. These issues, which have been summarized and prioritized in a treatment pathway (Scheeringa, 1999), include efforts to discuss directly the compliance issue, shelter, unemployment, education about psychiatric symptomatology, removal from ongoing life threats, day care, and parental symptomatology. As one can see, most of these issues are not therapy issues per se, but fall instead under the category of case management. Thus, case management is often critical to treatment success.

Once these barriers have been successfully addressed to the extent needed, or, in more fortunate cases in which the barriers never existed, therapy can be allowed to proceed relatively unimpeded. The extant treatment literature can be conveniently summarized into two categories: (1) anecdotal advice from a rich body of case studies and (2) a small, emerging literature of systematic efficacy trials using cognitive-behavioral treatment.

Advice from Case Studies

The vast majority of what is written about treatment for PTSD in preschool children can be categorized as individual, nondirective, psychodynamic play therapy with adjunctive supportive therapy with the caregivers. The many case studies reported in the literature are compelling stories in which children nearly always improve. Thus, these case studies provide invaluable templates from which others learn, and they demonstrate how complicated situations can be navigated successfully by careful, individualized attention, at least in the hands of skilled therapists. However, the timing and nature of interventions are idiosyncratic to each case; cases of failure are rarely, if ever, reported, and how such cases fare in the hands of less skilled therapists is undocumented. Most notably, the successes of reported case studies stand in contrast to our longitudinal data that preschool children receiving community treatment did not improve over 2 years (Scheeringa et al., 2005).

Nonetheless, the following lessons may be extracted from the case literature. First and foremost, it needs to be highlighted that despite concerns of caregivers and kindhearted advice from professionals, no case reports indicate that talking with children about their traumatic experiences is harmful. Of course, talking about the trauma events ought to be accomplished with appropriate sensitivity and timing. Young children are usually willing and even eager to engage spontaneously with therapists to recollect past traumatic experiences (Pruett, 1979). Minimal prodding with verbal prompts or toy props is needed. Therapists ought to focus their commentaries on the children's feelings about their past experiences, especially feelings of anger. The nature of interpretations that can be delivered to preschool children are, of course, less abstract than interpretations that are appropriate for older populations, but still appear to have potency (Gaensbauer, 1994).

When a parent has died, it seems best to give children concrete and honest answers to their questions about death rather than try to shield them with vague answers. This is true as a generality, because what people construct in their imaginations is usually worse than reality. Also, children usually know more than parents suspect they know, and giving them false answers may be more confusing than helpful. For example, when a preschool child anxiously wants to know where his or her deceased parent has gone, the answer "to heaven" may be too abstract for them, and the child's anxiety is relieved only when he or she is told the parent is buried in the ground (Bevin, 2002). In fact, despite the anxiety of many grandparent caregivers, the practice of allowing young children to visit gravesites for deceased parents seems uniformly helpful in the case literature. When children have witnessed the extreme violence of their fathers killing their mothers, they seem to need an adult's validation of what they saw. Children can be reassured, and their memories can be validated by confirming to them that their fathers did it (Pruett, 1979).

Important family dynamics may be missed if the therapist's attention is limited to individual therapy (MacLean, 1977, 1980; Pruett, 1979). Two common parental themes that need to be addressed are parental guilt and subsequent leniency with discipline, and overprotectiveness that transmits anxiety to the children (Scheeringa & Zeanah, 2001). A first step in therapy is simply to point out these dynamics to parents and give them direct advice to change their practices. Parents who cannot self-correct with this type of advice may need more intensive coaching from therapists.

Emerging Success with Cognitive-Behavioral Treatment

Cognitive-behavioral therapy (CBT) is an effective treatment modality for PTSD because of the focus on learning theories and cognitive distortions. Although it is not known what causes PTSD at the neurocircuitry level, it is evident that these new behaviors, thoughts, and feelings that were not present prior to a traumatic event seem to be driven by magnified and automatic cognitive processes. A review of studies of CBT in trauma populations identified three crucial factors for successful treatment: (1) emotional engagement with the trauma memory, (2) organization and articulation of a trauma narrative, and (3) modification of basic core beliefs about the world and about oneself (Zoellner, Fitzgibbons, & Foa, 2001). The challenge in working with younger children is how to apply these techniques in a developmentally sensitive fashion.

In older children, four studies have now demonstrated the effectiveness of CBT for traumatized samples. Copping, Warling, and Benner (2001) treated 27 traumatized 3- to 17-year-old children in an uncontrolled 21-week protocol that included CBT plus relational work based on attachment theory. Significant pre- to posttreatment improvements were shown for conduct disorder, social relations, and caregiver depression. King, Tonge, and Mullen (2000) randomly assigned 36 5- to 17-year-old sexually abused children to 20 sessions of child-alone CBT, family CBT, or a wait-list control condition. Both treatment groups significantly improved, but family CBT did not show an added benefit compared to child-alone CBT. Group CBT formats have also shown promise in a 10-week, randomized study of sixth-grade students (Stein, Jaycox, & Kataoka, 2003), and in an 18-week uncontrolled study of 10- to 15-year-old children (March, Amaya-Jackson, & Murry, 1998).

Only two controlled psychotherapy studies have focused on the preschool population, and both protocols were restricted to sexual abuse issues. Cohen and Mannarino (1996a) treated sexually abused 3- to 6-year-old children, who did not need to have PTSD to be in the study. Thirty-nine children were randomized to CBT and 28 children to nondirective supportive treatment (NST). This study provided strong support to show that traumatized children as young as 3 years of age can understand and utilize cognitive-behavioral techniques, and that CBT treatment is superior to nondirective treatment. Maternal depression was also shown to be a significant mediator of child outcome; specifically, higher initial maternal depression scores predicted less successful child outcomes (Cohen & Mannarino, 1996b). Deblinger, Stauffer, and Steer (2001) also demonstrated the effectiveness of CBT treatment for sexually abused young children in a randomized trial, but this not exclusively preschool sample included children ages 2–8 years. In addition, Stauffer and Deblinger (1996) demonstrated the effectiveness of a CBT protocol for 19 sexually abused 2- to 6-year-old children in an uncontrolled trial.

A gap exists because of the lack of a CBT protocol that can be used for any type of traumatic event. A trial is underway, funded by the NIMH, to test our new 12-session manual that is equal parts CBT and parent–child relationship treatment. The CBT techniques include a toolkit of relaxation techniques, detection of cognitive distortions, creation of a stimulus hierarchy of fears, and graded exposure in the lab and in the community. The importance of attending to parent–child relationship dynamics has been previously reviewed (Scheeringa & Zeanah, 2001), and cannot be summarized in detail in this space. Parent–child relationship issues are addressed by attending to the parents' own abuse and trauma histories, feelings of guilt, and disciplinary measures, and children's perceptions of their parents' roles in their traumas (manual available upon request from the author).

RISK AND PROTECTIVE FACTORS

Gender

Female gender has been associated with significantly greater levels of PTSD symptomatology following traumas in multiple studies of older children (Gerring, Slomine, & Vasa, 2002). However, gender was not a significant predictor in other studies of older children (McDermott & Palmer, 2002) or in preschool samples (Scheeringa & Zeanah, 1995). What tips the balance in considering female gender as a risk factor is that male gender is rarely a significant risk factor for PTSD (Dykman et al., 1997). Also, community representative studies, which presumably have little or no selection bias to recruit more symptomatic females for any reason, tend to identify female gender as a risk factor (Cuffe, Addy, & Garrison, 1998; Purves & Erwin, 2002). However, it is not clear what it is about being female that confers vulnerability to PTSD.

Age

Multiple studies sampling a broad age range of children have shown that younger children are at greater risk for PTSD (Vila, Witowski, & Tondini, 2001). Although this finding is tempered by the fact that as many or more studies have failed to find an age effect (Terr, Bloch, & Michel, 1999), only two known studies have shown that older age confers a greater risk for PTSD (deVries et al., 1999; Goldstein, Wampler, & Wise, 1997). All of these studies were of children 6 years or older, but the overall trend is that younger age confers a vulnerability, at least in some situations. Although this is interesting, age is an enormously vague proxy measure for developmental capacities. Unfortunately, no known studies have attempted to probe further the age variable. Interestingly, the studies that found an effect for younger age have so far involved only two types of traumatic events—natural disasters (Vila et al., 2001) and man-made disasters (Terr et al., 1999). It is tempting to speculate that large-scale disasters are qualitatively different from other traumatic events, because they trigger more basic survival instincts in parents. Vital survival issues become paramount, such as how to provide shelter, food, water, and protection each day. Caregivers may enter a "survival parenting" mode in which the finer daily moments of sensitivity, play, and attunement with their children are sacrificed (Chemtob, personal communication, 2005). This would logically have greater implications for younger than for older, more self-sufficient children.

Immediate Emotional and Cognitive Reactions

In contrast to most of the studied risk factors, which have inconsistent track records for being significant predictors of PTSD, emotional and cognitive reactions in the immediate peritraumatic period have emerged as perhaps the most consistent predictors of later posttraumatic symptomatology. These types of reactions include degree of fear, degree of perceived life threat, and peritraumatic dissociation (Ehlers & Clark, 2000). Unfortunately, these peritraumatic reactions are enormously difficult, if not impossible, to study in preschool children, who are not capable of self-reporting on symptomatology, much less on highly internalized, abstract phenomena.

Injury Severity

It seems likely that the salience of injury severity lies in how much individuals feared for their lives; therefore, injury severity is perhaps best thought of as a proxy for a cognitive variable—degree of perceived life threat. It is doubtful that the salience of injury severity lies in the ability of bone and soft tissue damage to translate mechanically into PTSD symptoms, although distantly related data indicate that immune functioning may be related to PTSD, and it is plausible that injury severity may be correlated to immune response. Nevertheless, injury severity has been an inconsistent predictor of PTSD. Injury severity is more often not a significant predictor (deVries et al., 1999) than a significant predictor of PTSD (Gerring et al., 2002).

Cognitive Strategies

Cognitive strategies have been proposed as key variables in the development and maintenance of PTSD symptoms (Ehlers & Clark, 2000). These strategies include, among other things, internal causal attributions (Runyon & Kenny, 2002), thought suppression (Ehlers, Mayou, & Bryant, 2003), and avoidant coping (Bal, van Oost, & de Bourdeaudhuij, 2003). However, little attention has been paid to whether these strategies are preexisting and stable traits of individuals, or are caused by the traumatic events. Theoretically, these seem more likely to be stable traits, although there is a lack of consensus on this issue (Bal et al., 2003). Overall, the evidence for the importance of cognitive strategies is in its early stages but is highly promising. However, due to the enormous measurement problem of young children not being able to self-report on these types of phenomena, little can be said so far with certainty about the preschool population.

Comorbid Disorders

Comorbid disorders may act in several different capacities. If preexistent to the traumatic events, comorbid disorders may act as vulnerability factors. If caused by the traumatic events, comorbid disorders may be unrelated to the course of PTSD, or they may increase the burden of mental illness in a way that prolongs all symptomatology, including PTSD. It is also plausible that comorbid disorders develop immediately after traumas when PTSD does not, but then act as vulnerability factors for delayed-onset PTSD.

Preexisting comorbid psychopathology has predicted the development of PTSD when that psychopathology was general (Daviss et al., 2000; Udwin, Boyle, & Yule, 2000) or internalizing (Gerring et al., 2002), but not when it was externalizing (Aaron, Zaglu, & Emery, 1999). None of these studies focused on preschool children.

Comorbid psychopathology caused by traumatic events has been little studied in relation to the development of PTSD in children.

What we do know about preschool children is that at least one comorbid disorder is present at least 90% of the time with PTSD (Scheeringa et al., 2003), exactly as in adult studies. However, the types of comorbid disorders that are present may be vastly different. For example, adult studies have shown consistently that major depressive disorder (MDD) and substance abuse disorders are the most common comorbid disorders. However, out of four disorders examined by Scheeringa and colleagues (2003), oppositional defiant disorder (ODD; 75%) was the most common, followed by separation anxiety disorder (SAD; 63%), and attention-deficit/hyperactivity disorder (ADHD; 38%), but MDD (6%) was uncommon. Substantially more research is needed, with a wider array of comorbid disorders and a prospective design that can track the sequence of development of each disorder.

Parental Factors

Our recent findings have led to a marked reconceptualization of the role of parental factors. A relatively large body of evidence has consistently shown that parental and family factors are significantly associated with PTSD in children (reviewed in Scheeringa & Zeanah, 2001). These factors include parents with elevated PTSD and general symptomatology, overprotectiveness, elevated parenting stress, less family cohesion, and elevated mother–father conflict. In the few studies that have focused exclusively on infant or preschool children, destruction of one's home by missile attacks, inadequate family cohesion (Laor et al., 1996), the mother's avoidant symptoms (Laor et al., 1997), and witnessing a threat to the caregiver (Scheeringa & Zeanah, 1995) predicted more posttraumatic stress symptoms. Unfortunately, none of these studies directly investigated mechanisms of how these factors might transmit their effects to children.

We conducted the first known study to investigate these factors at the mechanism level by actually measuring the parent–child relationship quality with both an observational measure and a prospective design. In the sample I mentioned previously, we videotaped mothers interacting with their children during a standardized sequence of activities designed to put some stress on the dyad and to force mother and child to work collaboratively (cleaning up toys and a series of four puzzle-solving tasks). The mothers were rated on a variety of scales that measured warmth and sensitivity. We had hypothesized that children with PTSD would have mothers who scored lower on warmth and sensitivity during this procedure. Contrary to expectations, we found the opposite to be true. Mothers of children with the diagnosis of PTSD had more sensitivity compared to mothers of children with subthreshold PTSD symptomatology (Scheeringa, 2004).

This unexpected finding has led us to reconceptualize our thinking in terms of whether standardized laboratory assessments adequately capture naturalistic parent–child relationships, and whether the behaviors that appear to be sensitivity in a laboratory might really be indicators of intrusive and overcompensating parenting behaviors at home. Alternatively, this finding could also be interpreted to mean that parents are adapting to their children, rather than to mean children are responding to the parents; that is, as children become more symptomatic, parents adapt by becoming truly more sensitive to their needs. These competing interpretations may have vastly different implications for treatment, and research aimed at understanding these issues is much needed.

Witnessing Threats to Caregivers

In the only study of infant and preschool children to assess vulnerability factors in relation to PTSD, witnessing a threat to a caregiver was the only significant predictor of PTSD symptomatology (Scheeringa & Zeanah, 1995). Children who witnessed threats developed more PTSD symptoms than children who themselves experienced traumas. However, it is not clear how the experience of witnessing translates into PTSD symptomatology. Is the mechanism child-driven? For example, do children who witness threats to their caregivers feel a greater sense of danger, or a greater loss of security? Or is the mechanism parent-driven? For example, do the parents who have been threatened become symptomatic and subsequently impaired in their sensitivity and warmth toward their children? This preliminary finding clearly needs replication, and competing hypotheses about the mechanism need to be tested.

Psychophysiology

Numerous studies of adults with PTSD have established that they show a variety of associated psychophysiological differences, including increased heart rate response to trauma stimuli, disturbed regulation of the hypothalamic–pituitary–adrenal axis that produces cortisol, reduced size of the hippocampal structures, and increased activity of the amygdala, coupled with decreased activity of the anterior cingulate cortex and prefrontal cortex in response to trauma stimuli (Vermetten & Bremner, 2002). However, important departures from adult findings have already been found in studies of older children and adolescents (DeBellis et al., 2002).

The only known psychophysiological study in preschool children with PTSD symptomatology showed that contrary to adult studies, the majority of highly symptomatic children did not experience increased heart rate in response to trauma stimuli (Scheeringa, Zeanah, Myers, & Putnam, 2004). Instead, an interaction effect was found, in which the most symptomatic children had increased heart rates only if they also had caregivers who employed more negative discipline when trying to get their children to clean up the toys in a lab procedure. This interaction effect was also found with a measure of parasympathetic activity (respiratory sinus arrhythmia, which is basically equivalent to vagal tone).

Overall, these early findings suggest that psychophysiological variables are important, just as they are in adult studies, but the findings may vary due to developmental differences and need to be analyzed in conjunction with parent–child relationship measurements.

CONCLUSION

Despite the preliminary, ominous picture of unremitting PTSD symptoms in young children, case studies and emerging evidence-based (CBT) treatments have demonstrated that PTSD in young children can be highly treatable. The wide variety of variables that appear to function as risk or vulnerability factors, plus the lack of consistency in significant findings across studies, suggests that one model of vulnerability does not fit all individuals; that is, it may be that the paths to PTSD are so idiosyncratic for each individual that the statistical analyses required to account for each possible path in a sample would be mind-boggling, not to mention the prohibitively large sample size required for such an analysis. The challenges of constructing an evidence-based PTSD model for preschoolers are three times greater than those for older children and adults, because of the necessity to consider emerging developmental capacities and high-quality measures of the unique salience of parent–child relationships.

REFERENCES

Aaron, J., Zaglu, H., & Emery, R. (1999). Posttraumatic stress in children following acute physical injury. *Journal of Pediatric Psychology, 24,* 335–343.
American Psychiatric Association. (1994). *Diagnostic and statistical manual of mental disorders* (4th ed.). Washington, DC: Author.
Bal, S., van Oost, P., & de Bourdeaudhuij, I. (2003). Avoidant coping as a mediator between self-reported sexual abuse and stress-related symptoms in adolescents. *Child Abuse and Neglect, 27*(8), 883–897.
Bevin, T. (2002). Violent deaths of both parents: Case of Marty, age 2½. In N. Webb (Ed.), *Helping bereaved children* (pp. 149–164). New York: Guilford Press.
Briere, J., Johnson, K., Bissada, A., Damon, L., Crouch, J., Gil, E., et al. (2001). The Trauma Symptom Checklist for Young Children (TSCYC): Reliability and association with abuse exposure in a multi-site study. *Child Abuse and Neglect, 25,* 1001–1014.
Cohen, J., & Mannarino, A. (1996a). A treatment outcome study for sexually abused preschool children: Initial findings. *Journal of the American Academy of Child and Adolescent Psychiatry, 35,* 42–50.
Cohen, J., & Mannarino, A. (1996b). Factors that mediate treatment outcome of sexually abused preschool children. *Journal of the American Academy of Child and Adolescent Psychiatry, 35,* 1402–1410.
Copping, V., Warling, D., & Benner, D. (2001). A child trauma treatment pilot study. *Journal of Child and Family Studies, 10*(4), 467–475.
Cuffe, S., Addy, C., & Garrison, C. (1998). Prevalence of PTSD in a community sample of older adolescents. *Journal of the American Academy of Child and Adolescent Psychiatry, 37*(2), 147–154.
Daviss, W., Mooney, D., Racusin, R., Ford, J., Fleischer, A., & McHugo, G. (2000). Predicting posttraumatic stress after hospitalization for pediatric injury. *Journal of the American Academy of Child and Adolescent Psychiatry, 39,* 576–583.
DeBellis, M., Keshavan, M., Shifflett, H., Iyengar, S., Beers, S., Hall, J., et al. (2002). Brain structures in pediatric maltreatment-related posttraumatic stress disorder: A sociodemographically matched study. *Biological Psychiatry, 52*(11), 1066–1078.
Deblinger, E., Stauffer, L., & Steer, R. (2001). Comparative efficacies of supportive and cognitive behavioral group therapies for young children who have been sexually abused and their nonoffending mothers. *Child Maltreatment, 6,* 332–343.
deVries, A., Kassam-Adams, N., Cnaan, A., Sherman-Slate, E., Gallagher, P., & Winston, F. (1999). Looking beyond the physical injury: Posttraumatic stress disorder in children and parents after pediatric traffic injury. *Pediatrics, 104*(6), 1293–1299.
Dykman, R., McPherson, B., Ackerman, P., Newton, J., Mooney, D., Wherry, J., et al. (1997). Internalizing and externalizing characteristics of sexually and/or physically abused children. *Integrative Physiological and Behavioral Science, 32*(1), 62–74.
Egger, H., Ascher, B., & Angold, A. (2002). *Preschool age psychiatric assessment.* Durham, NC: Duke University Medical Center.
Ehlers, A., & Clark, D. (2000). A cognitive model of posttraumatic stress disorder. *Behaviour Research and Therapy, 38,* 319–345.
Ehlers, A., Mayou, R., & Bryant, B. (2003). Cognitive predictors of posttraumatic stress dis-

order in children: Results of a prospective longitudinal study. *Behaviour Research and Therapy, 41*, 1–10.

Gaensbauer, T. (1994). Therapeutic work with a traumatized toddler. *Psychoanalytic Study of the Child, 49*, 412–433.

Gerring, J., Slomine, B., & Vasa, R. (2002). Clinical predictors of posttraumatic stress disorder after closed head injury in children. *Journal of the American Academy of Child and Adolescent Psychiatry, 41*(2), 157–165.

Ghosh-Ippen, C., Briscoe-Smith, A., & Lieberman, A. (2004). *PTSD symptomatology in young children.* Paper presented at the 20th annual meeting of the International Society for Traumatic Stress Studies, New Orleans, LA.

Ghosh-Ippen, C., Ford, J., Racusin, R., Acker, M., Bosquet, M., Rogers, K., et al. (2002). *Traumatic Events Screening Inventory—Parent Report Revised.* Unpublished manuscript, University of California, San Francisco.

Goldstein, R., Wampler, N., & Wise, P. (1997). War experiences and distress symptoms of Bosnian children. *Pediatrics, 100*(5), 873–878.

King, N., Tonge, B., & Mullen, P. (2000). Treating sexually abused children with posttraumatic stress symptoms: A randomized clinical trial. *Journal of the American Academy of Child and Adolescent Psychiatry, 39*(11), 1347–1355.

Laor, N., Wolmer, L., Mayes, L., & Gershon, A. (1997). Israeli preschool children under SCUDS: A 30-month follow-up. *Journal of the American Academy of Child and Adolescent Psychiatry, 36*, 349–356.

Laor, N., Wolmer, L., Mayes, L., Golomb, A., Silverberg, D., Weizman, R., et al. (1996). Israeli preschoolers under SCUD missile attacks. *Archives of General Psychiatry, 53*, 416–423.

Levendosky, A., Huth-Bocks, A., Semel, M., & Shapiro, D. (2002). Trauma symptoms in preschool-age children exposed to domestic violence. *Journal of Interpersonal Violence, 17*(2), 150–164.

MacLean, G. (1977). Psychic trauma and traumatic neurosis: Play therapy with a four-year-old boy. *Canadian Psychiatric Association Journal, 22*, 71–75.

MacLean, G. (1980). Addendum to a case of traumatic neurosis: Consideration of family dynamics. *Canadian Journal of Psychiatry, 25*, 506–508.

March, J., Amaya-Jackson, L., & Murry, M. (1998). Cognitive-behavioral psychotherapy for children and adolescents with posttraumatic stress disorder after a single-incident stressor. *Journal of the American Academy of Child and Adolescent Psychiatry, 37*(6), 585–593.

McDermott, B., & Palmer, L. (2002). Postdisaster emotional distress, depression and event-related variables: Findings across child and adolescent developmental stages. *Australian and New Zealand Journal of Psychiatry, 36*(6), 754–761.

McFarlane, A. (1987). Posttraumatic phenomena in a longitudinal study of children following a natural disaster. *Journal of the American Academy of Child and Adolescent Psychiatry, 26*, 764–769.

Ohmi, H., Kojima, S., Awai, Y., Kamata, S., Sasaki, K., Tanaka, Y., et al. (2002). Post-traumatic stress disorder in pre-school aged children after a gas explosion. *European Journal of Pediatrics, 161*, 643–648.

Pruett, K. (1979). Home treatment for two infants who witnessed their mother's murder. *Journal of the American Academy of Child Psychiatry, 18*, 647–657.

Purves, D., & Erwin, P. (2002). A study of posttraumatic stress in a student population. *Journal of Genetic Psychology, 163*(1), 89–96.

Runyon, M., & Kenny, M. (2002). Relationship of attributional style, depression, and posttrauma distress among children who suffered physical or sexual abuse. *Child Maltreatment, 7*(3), 254–264.

Scheeringa, M. (1999). Treatment for posttraumatic stress disorder in infants and toddlers. *Journal of Systemic Therapies, 18*(2), 20–31.

Scheeringa, M. (2004). *Mediation of PTSD course in young children by parental responsivity.*

Presentation at the 20th annual meeting of the International Society for Traumatic Stress Studies, New Orleans, LA.

Scheeringa, M., Peebles, C., Cook, C., & Zeanah, C. (2001). Toward establishing procedural, criterion, and discriminant validity for PTSD in early childhood. *Journal of the American Academy of Child and Adolescent Psychiatry, 40*(1), 52–60.

Scheeringa, M., & Zeanah, C. (1994). *Posttraumatic Stress Disorder Semi-Structured Interview and Observational Record for Infants and Young Children*. New Orleans, LA: Tulane University.

Scheeringa, M., & Zeanah, C. (1995). Symptom expression and trauma variables in children under 48 months of age. *Infant Mental Health Journal, 16*(4), 259–270.

Scheeringa, M., & Zeanah, C. (2001). A relational perspective on PTSD in early childhood. *Journal of Traumatic Stress, 14*(4), 799–815.

Scheeringa, M., Zeanah, C., Drell, M., & Larrieu, J. (1995). Two approaches to the diagnosis of posttraumatic stress disorder in infancy and early childhood. *Journal of the American Academy of Child and Adolescent Psychiatry, 34*(2), 191–200.

Scheeringa, M., Zeanah, C., Myers, L., & Putnam, F. (2003). New findings on alternative criteria for PTSD in preschool children. *Journal of the American Academy of Child and Adolescent Psychiatry, 42*(5), 561–570.

Scheeringa, M., Zeanah, C., Myers, L., & Putnam, F. (2004). Heart period and variability findings in preschool children with posttraumatic stress symptoms. *Biological Psychiatry, 55*(7), 685–691.

Scheeringa, M., Zeanah, C., Myers, L., & Putnam, F. (2005). Predictive validity in a prospective follow-up of PTSD in preschool children. *Journal of the American Academy of Child and Adolescent Psychiatry, 44*(9), 899–906.

Schore, A. (2002). Dysregulation of the right brain: A fundamental mechanism of traumatic attachment and the psychogenesis of posttraumatic stress disorder. *Australian and New Zealand Journal of Psychiatry, 36*, 9–30.

Shaffer, D., Fisher, P., & Lucas, C. (2000). NIMH Diagnostic Interview Schedule for Children Version IV (NIMH DISC-IV): Description, differences from previous versions, and reliability of some common diagnoses. *Journal of the American Academy of Child and Adolescent Psychiatry, 39*(1), 28–38.

Spitzer, R., & Williams, J. (1980). Classification of mental disorders and DSM-III. In H. Kaplan, A. Freedman, & B. Sadock (Eds.), *Comprehensive textbook of psychiatry* (Vol. 4, pp. 1035–1072). Baltimore: Williams & Wilkins.

Stauffer, L., & Deblinger, E. (1996). Cognitive behavioral groups for nonoffending mothers and their young sexually abused children: A preliminary treatment outcome study. *Child Maltreatment, 1*(1), 65–76.

Stein, B., Jaycox, L., & Kataoka, S. (2003). A mental health intervention for schoolchildren exposed to violence: A randomized controlled trial. *Journal of the American Medical Association, 290*(5), 603–611.

Stuber, M., Nader, K., & Yasuda, P. (1991). Stress responses after pediatric bone marrow transplantation: Preliminary results of a prospective longitudinal study. *Journal of the American Academy of Child and Adolescent Psychiatry, 30*(6), 952–957.

Terr, L. (1988). What happens to early memories of trauma?: A study of twenty children under age five at the time of documented traumatic events. *Journal of the American Academy of Child and Adolescent Psychiatry, 27*(1), 96–104.

Terr, L., Bloch, D., & Michel, B. (1999). Children's symptoms in the wake of Challenger: A field study of distant-traumatic effects and an outline of related conditions. *American Journal of Psychiatry, 156*(10), 1536–1544.

Udwin, O., Boyle, S., & Yule, W. (2000). Risk factors for long-term psychological effects of a disaster experienced in adolescence: Predictors of posttraumatic stress disorder. *Journal of Child Psychology and Psychiatry, 41*(8), 969–979.

van der Kolk, B. (2005). Developmental trauma disorder. *Psychiatric Annals, 35*(5), 401–408.

Vermetten, E., & Bremner, J. (2002). Circuits and systems in stress: II. Applications to neurobiology and treatment in posttraumatic stress disorder. *Depression and Anxiety, 16*(1), 14–38.

Vila, G., Witowski, P., & Tondini, M. (2001). A study of posttraumatic disorders in children who experienced an industrial disaster in the Briey region. *European Child and Adolescent Psychiatry, 10*(1), 10–18.

Zero to Three. (1994). *Diagnostic classification of mental health and developmental disorders in infancy and early childhood.* Washington, DC: Zero to Three: National Center for Infants, Toddlers and Families.

Zoellner, L., Fitzgibbons, L., & Foa, E. (2001). Cognitive-behavioral approaches to PTSD. In J. Wilson, M. Friedman, & J. Lindy (Eds.), *Treating psychological trauma and PTSD* (pp. 159–182). New York: Guilford Press.

9

Sleep Disorders

Melissa M. Burnham, Erika E. Gaylor,
and Thomas F. Anders

It is 2:00 in the morning and the family is exhausted. Two-year-old James is still screaming. He cannot get to sleep. His parents, sleep-deprived themselves, are at their wits' end. They have not had a good night's sleep since his birth. They argue about what to do, especially since all of the advice they have received from parents, friends, and even their physician has been to no avail. What to do? Let him scream? Take him into their bed to comfort him? What else?

This chapter reviews empirical data and clinical experience about young children's sleep problems to better inform clinicians who treat these youngsters and their families. We first review normal development of sleep–wake patterns, with a focus on the interaction of biological and maturational factors with psychosocial and environmental factors. Next, we review the types of sleep problems in this age group and some of the suspected daytime behavioral concomitants of nighttime sleep disruption. We discuss some of the issues related to classification of sleep disorders at these ages and present our own classification scheme as a potential new nosology requiring further research. Finally, we briefly discuss and conclude with some suggestions for best practices regarding both prevention and treatment of sleep problems in this age group.

NORMAL DEVELOPMENT OF SLEEP–WAKE PATTERNS
FROM BIRTH THROUGH THE PRESCHOOL YEARS

The relatively short period between birth and the preschool years involves considerable changes in sleep and wakefulness. Not only does diurnal rhythmicity emerge but also changes occur in the proportions of time young children spend in each sleep state and in the amount of time they spend asleep. Although many of these changes are maturational, the environmental context to which young children are exposed has been shown to impact the development of sleep and waking patterns. For instance, maternal well-being, parental ideology, and cultural beliefs impact the sleep setting, as well as the quality and development of typical sleep–wake patterns. Therefore, a large degree of individual variability marks the development of sleep, making it somewhat complicated to describe what is "normal." Each of these developmental and environmental factors is discussed briefly in an effort to describe the range of normal development in sleep over the course of the first 5 years of life.

Changes in Sleep Patterns and Sleep Structure

Research over the past 50 years has shown that the characteristics of sleep change with development. These changes occur in not only the amount of sleep but also sleep structure. Detailed study of infant sleep in the 1950s served to supplant several myths that prevailed in the early part of the century. For example, researchers discovered that during the newborn period, infants sleep approximately 16–17 hours per day, in sharp contrast to the estimated 20–22 hours reported in pediatric textbooks prior to the 1950s (Kleitman & Engelmann, 1953; Parmelee, Schulz, & Disbrow, 1961). It also had been generally accepted that the infant's total amount of sleep declines early in infancy. Kleitman and Engelmann's (1953) seminal longitudinal work, however, showed that the total duration of sleep did not differ over the first 3–6 months of life; rather, the distribution of sleep over the 24-hour day changed. This finding has been substantiated in subsequent investigations (Anders & Keener, 1985; Parmelee, 1961; Parmelee, Wenner, & Schulz, 1964). Although the total amount of 24-hour sleep has been found to remain quite stable, the longest continuous sleep period has been found to increase during this time period, from 3–4 hours at birth to 6 hours on average by age 6 months (Anders & Keener, 1985; Burnham, Goodlin-Jones, Gaylor, & Anders, 2002; Campbell, 1986; Coons & Guilleminault, 1984; Parmelee et al., 1964). Beyond the first 3–6 months, total sleep time decreases to 14–15 hours in 24 hours by the age of 1 year. In contrast, the longest continuous sleep period remains constant at 6–7 hours for the remainder of the first year (Anders & Keener, 1985; de Roquefeuil, Djakovic, & Montagner, 1993; Jacklin, Snow, Gahart, & Maccoby, 1980; Parmelee, 1961). This general pattern of change in amount and consolidation of sleep has held across a number of studies using different methodologies. During the toddler and preschool period, as naps are given up, total 24-hour sleep time is reduced even more. However, nighttime sleep remains constant.

Developmental research has revealed not only these changes in sleep patterns but also changes in sleep structure during infancy. Interestingly, the oscillations between active and quiet sleep were first observed in infants as early as 1924 by Denisova and Figurin (Anders, 1975). Their publication in an obscure European journal, however, precluded wide dissemination of these findings. In the 1960s, polysomnographic equipment and sleep-scoring procedures were adapted for use with infants and confirmed the findings derived from behavioral observations indicating developmental patterns in the amount and distribution of active and quiet sleep periods (e.g., Roffwarg, Dement, & Fisher, 1964; Roffwarg, Muzio, & Dement, 1966). These early studies revealed the unanticipated finding that newborns spend a much larger proportion of time in active sleep compared to adults (Roffwarg et al., 1966). Both behavioral and physiological measures of infant sleep have revealed that whereas the percentage of time spent in active sleep decreases over the first year of life, there is a concomitant increase in quiet sleep (Anders & Keener, 1985; Burnham et al., 2002; Dittrichová, 1966; Emde & Walker, 1976; Fagioli & Salzarulo, 1982; Harper et al., 1981; Louis, Cannard, Bastuji, & Challamel, 1997; Navelet, Benoit, & Bouard, 1982; Thoman & Whitney, 1989). Furthermore, the cycle length between active and quiet sleep is shorter than the 90-minute cycle characteristic of adult sleep. Cycling between active and quiet sleep occurs approximately every 50–60 minutes in infancy (Aserinsky & Kleitman, 1955; Dittrichová, 1966; Harper et al., 1981). The 90-minute pattern is not evident even by 2 years of age (Louis et al., 1997). Roffwarg and colleagues (1964) reported that the adult cycle length begins to appear in middle childhood, indicating a prolonged period of maturation.

Sleep Consolidation

Perhaps the most explicit change occurring in infant sleep is the consolidation of sleep to the nighttime period, which occurs in the first few months of life. A good base of literature has examined the development of the sleep–wake rhythm during early infancy. The bulk of these studies suggest that diurnal variation between sleep and waking, with sleep becoming consolidated to the nighttime hours, is well-established by the age of 3 months (Bamford, Bannister, Benjamin, Millier, Ward, & Moore, 1990; Burnham, in press; Coons & Guilleminault, 1984; Hellbrügge, Lange, Rutenfranz, & Stehr, 1964; Kleitman & Engelmann, 1953; McGraw, Hoffmann, Harker, & Herman, 1999; McMillen, Kok, Adamson, Deayton, & Nowak, 1991; Meier-Koll, Hall, Hellwig, Kott, & Meier-Koll, 1978; Parmelee et al., 1964; Shimada, Takahashi, Segawa, Higurashi, Samejim, & Horiuchi, 1999; Sostek, Anders, & Sostek, 1976; Spangler, 1991; Yokochi, Shiroiwa, Inukai, Kito, & Ogawa, 1989), if not earlier (Freudigman & Thoman, 1994; Sadeh, Dark, & Vohr, 1996). Thus, after a period of maturation during the first weeks of life, on average, sleep becomes consolidated to the nighttime hours by the age of 3 months. It is likely that there are individual differences in the development of sleep–wake rhythmicity, as well as sleep times, that may be either endogenous or environmentally induced (e.g., Parmelee et al., 1961; Menna-Barreto, Isola, Louzada,

Benedito-Silva, & Mello, 1996; Sander, Julia, Stechler, & Burns, 1972). Although infants do shift their sleep to the nighttime and begin to sleep for longer stretches of time, it is inaccurate to conclude that they "sleep through the night." Indeed, the vast majority of infants continue to awaken during the night, even at 12 months of age (Burnham et al., 2002; Goodlin-Jones, Burnham, Gaylor, & Anders, 2001). What appears to develop over time is infants' ability to "self-soothe" or put themselves back to sleep upon awakening, without waking a parent (Burnham et al., 2002).

A TRANSACTIONAL MODEL OF SLEEP–WAKE REGULATION

Nightly transitions between sleep and waking at bedtime and during the middle of the night offer opportunities for homeostatic regulation (e.g., hunger, temperature) and social regulation (separation, reunion, comfort; Anders, Goodlin-Jones, & Sadeh, 2000). Contingent responsiveness during these transitions presumably facilitates the development of self-regulation and very likely contributes to the emergence of a secure attachment relationship (Ainsworth, Blehar, Waters, & Wall, 1978). Failure to respond consistently and predictably to aid the child during these transitions is associated with less optimal regulation. An assessment of sleep in the infant, toddler, and preschool-age child therefore necessarily involves assessment of the emerging parent–child relationship and the psychosocial factors that impact that relationship, as depicted in Figure 9.1.

Proximal influences on the relationship include the primary caregiver's current state of physical and psychological well-being; the primary caregiver's own childhood experiences of being parented, including his or her experi-

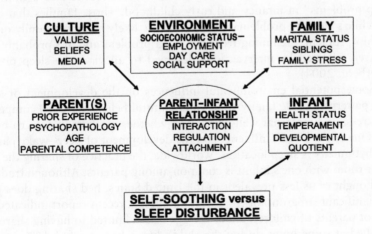

FIGURE 9.1. The transactional model, illustrating the context within which children's sleep develops.

ences around sleep; current social support networks; the family's economic and household conditions; and the infant's temperament and physical health. More distal factors in the transactional model include the broader cultural context of the family and indirect environmental influences. According to this model, proximal stressors, such as infant physical illness or maternal depression directly impact parent–child interactions surrounding regulation of sleep and, in turn, these altered interactions affect the family. A more thorough discussion of these influential factors is published elsewhere (Goodlin-Jones, Burnham, & Anders, 2000).

Thus, although in the past sleep was thought of as a characteristic of the individual, for young children, it is necessary to consider the larger context of their family and sleep environments to understand both the development of sleep–wake patterns and the emergence of sleep problems; that is, at this age, a sleep problem often is specific to a particular relationship or setting. A child will nap at the day care center but not at home (or vice versa), or a child will fall asleep more easily when the babysitter puts the infant to bed than when the parent does (or vice versa). Also, sometimes infants and young children respond differentially to mothers and fathers.

Conversely, but not empirically verified, is the possible impact of childhood sleep problems on the parent–child relationship and/or on the relationship between parents (see Richdale, Francis, Gavidia-Payne, & Cotton, 2000, for an example of families having a child with a disability). For instance, it is certainly possible that bed sharing as a reaction to a young child's sleep problems may have a negative impact on family relationships (Ramos, 2003). On the other hand, Ball, Hooker, and Kelly (2000) have reported positive effects of bed sharing on paternal nighttime caregiving involvement among a group of parents that did not originally plan to bed-share. It is likely that there is a large degree of individual variability in families' tolerance and definition of "sleep problems" in infancy and early childhood. Those families that define their child's sleep as problematic may be more likely to report family or relationship problems stemming from the sleep problem and are probably most positively affected by interventions designed to alleviate the sleep problem (Eckerberg, 2004).

Some potential environmental influences on the development of sleep–wake patterns include family values and cultural beliefs; parental competence and stress, and maternal well-being; and whether mothers choose to breastfeed. One of the largest influences on the development of sleep–wake patterns and rhythmicity is sleep location. Worldwide, the practice of sharing the same bed or room with one's infant is common among parents. Although traditionally thought of as less prevalent in the United States, bed sharing does occur in a significant subgroup of American families. A recent report indicated that 88% of parents of children under the age of 5 admitted to having shared the same bed at some point during the child's life, whereas a full 46% reported bed sharing for the majority of days during the past month (Weimer et al., 2002). Regardless of whether bed-sharing occurs in the United States as a preferred choice of parents or as the reaction to a "problem" with the child's sleep (cf. Ramos, 2003), it is clear that bed sharing is quite prevalent, especially during early infancy.

There is some evidence that the practice of bed sharing influences the development of sleep. For example, using polysomnography, Mosko, Richard, McKenna, and Drummond (1996) found that infants spend less time in deep sleep (non-rapid-eye-movement [NREM] Stage 3–4) and more time in shallower stages of sleep (NREM Stage 1–2) when bed sharing in a laboratory, regardless of the infant's routine sleeping environment. Richard and Mosko (2004) also have reported heart rate differences related to the sleep environment in these infants. They suggest that sensory differences between the two sleeping environments may account for these differences. Both arousability thresholds and heart rates appear to differ during bed sharing versus solitary sleeping, suggesting that the practice of bed sharing induces a physiologically based response in the infant. Bed sharing also tends to co-occur with the practice of breast-feeding (Ball, 2003; McKenna, Mosko, & Richard, 1997). Breast-feeding has been related to sleep patterns, with infants who are breast-fed during the night waking more and requiring more parental interventions upon awakening in the night than those who have been weaned (Burnham et al., 2002).

In addition to differences induced by the sleeping context, young children's sleep also may be influenced by family beliefs regarding children's use of sleep aids (e.g., a blanket or objects used for nighttime comfort) or when and how to respond to a crying infant. Several studies have shown that young children who use a sleep aid are more likely to soothe themselves to sleep during the night (Anders, Halpern, & Hua, 1992; Goodlin-Jones, Eiben, & Anders, 1997; Keener, Zeanah, & Anders, 1988); and that infants whose parents delay slightly their response to nighttime crying after 3 months of age, tend to be self-soothing infants at 1 year (Burnham et al., 2002). With regard to maternal well-being, Seifer, Sameroff, Dickstein, Hayden, and Schiller (1996) reported an association between young children's sleep patterns and maternal mental illness, as well as low levels of family functioning. Benoit, Zeanah, Boucher, and Minde (1992) reported a relationship between maternal attachment insecurity and sleep problems in toddlers.

IDENTIFICATION OF SLEEP DISORDERS IN YOUNG CHILDREN AND EFFECTS ON DAYTIME BEHAVIOR

In general, studies using various criteria to define a sleep problem, and provided by parental report questionnaires and diary methods, demonstrate that approximately 30% of young children have some kind of sleep problem, ranging from mild, time-limited difficulties with bedtime to chronic, serious sleep disorders, such as obstructive sleep apnea (Archbold, Pituch, Panahi, & Chervin, 2002; Armstrong, Quinn, & Dadds, 1994; Earls, 1980; Jenkins,

Bax, & Hart, 1980; Kataria, Swanson, & Trevathan, 1987; Richman, 1981; Ottaviano, Giannoti, Cortesi, Bruni, & Orraviano, 1996). When parents were asked whether they thought their child had a sleep problem, an epidemiological telephone survey conducted by the National Sleep Foundation (2004) noted that only 10% of parents report a sleep problem in their preschool-age child. Perhaps this discrepancy represents the individual variation in young children's sleep patterns, which in a transactional model interacts with parental belief systems about what is "problem" sleep and how to respond to nighttime difficulties. Although difficulties falling asleep at bedtime and frequent and/or prolonged night awakenings are the most common sleep disorders in young children, identification of excessive daytime sleepiness, in transigent behavioral sleep disorders, and more severe, medically based disorders, such as obstructive sleep apnea, are extremely important to recognize, because these disorders can impair physical, cognitive, and psychosocial development. Although it is possible that young children with bedtime settling and nighttime awakening problems also experience impaired daytime functioning, research in this area is, unfortunately, lacking.

Types of Sleep Disorders in Childhood

Dysomnia, a general category of sleep disorder defined by disruptions of sleep, includes *intrinsic dysomnias* (narcolepsy, sleep apnea, and restless leg syndrome) and *extrinsic dysomnias*, or behavioral sleep disorders (limit-setting sleep disorder and sleep-onset association disorder). A third category of sleep disorders that affects the preschool-age child is the *parasomnias*, which are defined as episodic nocturnal behaviors that interrupt sleep but do not affect the architecture of the active and quiet sleep cycles. They often involve cognitive disorientation, autonomic, and skeletal muscle disturbances, and are believed to be related to central nervous system (CNS) maturity (Mindell & Owens, 2003). NREM parasomnias appear to decrease with age, have a familial component, and occur at the transition out of deep sleep (NREM Stage 3–4). Night terrors are the most common parasomnia among preschool-age children who have high percentages of deep sleep. Any factor that increases the percentage of deep sleep (e.g., medications, sleep deprivation) has the potential to increase the frequency of these NREM parasomnia episodes (Klackenberg, 1982).

Night terrors (NREM parasomnia) should be distinguished from nightmares (REM parasomnia), which can also become problematic in this age group. Dreams are normally reported by children after age 3 years (Foulkes, 1982) and nightmares, shortly thereafter. Dream content before children are age 8 years is usually short and concrete. Dream symbolization and elaboration are uncommon. Nightmares, anxiety dreams that awaken the sleeping child, occur during active (REM) sleep and result in a fully awake and oriented child who remembers and recounts the content of the dream. Because active sleep occurs most commonly in the latter third of the night, nightmares generally are noted in the early morning hours, after 2:00 A.M., in comparison to night terrors, which occur in the beginning of the night and involve disorientation.

Sleep-disordered breathing is considered an *intrinsic dysomnia* and can, but does not necessarily, include obstructive sleep apnea syndrome (OSAS). Snoring and/or prolonged mouth breathing during sleep are two cardinal signs that should alert clinicians to this sleep disorder. Obstructed breathing in this age group is most likely due to enlarged tonsils and adenoids, and surgery most often leads to alleviation of the symptoms. OSAS peaks between ages 2 and 6 years, when approximately 2% of children are diagnosed (Schecter et al., 2002). An even greater percentage (8%) of preschool-age children have sleep-disordered breathing (Archbold et al., 2002; Redline et al., 1999). Identifying and treating sleep-disordered breathing may not only alleviate symptoms and improve the child's sleep but there is also evidence that sleep-disordered breathing is associated with a multitude of daytime problem behaviors (attention problems, anxiety/depression, hyperactivity, aggressiveness, and deficits in memory and language abilities) for preschool-age children (Ali, Pitson, & Stradling, 1993; Gottlieb et al., 2003; Kohyama, Furushima, & Hasegawa, 2003; O'Brien, Tauman, & Gozal, 2004). Treatment of the sleep-disordered breathing may indirectly mitigate these behavioral correlates.

Sleep-onset association disorder, an *extrinsic dysomnia*, refers to the association of falling asleep with exogenous cues (e.g., feeding, falling asleep with parent) and typically leads to disorders of maintaining sleep, more commonly known as night waking. These problems tend to *decrease* with age (Crowell, Keener, Ginsburg, & Anders, 1987; Jenkins, Owens, Bax, & Hart, 1984; Salzarulo & Chevalier, 1983). Nonetheless, sleep fragmentation (night waking) is one of the most common complaints of parents bringing their infant for well-baby visits. As noted in the description of normal sleep, most infants learn within the context of nighttime interactions with parents how to soothe themselves to sleep following night awakenings. A significant subset of infants, however, continues to have multiple and prolonged bouts of night waking that begin shortly after sleep onset and persist until morning rise time. For parents who view this as problematic, these awakenings can become a major source of family tension and can be associated with significant parental conflict about managing the infant's sleep.

In contrast, the prevalence of limit-setting sleep disorder (typically occurring around bedtime) *increases* during the preschool period, making it a common problem in the preschool-age child (Crowell et al., 1987; Jenkins et al., 1984; Salzarulo & Chevalier, 1983). Limit setting refers to the reinforcement of undesirable habits at wake-to-sleep transitions, and includes bedtime resistance and lengthy bedtime routines that delay sleep onset. Preschoolers, especially if there are older siblings in the family, enjoy participating in the family's evening activities. They fervently deny being tired when asked. Because daytime experiences for preschoolers are frequently exciting and over-stimulating, calming down at bedtime may be difficult. Whatever the causes, the preschool child may protest vigorously, attempting to delay bedtime. Examples of protestation include requesting bedtime stories to be repeated, returning for more good night hugs and kisses, asking for another glass of water or snack, and pleading for "5 more minutes" until bedtime. A child may also insist on falling asleep in the parents' bed or while lying next to and holding the parents. These behaviors delay sleep onset and can considerably shorten total sleep duration (National Sleep Foundation, 2004).

Impact on Daytime Functioning

Without effective interventions, both limit-setting and sleep-onset association disorders tend to persist (Kataria et al., 1987; Pollock, 1994; Salzarulo & Chevalier, 1983; Smedje, Broman, & Hetta, 2001; Zuckerman, Stevenson, & Bailey, 1987) and may lead to excessive daytime sleepiness and consequently impair daytime functioning. For example, Brunim Lo Reto, Miano, and Ottaviano (2000) found that frequent nighttime awakenings were associated with higher externalizing scale scores, and greater bedtime resistance was related to higher internalizing scale and total scale scores in preschool-age children. Thunstrom (2002) demonstrated that severe and chronic night waking during infancy was associated with an attention-deficit/hyperactivity disorder (ADHD) diagnosis at 5 years. Other studies support this latter association between early childhood sleep problems and later psychosocial disorders of regulation (Gregory, Eley, O'Connor, & Plomin, 2004; Lam, Hiscock, & Wake, 2003; Wolke, Rizzo, & Woods, 2002; Wong, Brower, Fitzgerald, & Zucker, 2004), although often these associations are accounted for by common psychosocial risk factors. Experimental studies are needed to confirm the existence and direction of these associations in preschool-age children (e.g., in school-age children, experimentally induced sleep restriction leads to cognitive deficits; Randazzo, Muehlbach, Schweitzer, & Walsh, 1998). What is clear is that the degree of sleep disruption is associated with concomitant daytime impairment in functioning. Evaluating the degree of sleep disruption is thus critical.

A POTENTIAL NEW DIAGNOSTIC CLASSIFICATION

Currently available clinical diagnostic systems are problematic for various reasons. The *Diagnostic and Statistical Manual of Mental Disorders*, fourth edition (DSM-IV; American Psychiatric Association, 1994) defines "dysomnias" as a group of disorders characterized by difficulty in initiating or maintaining sleep. However, young children do not typically meet the impairment and/or severity criteria. *The International Classification of Sleep Disorders: Diagnostic and Coding Manual* (ICSD-DCM; American Sleep Disorders Association, 1990) defines "extrinsic sleep disorders" as sleep-onset association disorder or limit-setting sleep disorder, as we described earlier. These syndromes use criteria that are vague and neither empirically nor developmentally determined. More importantly, pediatricians and professionals who work with preschool-age children are typically not aware of, nor do they use, this manual. The *Diagnostic Classification of Mental Health and Developmental Disorders of Infancy and Early Childhood* (DC:0–3; Zero to Three, 1994) is yet another nosology developed by early childhood specialists that focuses on young children from birth to age 3 years. There are no empirically derived, quantitative metrics in the DC:0–3 to guide classification of sleep disorders. In addition, and importantly, none of these classification systems take into account the context within which the child is developing (see Figure 9.1).

Therefore, we have proposed a new classification system that can be applied in both research and clinical settings to identify sleep disorders in preschool-age children. We have developed this classification system based on clinical experience and empirical data (Gaylor, Goodlin-Jones, & Anders, 2001; Gaylor, Burnham, Goodlin-Jones, & Anders, 2005). In addition, a simultaneous effort by the Task Force on Research Diagnostic Criteria (2003) has pushed for developmentally appropriate diagnostic criteria of psychopathology for preschool-age children that are based on clinical evidence and considered useful for promoting research in clinical trials and epidemiologic surveys (Task Force on Research Diagnostic Criteria, 2003). The Task Force on Research Diagnostic Criteria: Infancy and Preschool has adopted our sleep disorders classification system for further testing.

We have attempted to bridge the gap between research and clinical definitions of sleep disorders by developing acceptable and accurate research diagnostic criteria that can be ascertained by standard questionnaires and interviews or by more objective measures, such as actigraphy and/or videosomnography. A classification system was needed that accounts for both normative sleep patterns and the caregiving diversity of contemporary society. The authors have described the classification system in detail elsewhere (Anders et al., 2000; Gaylor et al., 2001, 2005). In general, the system, as depicted in Table 9.1, describes two different disorders in young children: sleep onset (similar to limit-setting sleep disorder) and night waking (equivalent to sleep-onset association disorder). It is divided by severity criteria into three categories— perturbation, disturbance, and disorder—in an attempt to engage parents and professionals in deciding when an intervention is necessary (Anders, 1989). Thus, it addresses frequency and duration criteria and is culturally sensitive (e.g., it avoids using co-sleeping itself as a criterion for a sleep disorder as previous criteria have done; cf. Richman, 1981). The term "protodysomnia" was chosen because the classification criteria are derived from the adult dysomnia criteria for sleep disorders in DSM-IV. The scheme is developmentally sensitive, dividing the transitional period into early toddlerhood (12–23 months) and preschool age (24–48 months). Of note, this scheme does not classify a disorder before the child is 1 year of age. There are certainly children with problematic sleep before that age; however, the relationship, family, and envi-

TABLE 9.1. Classification Scheme for Sleep Protodysomnias in Infants–Toddlers and Preschoolers

Sleep-onset protodysomnia (Child must meet any 2 of the 3 criteria listed)	
12–24 months	(1) > 30 minutes to fall asleep; (2) parent remains in room for sleep onset; (3) more than three reunions[a].
> 24 months	(1) > 20 minutes to fall asleep; (2) parent remains in room for sleep onset; (3) more than two reunions.

Night-waking protodysomnia	
12–24 months	1 or more awakenings[b]/night, totaling ≥ 30 minutes.
> 24 months	1 or more awakenings/night, totaling ≥ 20 minutes.
> 36 months	1 or more awakenings/night, totaling ≥ 10 minutes.

Note. A protodysomnia is not diagnosed before 1 year of age. The criteria pertain to solitary sleeping infants. Duration criteria are subdivided. *Perturbations* (one episode/week for at least 1 month) are considered variations within normal development; *disturbances* (two to four episodes/week for at least 1 month) are considered as possible risk conditions that may be self-limiting; *disorders* (five to seven episodes/week for at least 1 month) most likely are continuous and require intervention.

[a]Reunions reflect resistances in going to bed (e.g., repeated bids, protests, struggles).

[b]Awakenings must require parental intervention and occur after the child has been asleep for > 10 minutes.

ronmental contexts may require more attention than the infant's sleep problem during this age period (see Figure 9.1).

Of course, it is important, especially at the younger ages, always to rule out other causes for sleep problems. For example, medical concerns must be excluded, such as middle ear infections, congestion, pain, or allergies. If any of these concerns are present, medical intervention and treatment must begin before treatment of the sleep problem itself. Sometimes, however, after successful medical treatment, the sleep problem may continue due to the parent–infant interaction patterns that emerged in the middle of the night during the course of the acute illness.

BEST PRACTICES/TREATMENT

There are two primary settings in which a preschool-age child with a sleep disorder might come into contact with a clinician: a pediatric/family physician well-child visit (Mindell, Moline, Zendell, Brown, & Fry, 1994; Chervin, Archbold, Panahi, & Pituch, 2001) and a mental health clinic visit. Approximately 10–47% of parents of children presenting to an infant psychiatry clinic report symptoms of sleep disturbances (Frankel, Boyum, & Harmon, 2004; Keren, Feldman, & Tyano, 2001). This symptom presentation translates into a diagnosis of a sleep disorder in 0–10% of patients attending infant psychiatry clinics (Emde & Wise, 2003) and up to 22% in community-based infant mental health clinics (Keren et al., 2001). Interestingly, the average age of the child at the time of evaluation in an "infant" psychiatry clinic is 31 months (Frankel et al., 2004). Although the pediatrician will have had numerous opportunities for prevention and intervention during the first 5 years of the child's life, some parents and professionals rely on the "wait and see approach" with many early childhood problems. Therefore, because there is a stated reluctance to identify and label infants as having sleep disturbances, clinicians often first address disordered sleep during the preschool years.

In an attempt to study both the precursors of these problems, and the sensitivity and specificity of our proposed classification system, we used videosomnography to record the sleep patterns of 80 children from a nonclinical, community sample, ages 1 month to 1 year. We then followed 68 of them annually, until they were 4 years of age using a structured parent phone interview. The videotapes were coded for specific sleep behaviors that are potentially predictive of problem sleep in toddlers and preschool children (e.g., non-self-soothed night awakenings, sleeping in close proximity to parents, requiring parental presence to fall asleep; Gaylor et al., 2005). During the follow-up period, parent report of a sleep problem ranged from 7 to 18%. In contrast, the classification system revealed that 3–9% of children met criteria for a sleep-onset disorder or a night waking disorder at any given time between 2 and 4 years of age. The classification scheme demonstrated adequate sensitivity and specificity at 2 years, but sensitivity declined substantially at 3 and 4 years.

Another objective of this study was to examine the predictive validity of early self-soothing patterns. Interestingly, we found that consistent non-self-soothers between ages 6 and 12 months (33% of the sample) were more likely to meet criteria for a sleep-onset disorder and to be co-sleeping at age 2 years. Sleeping in the parents' room at 12 months of age was predictive of night waking at 2 years of age (although not a full-blown night waking disorder). Approximately 25% of children were reported to be co-sleeping at each follow-up interview, but only 33% of their parents reported this behavior to be problematic.

Most common sleep disturbances, including nightmares and bedtime protestations, are transient, ordinary occurrences that do not seriously disrupt family functioning. Additionally, sleep disorders can occur as part of a comorbid presentation of more general dysregulation. For example, children with autism tend to have higher rates of behavioral sleep disorders and circadian rhythm disorders. In treating sleep disorders, the clinician must be prepared to explore sources of anxiety and interventions that can address, as well as possible, the child's needs for comfort, security, regularity of sleep habits, and protection from overstimulation.

Taking a Sleep History

It is important not only to obtain a careful sleep history when evaluating children with sleep problems but also to inquire about sleep habits in all children with behavior problems. Some attention deficit and hyperactivity symptoms may actually be manifestations of disordered sleep rather than actual syndromes; growth retardation also may be associated with sleep disorders (Stores & Wiggs, 1998).

A sleep history requires a detailed description of all sleep-related symptoms in the child and a thorough history of sleep problems and patterns in other family members. It is helpful to use the framework provided by the transactional model in gathering the data. There are four areas to focus on in the assessment, including (1) the specifics of the sleep problem and for whom it is a problem; (2) infant characteristics, such as temperament or illness; (3) parent–child interaction patterns (sensitive, consistent, controlling); and (4) contextual factors, including both proximal (parental characteristics and family context) and more distal factors, such as culture and environment (cf. Figure 9.1; Anders et al., 2000).

Other questions need to be addressed: What is the age at onset of the problem? What is the frequency of the symptom(s) in terms of events per week and per night, and what has been its course (stable, worsening, improving)? What time during the night or day does the symptom occur, in terms of both clock time and time since falling asleep? For example, parasomnias are related to sleep onset and not to clock time. They generally occur 90–120 minutes after falling asleep. Night terrors can be distinguished from nightmares in that the former occur during the first one-third of the sleep period in Stage 4 NREM sleep, and the latter occur later in the night, when REM sleep predominates.

The child's customary sleep habits, often referred to as "sleep hygiene" are important to establish. What is the usual bedtime and rise time? How regular are sleep habits? What are the sleeping arrangements? With whom does the child share a room or bed? Do the child's symptoms disturb others? Are bedtime rituals present? How common are dreams and nightmares? How common are night waking and bedwetting? All sleep histories need to gather data about breathing during sleep. In the absence of colds, is the child's breathing labored? Are pauses in breathing audible? Is snoring prominent, regular? Is mouth breathing common, regular? Finally, it is important to assess the caregivers' perception of the effects of a nighttime sleep problem on daytime functioning. Is the child sleepy during the day, or is the child alert and active? Does the child nap regularly? Do the nighttime symptoms encroach on normal social functions? For example, is the child embarrassed to sleep at a friend's house or away at camp because of the sleep problem?

Does a child's sleep schedule fit well with the family's schedule in a socially appropriate way, and are the child's need for sleep met by the current schedule? What is a typical day like in terms of rise time, naps, and bedtime? What type of interaction is typical at bedtime and naptime? How regular are the sleep patterns? How long does it take the child to fall asleep once in his or her sleeping place? Does the child fall asleep alone or with others? Does the child waken during the night and cry out for someone? How many times during the night, and how many nights during the week? Who usually responds? How long does it take the child to return to sleep? What soothing techniques are required? What sleep aids does the child use? What are middle-of-the-night interactions like?

Monitoring Sleep and Waking Behavior

A sleep diary or log should be completed for 1–2 weeks. The diary measures night-to-night stability of the problem(s) and includes information about sleeping, waking, and interactional behaviors. Structured questionnaires that identify sleep disorders and measure their severity are in short supply for this age group. Perhaps because preschool-age children fall somewhere in between the still developing infant/toddler (2- to 3-year-old) and the school-age child (6+ years old), this group has largely been ignored. However, in order for early detection of sleep problems to occur, age-appropriate screening and surveillance of pediatric populations are necessary. Screening tools for pediatricians are useful to detect severe problem sleep in a normative population (e.g., bedtime issues, excessive daytime sleepiness, night awakenings, regularity and duration of sleep, and snoring; BEARS; Owens et al., 2000; Bruni et al., 1996; Chervin, Aldrich, Pickett, & Guilleminault, 1997; Sadeh, 2004) and can help health practitioners who are in a position to identify sleep problems in children to implement education and intervention. The mental health clinician who is required to assess and treat multiple behavioral domains needs a well-validated measure to identify the impact of sleep disorders on behavior and functioning.

Parental report measures include the Children's Sleep Habits Questionnaire (CSHQ; Owens et al., 2000) and the Pediatric Sleep Questionnaire (PSQ; Chervin, Hedger, Dillon, & Pituch, 2000), both of which are dimensional scales of problem sleep behaviors (bedtime problems, sleep-disordered breathing, etc.). These questionnaires have demonstrated reliability and validity with respect to identifying both behaviorally based and medically based sleep disorders in children ages 2–18 years (Chervin et al., 2000) and 4–10 years (Owens et al., 2000). The CHSQ has been adapted for use in parental interviews in a younger population (1–4 years) by the authors (Gaylor et al., 2001, 2005), although psychometric data from the interview format have not been calculated.

Laboratory methods are indicated if the problem is believed to be an intrinsic dysomnia, if parental report is suspect, or if excessive daytime sleepiness is evident (Carroll & Loughlin, 1995). Polysomnography (PSG), a diagnostic tool that examines sleep architecture and shows details about breathing, movement, and arousals during sleep, is usually indicated to diagnose sleep-disordered breathing, periodic leg movement, and/or unexplained, excessive daytime sleepiness. For example, Gozal and colleagues (Tauman, O'Brien, Holbrook, & Gozal, 2004; O'Brien et al., 2004) recently used a sleep pressure score derived from PSG to demonstrate that the severity of sleep disordered breathing differentially predicts the level of day-time sleepiness and problem behavior in children ages 1–18 years. However, PSG studies are expensive and not always covered by insurance, especially for young children, nor are they always necessary (for a discussion of these issues, see Ramchandani, Wiggs, Webb, & Stores, 2000, and accompanying letters to the editor).

Promoting Sleep Hygiene and Treating Disorders

A specific treatment depends on a clear diagnosis. For example, a diagnosis of OSAS in this age group is most often relieved by a tonsillectomy and adenoidectomy. Similarly, a night terror disorder is best treated by parental reassurance and support. With maturation of sleep patterns, most para-somnias disappear spontaneously. However, for the more common night-waking and sleep-onset protodysomnias, a number of general behavioral strategies to assist families have been advised. These range from letting the child cry in his or her own sleep environment for five to seven nights, to with-drawing parental presence gradually by waiting a longer time before interven-ing (Ferber, 1985), to shaping bedtime behaviors, such as getting ready for bed and sleep (Moore & Ucko, 1957). From the perspective of the trans-actional model, however, interventions should be more relationship-based and focused on the factors that impact optimal parent–child regulation; that is, one should individualize each intervention to the particular child and fam-ily, keeping in mind the context within which the family exists.

The impact of parent–child interaction as a critical "regulator" of sleep–wake transitions, and the process of consolidation is clear. It is one of the most consistent findings for factors influencing sleep problems in early child-hood (Anders, 1994; Ferber & Kryger, 1995; Goodlin-Jones et al., 2000; Ware & Orr, 1992). The manner in which the parent conducts the bedtime routine influences how the child settles at the beginning of the night and his or her behavior after a nighttime awakening. A typical pattern of back rub-bing or rocking a child to sleep at sleep onset is then expected again in the middle of the night, if the child wakens again (Adair, Bauchner, Philipp, Levenson, & Zuckerman, 1991; Anders et al., 1992). Mothers rated as incon-sistent in their handling of the infant at bedtime and fluctuating between dif-ferent styles of interaction had infants who exhibited delays in falling asleep (Scher & Blumberg, 1999). According to the American Academy of Pediat-rics, it is best to place the drowsy but awake child in his or her own bed at the beginning of the night (Cohen, 1999). Children supposedly develop a "posi-tive sleep association" when they make the mental association between lying quietly in their bed by themselves and falling asleep. Parental presence at the beginning of the night also may discourage the child's use of a sleep aid (Wolf & Lozoff, 1989). Three- and 8-month-old infants who used a sleep aid were more likely to be placed in their bed awake and to use a sleep aid to self-soothe in the middle of the night (Anders et al., 1992). Last, the absence of a regular bedtime routine is associated with sleep problems (Cohen, 1999; Quine, Wade, & Hargreaves, 1991).

Given these data, it seems apparent that good sleep hygiene begins early in the infant's life, and the use of potentially "preventive" parenting practices around sleep may be useful. We have learned that there are significant differences in the way parents of 9- to 12-month-old night-waking infants who do not self-soothe handle their infants at bedtime by 4 months of age. In general, after 4 months of age, parents of non-self-soothing infants place their infants into the crib when the infants are already asleep. Infants who were able to self-soothe after a nighttime awakening were more likely to have been placed into their crib while awake from as early as 4 months of age, and allowed to fall asleep on their own at the beginning of the night. Prior to 4 months of age, almost all infants fall asleep while feeding and are put into their cribs already asleep. But by 4 months of age, the transition to wakeful sleep onset in the crib has begun (Burnham et al., 2002).

In addition, self-soothing infants are more likely to make use of a sleep aid, such as a pacifier, to help them fall asleep on their own. Non-self-soothing infants, in contrast, do not avail themselves or have access to a sleep aid, because they are already asleep. In the middle of the night, after an awakening, the process of falling asleep is repeated. Self-soothing infants, when they awaken for 3–5 minutes, fall asleep on their own; they frequently use their sleep aid. Non-self-soothing infants awaken, become fussy, and begin to cry. They seem to use their parents as their sleep aid (Anders et al., 1992).

From these observations, it appears that "preventive" sleep hygiene strategies should encourage infants to "learn" to fall asleep on their own after 4 months of age; that is, after 4 months of age, parents who want to encourage self-soothing should engage their babies in wakeful activity following a feeding for a few minutes, before putting them into their cribs while they are still awake. Letting the baby fall asleep by him- or herself at the beginning of the night enhances the likelihood of a repetition of that pattern following a nighttime awakening. Parents might also encourage the child's use of a sleep aid, such as a pacifier, thumb, or soft object when falling asleep. Finally, additional advice might include moving the crib/bassinet out of the parental bedroom after the child is 4 to 6 months of age. All of these suggestions, however, must be offered in the context of the family's values and beliefs, and the child's own characteristics and temperament. Both parents' (where applicable) agreement with the advice is essential. If these preventive measures are followed, night-waking problems during the first year of life and thereafter should be minimized. One important caveat is that nursing infants often require additional nighttime feedings following an awakening, so that some signaling is expected.

But what to do with 2-year-old James described at the beginning of this chapter, whose nighttime awakenings have totally disrupted his family? A careful history and 2-week sleep diary revealed that James was not really sleep-deprived, because he obtained most of his sleep napping during the day.

It was his parents who were severely sleep-deprived. James had not made the diurnal transition to consolidating daytime waking and nighttime sleep. Intervention in this case involved educating the parents about the importance of regular schedules, darkening the environment at night, establishing nighttime bedtime routines, and providing a calm, customary sleep environment for the child. A shaping protocol was instituted that shortened James's daytime naps gradually over a 2-week period. Day–night sleep diaries were closely monitored and daily phone calls with the mother provided encouragement and support. The mother was encouraged to sleep whenever the child slept and, for the duration of treatment, the father was encouraged to sleep in a separate room, so that he could get enough sleep to function at work. James's crib was moved into his mother's room, and when he awakened at night, she talked softly to him and rubbed his back, without feeding him or taking him out of his bed. Over a 2-week period, James shifted his diurnal sleep–wake rhythm and became much easier to calm. When he became a self-soother in his mother's room, his crib was returned to his own room and his mother slept on a bed next to his crib. She gradually moved farther away, until James was able to self-soothe in his own room. The mother and father were then reunited in their room and family harmony was restored. Within the month, James was taking two relatively brief daytime naps and slept alone in his own room at night.

FUTURE DIRECTIONS

We clearly need more information about sleep disorders in preschool-age children in clinical settings (Frankel et al., 2004; Dunitz, Scheer, Kvas, & Macari, 1996; Keren et al., 2001). Cultural changes in the demands on parents (e.g., increase in working mothers, use of child care) may affect the child's presentation and the parents' tolerance of certain behaviors (e.g., sleep symptoms, separation anxiety). Oftentimes studies do not include a representative sample or sufficient description of ethnic and cultural characteristics. We need more information about the effects and consequences of sleep loss for cognitive, learning/memory, behavioral, and psychosocial development. And finally, we need more information about how the relationship patterns, as influenced by the factors that comprise the transactional model, affect sleep–wake state organization and the emergence of sleep problems in this age group.

REFERENCES

Adair, R., Bauchner, H., Philipp, B., Levenson, S., & Zuckerman, B. (1991). Night waking during infancy: Role of parental presence at bedtime. *Pediatrics, 87,* 500–504.
Ainsworth, M., Blehar, M., Waters, E., & Wall, S. (1978). *Patterns of attachment: A psychological study of the Strange Situation.* Hillsdale, NJ: Erlbaum.

Ali, N. J., Pitson, D. J., & Stradling, J. R. (1993). Snoring, sleep disturbance, and behaviour in 4–5-year-olds. *Archives of Disease in Childhood, 68,* 360–366.

American Psychiatric Association. (1994). *Diagnostic and statistical manual of mental disorders* (4th ed.). Washington, DC: Author.

American Sleep Disorders Association. (1990). *The international classification of sleep disorders: Diagnostic and coding manual (ICSD:DSM).* Kansas City, KS: Allen Press.

Anders, T. (1989). Clinical syndromes, relationship disturbances, and their assessment. In A. J. Sameroff (Ed.), *Relationship disturbances in early childhood: A developmental approach* (pp. 125–144). New York: Basic Books.

Anders, T. F. (1975). Maturation of sleep patterns in the newborn infant. *Advances in Sleep Research, 2,* 43–66.

Anders, T. F. (1994). Infant sleep, nighttime relationships, and attachment. *Psychiatry, 57,* 11–21.

Anders, T. F., Goodlin-Jones, B. L., & Sadeh, A. (2000). Sleep disorders. In J. C. H. Zeanah (Ed.), *Handbook of infant mental health* (2nd ed., pp. 326–338). New York: Guilford Press.

Anders, T. F., Halpern, L. F., & Hua, J. (1992). Sleeping through the night: A developmental perspective. *Pediatrics, 90,* 554–560.

Anders, T. F., & Keener, M. (1985). Developmental course of nighttime sleep–wake patterns in full-term and premature infants during the first year of life: I. *Sleep, 8*(3), 173–192.

Archbold, K. H., Pituch, K. J., Panahi, P., & Chervin, R. D. (2002). Symptoms of sleep disturbances among children at two general pediatric clinics. *Journal of Pediatrics, 140,* 97–102.

Armstrong, K., Quinn, R., & Dadds, M. (1994). The sleep patterns of normal children. *Medical Journal of Australia, 161,* 202–206.

Aserinsky, E., & Kleitman, N. (1955). A motility cycle in sleeping infants as manifested by ocular and gross bodily activity. *Journal of Applied Physiology, 8,* 11–18.

Ball, H. L. (2003). Breastfeeding, bed-sharing, and infant sleep. *Birth: Issues in Perinatal Care, 30,* 181–188.

Ball, H. L., Hooker, E., & Kelly, P. J. (2000). Parent–infant co-sleeping: Fathers' roles and perspectives. *Infant and Child Development, 9,* 67–74.

Bamford, F. N., Bannister, R. P., Benjamin, C. M., Hillier, V. F., Ward, B. S., & Moore, W. M. O. (1990). Sleep in the first year of life. *Developmental Medicine and Child Neurology, 32,* 718–724.

Benoit, D., Zeanah, C. H., Boucher, C., & Minde, K. (1992). Sleep disorders in early childhood: Association with insecure maternal attachment. *Journal of the American Academy of Child and Adolescent Psychiatry, 31,* 86–93.

Bruni, O., Lo Reto, F., Miano, S., & Ottaviano, S. (2000). Daytime behavioral correlates of awakenings and bedtime resistance in preschool children. *Supplements to Clinical Neurophysiology, 53,* 358–361.

Bruni, O., Ottaviano, S., Guidetti, V., Romoli, M., Innocenzi, M., Cortesi, F., et al. (1996). The Sleep Disturbance Scale for Children (SDSC): Construction and validation of an instrument to evaluate sleep disturbances in childhood and adolescence. *Journal of Sleep Research, 5,* 251–261.

Burnham, M. M. (in press). The ontogeny of diurnal rhythmicity in bed-sharing and solitary-sleeping infants: A preliminary report. *Infant and Child Development.*

Burnham, M. M., Goodlin-Jones, B. L., Gaylor, E. E., & Anders, T. F. (2002). Nighttime sleep–wake patterns and self-soothing from birth to one year of age: A longitudinal intervention study. *Journal of Child Psychology and Psychiatry, 43,* 713–725.

Campbell, I. (1986). Postpartum sleep patterns of mother–baby pairs. *Midwifery, 2,* 193–201.

Carroll, J., & Loughlin, G. (1995). Obstructive sleep apnea syndrome in infants and children: Clinical features and pathophysiology. In R. Ferber & M. Kryger (Eds.), *Principles and practice of sleep medicine in the child* (pp. 163–191). Philadelphia: Saunders.

Chervin, R., Archbold, K., Panahi, P., & Pituch, K. (2001). Sleep problems seldom addressed at two general pediatric clinics. *Pediatrics, 107,* 1375–1380.

Chervin, R., Hedger, K., Dillon, J., & Pituch, K. J. (2000). Pediatric Sleep Questionnaire (PSQ): Validity and reliability of scales for sleep-disordered breathing, snoring, sleepiness, and behavioral problems. *Sleep Medicine, 1*(1), 21–32.

Chervin, R. D., Aldrich, M. S., Pickett, R., & Guilleminault, C. (1997). Comparison of the results of the Epworth Sleepiness Scale and the Multiple Sleep Latency Test. *Journal of Psychosomatic Research, 42,* 145–155.

Cohen, G. J. (1999). *American Academy of Pediatrics guide to your child's sleep: Birth through adolescence.* New York: Villard.

Coons, S., & Guilleminault, C. (1984). Development of consolidated sleep and wakeful periods in relation to the day/night cycle in infancy. *Developmental Medicine and Child Neurology, 26,* 169–176.

Crowell, J., Keener, M., Ginsburg, N., & Anders, T. (1987). Sleep habits in toddlers 18 to 36 months old. *Journal of the American Academy of Child and Adolescent Psychiatry, 26,* 510–515.

de Roquefeuil, G., Djakovic, M., & Montagner, H. (1993). New data on the ontogeny of the child's sleep–wake rhythm. *Chronobiology International, 10*(1), 43–53.

Dittrichová, J. (1966). Development of sleep in infancy. *Journal of Applied Physiology, 21*(4), 1243–1246.

Dunitz, M., Scheer, P., Kvas, E., & Macari, S. (1996). Psychiatric diagnoses in infancy: A comparison. *Infant Mental Health Journal, 17,* 12–23.

Earls, F. (1980). Prevalence of behavior problems in 3-year-old children. *Archives of General Psychiatry, 37,* 1153–1157.

Eckerberg, B. (2004). Treatment of sleep problems in families with young children: Effects of treatment on family well-being. *Acta Paediatrica, 93,* 126–134.

Emde, R., & Wise, B. (2003). The cup is half full: Initial clinical trials of DC: 0–3 and a recommendation for revision. *Infant Mental Health Journal, 24*(4), 437–446.

Emde, R. N., & Walker, S. (1976). Longitudinal study of infant sleep: Results of 14 subjects studied at monthly intervals. *Psychophysiology, 13*(5), 456–461.

Fagioli, I., & Salzarulo, P. (1982). Sleep states development in the first year of life assessed through 24-h recordings. *Early Human Development, 6,* 215–228.

Ferber, R. (1985). *Solve your child's sleep problems.* New York: Simon & Schuster.

Ferber, R., & Kryger, M. (Eds.). (1995). *Principles and practice of sleep medicine in the child.* Philadelphia: Saunders.

Foulkes, D. (1982). A cognitive–psychological model of REM dream production. *Sleep, 5,* 169–187.

Frankel, K., Boyum, L., & Harmon, R. (2004). Diagnoses and presenting symptoms in an infant psychiatry clinic: Comparisons of two diagnostic systems. *Journal of the American Academy of Child and Adolescent Psychiatry, 43*(5), 578–587.

Freudigman, K., & Thoman, E. B. (1994). Ultradian and diurnal cyclicity in the sleep states of newborn infants during the first two postnatal days. *Early Human Development, 38,* 67–80.

Gaylor, E. E., Burnham, M. M., Goodlin-Jones, B. L., & Anders, T. F. (2005). A longitudinal follow-up study of young children's sleep patterns using a developmental classification system. *Behavioral Sleep Medicine, 3,* 44–61.

Gaylor, E. E., Goodlin-Jones, B. L., & Anders, T. F. (2001). Classification of young children's sleep problems: A pilot study. *Journal of American Academy of Child and Adolescent Psychiatry, 40*(1), 61–67.

Goodlin-Jones, B., Burnham, M., & Anders, T. (2000). Sleep and sleep disturbances: Regulatory processes in infancy. In A. Sameroff, M. Lewis, & S. Miller (Eds.), *Handbook of developmental psychopathology* (2nd ed., pp. 309–325). New York: Kluwer Academic/Plenum Press.

Goodlin-Jones, B., Burnham, M., Gaylor, E., & Anders, T. (2001). Night waking, sleep–wake organization, and self-soothing in the first year of life. *Journal of Developmental and Behavioral Pediatrics, 22*(4), 226–233.

Goodlin-Jones, B., Eiben, L., & Anders, T. (1997). Maternal well-being and sleep–wake behaviors in infants: An intervention using maternal odor. *Infant Mental Health Journal, 18*(4), 378–393.

Gottlieb, D. J., Vezina, R. M., Chase, C., Lesko, S. M., Heeren, T. C., Weese-Mayer, D. E., et al. (2003). Symptoms of sleep-disordered breathing in 5-year-old children are associated with sleepiness and problem behaviors. *Pediatrics, 112,* 870–877.

Gozal, D. (1998). Sleep-disordered breathing and school performance in children. *Pediatrics, 102*(3), 616–620.

Gregory, A. M., Eley, T. C., O'Connor, T. G., & Plomin, R. (2004). Etiologies of associations between childhood sleep and behavioral problems in a large twin sample. *Journal of the American Academy of Child and Adolescent Psychiatry, 43,* 744–751.

Harper, R. M., Leake, B., Miyahara, L., Mason, J., Hoppenbrouwers, T., Sterman, M. B., et al. (1981). Temporal sequencing in sleep and waking states during the first 6 months of life. *Experimental Neurology, 72,* 294–307.

Hellbrügge, T., Lange, J. E., Rutenfranz, J., & Stehr, K. (1964). Circadian periodicity of physiological functions in different stages of infancy and childhood. *Annals of the New York Academy of Sciences, 117,* 361–373.

Jacklin, C. N., Snow, M. E., Gahart, M., & Maccoby, E. E. (1980). Sleep pattern development from 6 through 33 months. *Journal of Pediatric Psychology, 5*(3), 295–303.

Jenkins, S., Bax, M., & Hart, H. (1980). Behaviour problems in pre-school children. *Journal of Child Psychology and Psychiatry, 21,* 5–17.

Jenkins, S., Owens, C., Bax, M., & Hart, H. (1984). Continuities of common behaviour problems in preschool children. *Journal of Child Psychology and Psychiatry, 25*(1), 75–89.

Kataria, S., Swanson, M., & Trevathan, G. (1987). Persistence of sleep disturbances in preschool children. *Journal of Pediatrics, 110,* 642–646.

Keener, M. A., Zeanah, C. H., & Anders, T. F. (1988). Infant temperament, sleep organization, and nighttime parental interventions. *Pediatrics, 81,* 762–771.

Keren, M., Feldman, R., & Tyano, S. (2001). Diagnoses and interactive patterns of infants referred to a community-based infant mental health clinic. *Journal of the American Academy of Child and Adolescent Psychiatry, 40*(1), 27–35.

Klackenberg, G. (1982). Somnambulism in childhood—Prevalence, course, and behavioral correlations. *Acta Paediatrica Scandinavica, 71,* 495–499.

Kleitman, N., & Engelmann, T. G. (1953). Sleep characteristics of infants. *Journal of Applied Physiology, 6,* 269–282.

Kohyama, J., Furushima, W., & Hasegawa, T. (2003). Behavioral problems in children evaluated for sleep disordered breathing. *Sleep and Hypnosis, 5,* 89–94.

Lam, P., Hiscock, H., & Wake, M. (2003). Outcomes of infant sleep problems: A longitudinal study of sleep, behavior, and maternal well-being. *Pediatrics, 111*(3), e203–e207.

Louis, J., Cannard, C., Bastuji, H., & Challamel, M. (1997). Sleep ontogenesis revisited: A longitudinal 24–hour home polysomnographic study on 15 normal infants during the first two years of life. *Sleep, 20*(5), 323–333.

McGraw, K., Hoffmann, R., Harker, C., & Herman, J. H. (1999). The development of circadian rhythms in a human infant. *Sleep, 22,* 303–310.

McKenna, J. J., Mosko, S. S., & Richard, C. A. (1997). Bedsharing promotes breastfeeding. *Pediatrics, 100*(2), 214–219.

McMillen, I. C., Kok, J. S. M., Adamson, T. M., Deayton, J. M., & Nowak, R. (1991). Development of circadian sleep–wake rhythms in preterm and full-term infants. *Pediatric Research, 29,* 381–384.

Meier-Koll, A., Hall, U., Hellwig, U., Kott, G., & Meier-Koll, V. (1978). A biological oscillator system and the development of sleep–waking behavior during early infancy. *Chronobiologia, 5,* 425–440.

Menna-Barreto, L., Isola, A., Louzada, F., Benedito-Silva, A. A., & Mello, L. (1996). Becoming circadian: A one-year study of the development of the sleep–wake cycle in children. *Brazilian Journal of Medical and Biological Research, 29,* 125–129.

Mindell, J., Moline, M., Zendell, S., Brown, L., & Fry, J. (1994). Pediatricians and sleep disorders: Training and practice. *Pediatrics, 94*(2), 194–200.

Mindell, J. A., & Owens, J. A. (2003). *A clinical guide to pediatric sleep: Diagnosis and management of sleep problems.* Philadelphia: Lippincott/Williams & Wilkins.

Moore, T., & Ucko, L. (1957). Night waking in early infancy: Part I. *Archives of Disease in Childhood, 32,* 333–342.

Mosko, S., Richard, C., McKenna, J., & Drummond, S. (1996). Infant sleep architecture during bedsharing and possible implications for SIDS. *Sleep, 19*(9), 677–684.

National Sleep Foundation. (2004). *Sleep in America poll 2004.* Retrieved on 1/27/06 from the National Sleep Foundation website, www.sleepfoundation.org/hottopics/index. php?secid=16&id=143

Navelet, Y., Benoit, O., & Bouard, G. (1982). Nocturnal sleep organization during the first months of life. *Electroencephalography and Clinical Neurophysiology, 54,* 71–78.

O'Brien, L., Mervis, C., Holbrook, C., Bruner, J., Klaus, C., Rutherford, J., Raffield, T., et al. (2004). Neurobehavioral implications of habitual snoring in children. *Pediatrics, 114*(1), 44–49.

O'Brien, L. M., Tauman, R., & Gozal, D. (2004). Sleep pressure correlates of cognitive and behavioral morbidity in snoring children. *Sleep, 27,* 279–282.

Ottaviano, S., Giannotti, F., Cortesi, F., Bruni, O., & Ottaviano, C. (1996). Sleep characteristics in healthy children from birth to 6 years of age in the urban area of Rome. *Sleep, 19,* 1–3.

Owens, J., Maxim, R., Nobile, C., McGuinn, M., & Msall, M. (2000). Parental and self-report of sleep in children with attention-deficit/hyperactivity disorder. *Archives of Pediatric and Adolescent Medicine, 154,* 549–555.

Owens, J., Spirito, A., & McGuinn, M. (2000). The Children's Sleep Habit Questionnaire (CSHQ): Psychometric properties of a survey instrument for school-age children. *Sleep, 23*(8), 1043–1051.

Parmelee, A. H. (1961). Sleep patterns in infancy: A study of one infant from birth to eight months of age. *Acta Paediatrica, 50,* 160–170.

Parmelee, A. H., Schulz, H. R., & Disbrow, M. A. (1961). Sleep patterns of the newborn. *Journal of Pediatrics, 58*(2), 241–250.

Parmelee, A. H., Wenner, W. H., & Schulz, H. R. (1964). Infant sleep patterns: From birth to 16 weeks of age. *Journal of Pediatrics, 65,* 576–582.

Pollock, J. (1994). Night-waking at five years of age: Predictors and prognosis. *Journal of Child Psychology and Psychiatry, 35*(4), 699–708.

Quine, L., Wade, K., & Hargreaves, R. (1991). Learning to sleep. *Nursing Times, 87,* 41–43.

Ramchandani, P., Wiggs, L., Webb, V., & Stores, G. (2000). A systematic review of treatments for settling problems and night waking in young children. *British Medical Journal, 320,* 209–213.

Ramos, K. D. (2003). Intentional versus reactive cosleeping. *Sleep Research Online, 5,* 141–147.

Randazzo, A., Muehlbach, M., Schweitzer, P., & Walsh, J. (1998). Cognitive function following acute sleep restriction in children ages 10–14. *Sleep, 21*(8), 861–868.

Redline, S., Tishler, P., Schluchter, M., Aylor, J., Clark, K., & Graham, G. (1999). Risk factors for sleep disordered breathing in children: Associations with obesity, race, and respiratory problems. *American Journal of Respiratory and Critical Care Medicine, 159,* 1527–1532.

Richard, C. A., & Mosko, S. S. (2004). Mother–infant bedsharing is associated with an increase in infant heart rate. *Sleep, 27,* 507–511.

Richdale, A., Francis, A., Gavidia-Payne, S., & Cotton, S. (2000). Stress, behaviour, and sleep problems in children with an intellectual disability. *Journal of Intellectual and Developmental Disability, 25*(2), 147–161.

Richman, N. (1981). A community survey of characteristics of one- to two-year-olds with sleep disruptions. *Journal of the American Academy of Child Psychiatry, 20,* 281–291.

Roffwarg, H. P., Dement, W. C., & Fisher, C. (1964). Preliminary observations of the sleep–dream pattern in neonates, infants, children and adults. In E. Harms (Ed.), *Problems of sleep and dream in children* (pp. 60–72). New York: Macmillan.

Roffwarg, H. P., Muzio, J. N., & Dement, W. C. (1966). Ontogenetic development of the human sleep–dream cycle. *Science, 152,* 604–619.

Sadeh, A. (2004). A brief screening questionnaire for infant sleep problems: Validation and findings for an Internet sample. *Pediatrics, 113*(6), e570–e577.

Sadeh, A., Dark, I., & Vohr, B. R. (1996). Newborns' sleep–wake patterns: The role of maternal, delivery and infant factors. *Early Human Development, 44,* 113–126.

Salzarulo, P., & Chevalier, A. (1983). Sleep problems in children and their relationship with early disturbances of the waking sleep–wake rhythms. *Sleep, 6*(1), 47–51.

Sander, L. W., Julia, H. L., Stechler, G., & Burns, P. (1972). Continuous 24-hour interactional monitoring in infants reared in two caretaking environments. *Psychosomatic Medicine, 34*(3), 270–282.

Schecter, M. S., and the American Academy of Pediatrics, Section on Pediatric Pulmonology, Subcommittee on Obstructive Sleep Apnea Syndrome. (2002). Technical report: Diagnosis and management of childhood obstructive sleep apnea syndrome. *Pediatrics, 109*(4). Available at www.pediatrics.orq/cqi/contentlfull/1 09/4/e69

Scher, A., & Blumberg, O. (1999). Night waking among 1-year-olds: A study of maternal separation anxiety. *Child: Care, Health and Development, 25*(5), 323–334.

Seifer, R., Sameroff, A. J., Dickstein, S., Hayden, L. C., & Schiller, M. (1996). Parental psychopathology and sleep variation in children. *Child and Adolescent Psychiatric Clinics of North America, 5*(3), 715–727.

Shimada, M., Takahashi, K., Segawa, M., Higurashi, M., Samejim, M., & Horiuchi, K. (1999). Emerging and entraining patterns of the sleep–wake rhythm in preterm and term infants. *Brain and Development, 21,* 468–473.

Smedje, H., Broman, J., & Hetta, J. (2001). Short-term prospective study of sleep disturbances in 5–8 year old children. *Acta Paediatrica, 90,* 1456–1463.

Sostek, A. M., Anders, T. F., & Sostek, A. J. (1976). Diurnal rhythms in 2– and 8-week-old infants: Sleep–waking state organization as a function of age and stress. *Psychosomatic Medicine, 38*(4), 250–256.

Spangler, G. (1991). The emergence of adrenocortical circadian function in newborns and infants and its relationship to sleep, feeding, and maternal adrenocortical activity. *Early Human Development, 25,* 197–208.

Stores, G., & Wiggs, L. (1998). Clinical services for sleep disorders. *Archives of Disease in Children, 79,* 495–497.

Task Force on Research Diagnostic Criteria: Infancy and Preschool. (2003). Research diagnostic criteria for infants and preschool children: The process and empirical support. *Journal of the American Academy of Child and Adolescent Psychiatry, 42*(12), 1504–1512.

Tauman, R., O'Brien, L., Holbrook, C., & Gozal, D. (2004). Sleep Pressure Score: A new index of sleep disruption in snoring children. *Sleep, 27*(2), 274–278.

Thoman, E. B., & Whitney, M. P. (1989). Sleep states of infants monitored in the home: Individual differences, developmental trends, and origins of diurnal cyclicity. *Infant Behavior and Development, 12,* 59–75.

Thunstrom, M. (2002). Severe sleep problems in infancy associated with subsequent development of attention-deficit/hyperactivity disorder at 5.5 years of age. *Acta Paediatrica Scandinavica, 91,* 584–592.

Ware, J., & Orr, W. (1992). Evaluation and treatment of sleep disorders in children. In C. E. Walker & M. C. Roberts (Eds.), *Handbook of clinical child psychology* (2nd ed., pp. 261–282). New York: Wiley.

Weimer, S., Dise, T., Evers, P., Ortiz, M., Welldaregay, W., & Steinman, W. (2002). Prevalence, predictors, and attitudes toward cosleeping in an urban pediatric center. *Clinical Pediatrics, 41*, 433–438.

Wolf, A., & Lozoff, B. (1989). Object attachment, thumbsucking, and the passage to sleep. *Journal of the American Academy of Child and Adolescent Psychiatry, 28*(2), 287–292.

Wolke, D., Rizzo, P., & Woods, S. (2002). Persistent infant crying and hyperactivity problems in middle childhood. *Pediatrics, 109*(6), 1054–1060.

Wong, M., Brower, K., Fitzgerald, H., & Zucker, R. (2004). Sleep problems in early childhood and early onset of alcohol and other drug use in adolescence. *Alcoholism: Clinical and Experimental Research, 28*(4), 578–587.

Yokochi, K., Shiroiwa, Y., Inukai, K., Kito, H., & Ogawa, J. (1989). Behavioral state distribution throughout 24–h video recordings in preterm infants at term with good prognosis. *Early Human Development, 19*, 183–190.

Zero to Three. (1994). *Diagnostic classification of mental health and developmental disorders of infancy and early childhood.* Washington, DC: Zero to Three: National Center for Infants, Toddlers, and Families.

Zuckerman, B., Stevenson, J., & Bailey, V. (1987). Sleep problems in early childhood: Continuities, predictive factors, and behavioral correlates. *Pediatrics, 80*(5), 664–671.

10

Mood Disorders

Phenomenology and a Developmental Emotion Reactivity Model

JOAN L. LUBY and ANDY C. BELDEN

In this chapter, we review the available empirical data on major mood disorders, specifically depression in preschool children. Preliminary data and speculation about the phenomenology of bipolar disorder are also reviewed. We place these findings in the historical context of the skepticism about the application of mood disorder diagnoses to young children and present early observations that provided the first descriptions of depressed affect arising very early in life. Examples of representative clinical cases of a preschool-age child with depression and one with presumptive bipolar disorder are presented to illustrate typical preschool symptom presentations.

Essential to understanding early-onset mood disorders is knowledge about the developmental trajectory of the related, basic emotional processes. Along these lines, we also review the available empirical data base, and its substantial gaps, related to the emotional development of joy and sadness, as well as the "complex and self-conscious" emotions of guilt and shame. These selected emotions are deemed key to understanding the developmental psychopathology of mood disorders. We also review developmental literature on "emotion dynamics" and "emotional competence," and propose an integration of these two emotion-development frameworks to create a new and testable developmental psychopathology model for understanding early-onset mood disorders (Campos, Campos, & Barrett, 1997; Saami, 1999; Thompson, 1994; Thompson & Calkins, 1996). We describe how the proposed model may be used to characterize and quantify "optimal" or "adaptive" emotional reactivity within the mood-related affective domains. Finally, we describe how this novel, emotion-based model of developmental psychopathology is testable and could inform future phenomenology prevention and treatment studies of early-onset mood psychopathology.

PHENOMENOLOGY OF MOOD DISORDERS IN THE PRESCHOOL PERIOD

The Idea of Mood "Disorder" in a Young Child

The concept of clinical mood disorders arising in young children is, in general, one that meets with strong social resistance. This may be because it is both disturbing and counterintuitive to imagine a young child suffering from a clinical mood disorder. The notion of an early-onset mood disorder conflicts with the wish that early childhood be an inherently joyful and carefree time of life. However, the normative extremes of emotional intensity, poorer differentiation, and organization of discrete emotional expressions in children create greater ambiguity in our efforts to distinguish clinical disorders from normative and transient developmental difficulties during this period of development. Due to the unfortunate social stigma that continues to surround mental disorders, it is important to avoid prematurely or inaccurately labeling young children with a mood disorder diagnosis. However, the potential for more effective intervention earlier in life, related to higher neuroplasticity of the brain during this period (Cicchetti & Toth, 1998; see Faja & Dawson, Chapter 17, this volume), makes it equally important to identify mood disturbances that cross the clinical threshold into impairing disorders at the earliest possible developmental point. Therefore, although the issue of wide normative developmental variation must be considered, this can be addressed with proper study methodology, so that the critical distinctions between the normative and transient emotional difficulties of development, and clinically significant signs and symptoms can be disentangled.

First Reports of Alterations in Infant Affect

As early as the mid-1940s the behaviors and emotional expressions of infants with a presumed depressive syndrome were described by pediatrician Renée Spitz. Spitz was among the first to identify remarkable alterations in affective expressions observed in human infants separated from their primary caregivers and maintained in institutional settings. These early observations represent the first and earliest identification of the expressions of depressed mood and related negative affect in human infants and contradicted prevailing developmental theory suggesting that it was impossible for these emotions to be experienced at this early developmental point. These observations were, however, consistent with psychoanalytic theory purposing that "anaclitic depression" could arise in infancy as a response to separation from the caregiver (Spitz, 1945, 1946, 1949).

Despite these compelling observations, Spitz's publications had little impact on the practice of mainstream child psychiatry or child development research for decades, until interest in high-risk studies of the infants of depressed mothers was initiated in the early 1980s. These studies, which set the groundwork for later clinical investigations of depression in young children, focused on normal and aberrant development of mood and affect in infants and toddlers at "high risk" for depression on the basis of having a depressed mother. "High-risk" studies utilized standardized observations of the infant offspring of mothers experiencing mood disturbances compared to the offspring of healthy mothers. This approach was compelling based on the known increased rate of affective disorders in the offspring of individuals with mood disorders (Kovacs, Devlin, Pollock, Richards, & Mukerji, 1997; Weissman et al., 1984).

Although Spitz focused on samples of institutionalized children experiencing emotional deprivation, these studies had clear implications for understanding and greater appreciation of the complexity of the early emotional experience of normally developing children. Since the time of Spitz's observations, research in developmental psychology has begun to investigate the expression of emotions in infancy and early childhood. Despite the ongoing interest in the role of emotion in early child development, much remains unknown about the normal development of specific emotions and associated emotional regulatory process during the preschool period of development.

Phenomenology of Depression in Preschoolers

Age-adjusted criteria for the identification of clinical depression in young children between the ages of 3 and 6 years have been described and validated in one sample of reasonable size to date (Luby et al., 2002, 2003b). Prior to the availability of these data, numerous case studies and data from smaller samples suggested that a depressive syndrome might be identifiable in preschool children (e.g., Kashani, 1982; Kashani & Carlson, 1985; Kashani, Holcomb, & Orvaschel, 1986; Kashani & Ray, 1983; Kashani, Ray, & Carlson, 1984; Poznanski & Zrull, 1970). Kashani et al. (1986) studied the third edition of the *Diagnostic and Statistical Manual of Mental Disorders* (DSM-III; American Psychiatric Association, 1980) symptoms of depression in community samples of preschoolers and identified "concerning symptoms" but few children who met formal criteria for major depressive disorder (MDD), and suggested the need for developmental modifications to the criteria for depression for preschoolers. Subsequently, Luby et al. (2002, 2003b) demonstrated that the "typical" symptoms of MDD could be identified in preschool children when symptom states were "translated" to describe age-appropriate manifestations of DSM MDD constructs. One tangible example of this was that anhedonia was described as the inability to enjoy activities and play.

A further developmental modification that was tested was that negative themes in play were considered as an adjusted manifestation of a depressive symptom in lieu of (or in addition to) direct expression of sadness, guilt, negative thoughts, or other related depressive symptoms. Taken together, numerous findings support the notion that the basic integrity of the core depressive constructs (the adult manifestation of which are described in DSM-IV) appear to apply as early as age 3. Early, prevailing developmental theory suggested that young children would manifest "masked" symptoms of depression instead of depressed affect. Refuting this theory, we found that, similar to findings from investigations of this issue in older depressed children, masked symptoms appeared in depressed young children but with much less frequency than "typical" symptoms such as sadness, irritability, or vegetative signs in addition to changes in activity, sleep, and appetite (Carlson & Cantwell, 1980; Luby et al., 2003b).

The sign/symptom of anhedonia emerged as a characteristic of a more severe and possibly biologically based putative melancholic subtype in young children (Luby, Mrakotsky, Heffelfinger, Brown, & Spitznagel, 2004). Furthermore, anhedonia also emerged as a highly specific symptom of depression (and was not observed in any child in the psychiatric or healthy comparison groups). Preschoolers with depressive symptoms characterized by anhedonia had higher depression severity, greater alterations in cortisol reactivity, and failure to brighten in response to joyful events, similar to characteristics demonstrated in adults with this depressive subtype. This distinction may be important for future treatment studies of young children, as melancholically depressed adults appear to be more responsive to pharmacological treatments (Klein, 1974). The notion that an inability to experience pleasure and joy from activities and play would be a clinical symptom in a preschooler and a marker of serious psychopathology is consistent with the concept that young children are inherently joyful and pleasure seeking. Therefore, impairments in the young child's ability to experience joy and pleasure could be a marker of a clinical problem. In keeping with this concept, preschoolers were more likely to appear and to describe themselves as "less happy" rather than as overtly "sad" than same-age nondepressed peers (Luby et al., 2002). (See Figure 10.1.)

As a result, the sign/symptom of anhedonia (in addition to or in combination with other key symptoms) appears to be a useful screening item for depression in large populations (Luby, Heffelfinger, Koenig-McNaught, Brown, & Spitznagel, 2004). To screen for depression among preschool-age children, the Preschool Feelings Checklist (PFC; Luby, Heffelfinger, Mrakotsky, & Hildebrand, 1999), a 16-item yes–no questionnaire, is suitable for use in primary care or other community-based settings, and has established reliability (Luby, Heffelfinger, et al., 2004). A score of 3 or greater on the checklist suggests that further clinical evaluation for a mood disorder is warranted. The feasibility and public health benefit of screening for depression in primary care settings has been recently established in adolescent populations (Asarnow, et al., 2005).

Findings from our cross-sectional study reveal that 98% of depressed children were described by their parents as "often appearing sad," or "often appearing grouchy," 6% had trouble thinking or concentrating, and 78%

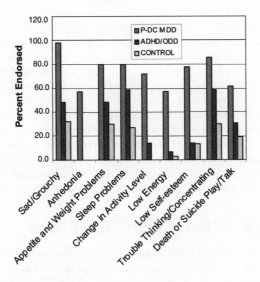

FIGURE 10.1. Typical symptoms of depression: Comparison of three groups.

were observed to have low self-esteem. Only 55% of depressed preschoolers in the study sample whined or cried excessively. The presence of neurovegetative signs in these very young depressed children was evidenced by the finding that 80% of depressed preschoolers showed changes in sleep, 80% had weight or appetite changes, and 71% demonstrated changes in activity. Highly notable was the finding that 74% of young children with MDD demonstrated play themes involving death or killing themselves, representing a significantly higher incidence than that observed in either of the two comparison groups. Regarding "masked" symptoms or "depressive equivalents" mentioned earlier, 51% had multiple somatic complaints, and only 37% of depressed preschoolers displayed the more nonspecific symptom of regression in development (Luby et al., 2002). (See Figure 10.1.)

Case Descriptions

A 5-year, 2-month-old Caucasian male presented to the clinic with irritability and aggression, and subsequent to the manifestations of these symptoms, the emergence of clear anhedonia. This symptom became evident to the mother as Halloween was nearing—the child's favorite holiday in years past. To his mother's surprise, he expressed no interest in, or excitement about, participating in dressing up, or trick or treating. He did not want to go out and play with neighborhood friends, an activity that he previously enjoyed and sought out. Because the child's irritability was more pronounced than his sadness, and this symptom was combined with aggression, a disruptive behavioral disorder rather than a mood disorder had been considered by previous clinicians. In addition to lack of interest in Halloween festivities and peer play, he also showed less interest in, and derived less pleasure from, his favorite foods.

A 3-year, 6-month-old African American male was referred to the infant/
preschool mental health clinic by his day care teacher due to sustained
nonparticipation in activities, isolated play, and social withdrawal. He
was described as having a "flat" and "serious" mood both at home and
at school. Although he did not appear to enjoy school, he did not display
separation anxiety. His behavior at home and at school was also described as very slow; it took an excessively long time for him to complete
a task. Although no weight loss was noted, his disinterest in food and
snacks was also evident in the school setting. A sustained preoccupation
with negative play themes was also described by his mother and observed
on clinical evaluation. A further family history revealed extensive anxiety
and mood disorders in first- and second-degree relatives.

Bipolar Disorder: Does It Arise during the Preschool Period?

Beyond case studies, there have been few controlled empirical investigations
of the nosology of bipolar disorder arising in preschool populations. Despite
this, there has been escalating clinical interest in the issue of whether mania
can arise, and if so, how it would manifest in such young children. The scientific debate on the existence and characteristics of bipolar disorder in children
over the age of 7 has been heated and controversial despite converging evidence about the presence of a very rapid-cycling phenotype from several independent samples (for review, see Nottelman et al., 2001).

In preschool-age children (< 6 years of age), several case reports and a
few very small-scale investigations focusing on treatment have been done
(e.g., Mota-Castillo et al., 2001; Poznanski et al., 1984; Scheffer, Niskala, &
Apps, 2004; Tumuluru, Weller, Fristad, & Weller, 2003; Tuzun, Zoroglu, &
Savas, 2002). Numerous clinical observations have suggested that mania may
manifest at least as early as 4 years of age and possibly younger. Appropriate
developmentally informed investigations of preschool bipolar disorder are
complicated by the fact that they must take into account the higher levels of
normative elevated mood and grandiose fantasy play that characterize this developmental period. Highly pertinent to these clinical questions are findings
on the normative development of self-concept during the preschool period. It
appears that a preschooler's concept of self begins to coalesce but is not yet
stable during the preschool period (see Thompson, Goodvin, & Meyer, Chapter 1, this volume). A clearer understanding of the developmental trajectory
of self-concept would be key to understanding whether true clinical grandiosity, comparable to that known in older children and adults, can arise in
preschool children. Related to the distinction between developmental norms
and clinical symptoms in this area is the need to distinguish putative "cycling"
from normative mood instability that is expected to be greater during this age
period.

    An exploratory study of mania symptoms in preschool children is in
progress at the Washington University Early Emotional Development Program. In this study, age-appropriate manifestations of putative mania symptoms are assessed in 3- to 6-year-old children using a newly developed mania

module of the Preschool Age Psychiatric Assessment (PAPA), for which test–retest reliability has been established (Luby & Belden, in press). Key issues to be addressed in this study focus on the distinction between age-appropriate fantasy play and grandiosity, as well as age-appropriate joy versus sustained elevated and impairing joy that could be classified as elated mood. In clinical practice, the presence of clear, persistent, fixed, and false grandiose delusions, as well as inappropriate and impairing elated mood, seem to be useful delineators of normative versus impairing symptoms in Luby's experience as a preschool clinician. Hypersexuality may also be a robust marker among preschool populations (since sexual interest or acting out is never age-appropriate for a preschool child), but sexual abuse or inappropriate early sexual stimulation may be a more common cause of this behavior and must therefore be carefully ruled out. Findings from the baseline wave of data collection in this ongoing study suggest that a valid and robust bipolar syndrome, that has discriminant validity from ADHD and is associated with high levels of impairment can be identified in preschoolers (Luby & Belden, in press).

Leibenluft and colleagues and Biermeyer and colleagues are two independent research groups currently assessing for the presence of mania precursors, or signs of risk in the preschool offspring of parents (or siblings) with bipolar disorders. Interest in such investigations is based on the observation that the parents of children with bipolar disorder often recall a much earlier onset of problems.

Despite the absence of sufficient data on the clinical criteria for bipolar disorders in preschool populations, several treatment studies of preschool bipolar disorder are being conducted. The collection of these data prior to the necessary data on the nosology of the disorder may be related to the widespread prescription of atypical antipsychotics in young children for nonspecific mood instability (Zito et al., 2000). Based on this prescribing phenomenon, data on the safety and efficacy of these medications in this age group is urgently needed. Kowatch and colleagues are currently conducting a placebo-controlled trial of valproate and risperidone in preschool bipolar disorder (R. Kowatch, personal communication, 2005). An open-label treatment study of olanzapine and risperidone in "bipolar" preschoolers was conducted by Beiderman et al. (2005). Although it is unclear how these investigations may inform our understanding of bipolar disorder per se, they may be informative about the safety of pharmacological interventions in these young populations, as well as their efficacy in the regulation of mood instability in general.

Case Descriptions

A 5-year-old white female was referred by her mother due to concerns about excessive energy, precocity, talkativeness, and periods of lack of need for sleep and, at times, food. The mother reported that the child wakes up routinely at 3 or 4 A.M. full of energy and wanting to play. She described her as talking incessantly at home, being inclined to engage complete strangers in a grocery store, and showing excessive talkativeness and directiveness both at school and at home. The mother described these symptoms as occurring on a daily basis. However, she noted that they are worse in the afternoon. In addition to this baseline behavior, there were periods during which the patient had a decreased need for sleep associated with a decreased interest in food, resulting in significant weight loss that caused health concerns. During these periods, the patient seemed to need to sleep only 3–4 hours a night and did not appear obviously fatigued during the day but did display increased irritability and activation. These periods were interrupted by periods in which normal eating and sleeping patterns returned. However, the patient had a persistent decreased need for sleep, which the parents believed had been present since birth.

During clinical observation, her behavior was remarkable for social precocity. For example, when the patient entered into the unfamiliar setting of the clinic, she immediately began to taunt an unfamiliar physician examiner. The child teased this doctor about "eating eyeballs for dinner" and tauntingly accused him of "asking the secretary out for a date," while laughing with great intensity and obviously amusing herself (despite her mother's obvious embarrassment and admonitions about appropriate social behavior). During the interview, when asked about her future plans, the child indicated that she was going to be a "better singer than Britney Spears" when she grew up, as she confidently explored the playroom, while periodically taunting the examiner further.

The family history revealed several individuals with unusually high levels of energy, decreased need for sleep, and histories of unusually bold behavior in early childhood but no formal psychiatric diagnoses. Most notable was the history of a paternal grandfather who at the age of 5 years, held on to the bumper of a stranger's car and rode 10 miles into town (sliding all the way) during a snowstorm. He had been known to "retile the kitchen floor at 3 A.M." and now, at age 75, routinely goes to the grocery store in the middle of the night to do his shopping.

A 4-year-old, white male was referred to the infant/preschool mental health clinic by his teacher. He had received the diagnosis of pervasive developmental disorder not otherwise specified from a pediatric neurologist. Although the teacher acknowledged significant behavioral problems in school, she was adamant that this diagnosis was not correct. The child was described as very active, constantly "on the go," and socially promiscuous, engaging family, friends, and strangers. He also had periods of decreased need for sleep. He had a history of going through periods in which he was constantly in need of physical contact with a parent. During these times, he had a seemingly persistent need to press his body up against his mother's body and expressed the need to be in constant physical contact with her. This was interspersed with periods in which he seemed relatively aloof, withdrawn, and uninterested in social or physical engagement. His parents also describe him as excessively friendly to strangers, both adults and children.

During a mental status exam, he immediately jumped into the unfamiliar examiner's lap within seconds after she entered the room. After just meeting her, he began to hug her, to tell her that he loved her, and to attempt kissing her on the face and lips. Despite this intrusive behavior, he had an engaging, charming, and charismatic demeanor. There was no history of sexual abuse or premature sexual stimulation. His mother was being treated for "depression," but she also described periods of elevated mood and excessive energy, with decreased need for sleep.

Although case studies and clinical observations and preliminary findings are highly suggestive of the existence of early-onset mania, more data is needed to clarify the characteristics of clinical bipolar disorder in preschool children. Several ongoing studies show promise in helping to inform this area. Data about the specific, sensitive signs and symptoms of clinical bipolar disorders, if arising in the preschool period, are urgently needed to guide clinical care.

EMOTIONAL DEVELOPMENT AND MOOD DISORDERS: A PROPOSED EMOTION REACTIVITY MODEL

The previous sections demonstrate that whereas some data on the phenomenology of preschool mood disorders are now available, defining the characteristics of these disorders and distinguishing these from normative developmental manifestations of emotions and mood during this period are important areas for future research. Future investigations must account for two critical developmental issues. The first is whether sufficient emotional development has taken place for the specific mood symptoms to manifest. For example, it is not possible at this time to diagnose autistim spectrum disorder earlier than 18 months of age, because the social developmental milestones of interest that serve as key markers and are known to be impaired in these disorders have not yet developed. The second issue is the need to distinguish between normative difficulties of emotional development and clinically significant phenomena. This task is complicated by the presence of major gaps in the empirical literature in the area of preschool emotional development pertinent to mood disorders. In an attempt to elucidate some of these issues, we provide in this section a brief review of the development of emotions pertinent to mood disorders and propose a model for future investigations of normative and disordered development of emotion reactivity and mood states.

Defining Emotion

Emotions are a rich and complex part of the human experience. and their role in intrapsychic, interpersonal, and social functioning is of paramount importance to understanding developmental psychopathology in general and mood disorders in particular. However, defining "emotion" is a surprisingly difficult task. Emotion is a construct that seems to elude definition, without invoking a related construct or synonym (e.g., feeling or affect). Despite this, emotion itself is a universal human experience the meaning of which is self-evident. Most standard definitions describe the sources, outcomes, and correlates of emotion but seemingly fail to capture the essence of what qualifies as a true emotion. The functionalist approach to emotion development outlines the useful and cogent rationale that emotions serve to create, preserve, or disrupt relations between an individual and his or her internal and external environment, when such relations are deemed significant (Campos, Mumme, Kermoian, & Campos, 1994; Frijda, 1986).

Normative Developmental Trajectory of Emotion States Pertinent to Mood Psychopathology

Our ability to define and understand early mood psychopathology is inextricably linked to and limited by our understanding of the normative development of basic, as well as complex, emotions related to mood disorders, such as joy, sadness, guilt, and shame. Whereas previous studies (e.g., Kochanska, Gross, Lin, & Nichols, 2002; Tangney, Wagner, & Gramzow, 1992) have examined the development of complex emotions such as guilt and shame, there is a dearth of investigations on the normative experiences and expressions of basic emotions such as joy and sadness during the preschool period. Surprisingly, gaps in the emotion development literature pertaining to the experience of basic emotions during the preschool years remain despite the many useful frameworks and theoretical approaches to emotion development that have been proposed but remain insufficiently tested (Campos et al., 1994; Sroufe, 1979, 1995; Thompson, 1990, 1991).

A Brief Overview of the Development of Joy, Sadness, Guilt, and Shame

The Development of Joy

Previous emotion research examining the development of joy has focused on children from birth to approximately 2 years of age. For example, observational studies of facial expression have shown that the human infant begins to express joy and happiness during the first 6–8 weeks of life (White, 1985). Social smiles during interaction with caregivers during this period mark the infant's first expressions of joy. Shortly after their first social smiles, infants begin to show happiness in both social and nonsocial contexts when able to manipulate a particular event or object (Lewis, Alessandri, & Sullivan, 1990). At 7 months, infants begin to smile and laugh while interacting with familiar adults. As children mature cognitively, they begin to take pleasure (as evidenced by increased smiling and laughing) in unexpected or discrepant events, such as in response to a funny noise or face (Kagan, Lapidus, & Moore, 1978).

Research on the experience and expressions of joy in older children often emphasizes their ability to recognize joy in self and others, explains the causes of joyful feelings, and examines children's expressions of joy. For instance, by 2 years of age, children are able to amuse themselves and become interested in their ability to elicit laughter from others. At 3 years of age, children begin to report feelings of joy in response to gratifying experiences (Denham & Zoller, 1991). For instance, young children may report being joyful when playing at the park or when a parent gives them a special toy or treat. Children between 3 and 7 years of age also report physical stimuli (e.g., being tickled or receiving hugs) as a source for joy (Denham & Zoller, 1991). Starting around age 3, children begin to recognize ways to maintain feelings of joy and happiness. For example, young children often report knowing that because physical and social aggression can cause feelings of happiness to change to sadness, aggression is to be avoided to maintain positive affect (McCoy & Masters, 1985).

The Development of Sadness

Izard, Hembree, and Huebner (1987) found that sadness can be reliably differentiated from other negative emotions in the human infant as early as 2 months of age, detected by inference from facial expressions. Between 2 and 6 months of age, facial expressions of sadness arise congruent with negative incentive events, providing further evidence for the presence of sorrowful emotion at this early point in development (Izard et al., 1995). Bowlby (1980) theorized that, related to the development of attachment, sadness arising during the first 2 years of life is most commonly due to prolonged periods of separation from primary caregivers. Starting at around 4 years of age, children begin to experience sadness as a result of more complex social events. For example, children between 4 and 12 years of age reported the loss of relationships, the occurrence of undesirable events, experiences of powerlessness, or the possibility of being harmed as reasons for their feelings of sadness (Denham & Zoller, 1991).

By 4 years of age, children begin to demonstrate an ability to regulate their feelings of sadness. This is evidenced by the findings that children often during this period suggest that physical nurturing (i.e., receiving/giving hugs or kisses) is helpful in reducing their own, as well as others', feelings of sadness (Denham, 1998). In one of the few studies explicitly examining the development of sadness, Rotenberg, Mars, and Crick (1987) found that younger children typically take an egocentric approach to explaining sadness. Specifically, young children most frequently reported sadness being caused by harm to one's self, whereas older children were more able to recognize that harm to others was also a cause for sadness. An increase in the child's sophistication in the understanding of emotions is also evidenced by the finding of an increased awareness and understanding of children's perceived motives for emotions. For example, older children were more likely to understand the motives of emotion as attempts to get others to understand their point of view (Rotenberg et al., 1987).

Developmental changes in the intensity of the emotional experience of sadness with increasing age may also be present. Rotenberg et al. (1987) found a trend for young children to report less intense experiences of sadness. Interestingly, children of all ages report infrequently verbalizing their sadness to others, and often do not show their sadness at all. This is in keeping with the clinical observation and empirical evidence of depressed young children reporting themselves as "less happy" rather than as overtly "sad" on an age-appropriate puppet interview (Luby et al., 2002). These findings suggest that young children may have more subtle manifestations of sadness. We have posited that this greater subtlety may contribute to the underrecognition of depressed mood states in young children.

The Development of Guilt and Shame

Emotions that require the ability to make the distinction between the expectations (i.e., goals, motivation, and behaviors) of self and others are referred to as "self-conscious" and/or "complex" emotions (Tangney et al., 1992). Young children's self-evaluations of performance in relation to the social standards and the expectations of others are prerequisites for the emotions of guilt and shame. The development of these emotions may be of particular interest for understanding early-onset mood psychopathology, because they are core features of mood disorders in adult populations. Self-conscious emotions such as guilt and shame are salient in depressive states and theoretically could also be important in manic states if absent or occurring at low levels. Although the ability to experience complex emotions requires more sophisticated cognitive processes paired with advancing social skills, more recent data suggest that children as young as 2 years old have the ability to experience an array of complex emotions, including self-conscious emotions (Zahn-Waxler & Robinson, 1995). Using narrative techniques, Zahn-Waxler, Cole, and Barrett (1991) have shown that children as young as 3 years of age understand and experience guilt.

The clinical depression literature based on studies of older populations links depression to the chronic tendency to make internal, stable, and global self-blaming attributions (i.e., guilt and shame) in the face of negative events (Robins & Block, 1988). However, the role and salience of guilt and/or shame in depression in young children remains unexplored. Young children's ability to regulate their expression of intense positive and negative emotions, such as sadness and joy, as well as the complex emotions of guilt and shame, is an important factor in the boundary between adaptive expressions of these emotions and maladaptive expressions that cross the threshold into "symptom states." For example, preschool children with the inability to control the intensity or duration of their feelings of sadness, in addition to having proneness for shame and guilt, may be at much greater risk for depression compared to emotionally well-regulated same-age peers who experience shame and guilt more rarely and only in extreme and/or appropriate circumstances.

Despite some specific data on children's experience, understanding, and expressions of joy, sadness, guilt, and shame, to date we are lacking systematic literature that elucidates and tracks the normative trajectory of emotion development during the preschool period. Such information could have important clinical applications to understanding the early development of mood disorders. For instance, we do not know how often normally developing preschoolers become joyful or sad during a typical day, week, or month. The "normative" expression of guilt or shame after a wrongdoing (encompassing duration, intensity, and appropriate circumstances) remains unclear. The parameters of the healthy range and peak of intensity in a preschooler's experience and expression of joy and sadness also remain unclear. Data defining these parameters would allow clinicians to determine whether a child is falling outside of the normative range for specific emotions and crossing into the clinical range. Such data could further clarify developmental psychopathology in young children.

Emotion Regulation

In addition to the importance of understanding the normative experience and expression of specific emotions during the preschool period is the tracking of normative trajectories of young children's capacities to control and modulate their emotional expressions. Children who develop the ability to monitor, appraise, and, if necessary, modulate their emotional reactions to emotionally laden stimuli, allowing them to achieve goals and function appropriately within their social environments, are thought to be able to engage in effective *emotion regulation* (Campos et al., 1997; Thompson, 1994). The capacity to regulate varying intensities, durations, and specific types of emotion experiences and expressions (e.g., joy and sadness) is critical for achieving social and emotional competence and is a key component of early emotional development (Saarni, 1999).

Previous studies examining normally developing children suggest that preschoolers who are better able to regulate inappropriate expressions of emotions, delay gratification, and use cognitive strategies to monitor their emotions and subsequent reactions tend to be more socially competent, more well-liked by peers, and are perceived as being more well-adjusted (Lemery, Essex, & Snider, 2002; Lengua, 2002). Conversely, the inability to adaptively regulate emotional experiences and expressions has been shown to place children at an increased risk for childhood psychopathology (Cicchetti, Ackerman, & Izard, 1995). Along these lines and potentially pertinent to depressive syndromes, Zeman, Shipman, and Suveg (2002) found that school-age children's inability to regulate feelings of sadness predicted an increase in their internalizing symptoms, placing these children at a heightened risk for psychopathology. Despite growing interest in the relationship between emotion regulation and childhood psychopathology, relatively few studies to date have addressed these constructs in a sufficiently detailed manner for application to specific clinical mental disorders.

An Emotion Reactivity Model for Defining Mood Disorders in Young Children

Thompson (1994) outlines how an individual's emotional response to incentive events (e.g., situation or experience) evoking emotions such as joy or sadness can be quantified by measuring the following key dynamic features: (1) latency to respond, (2) time from initial arousal to peak arousal intensity, (3) peak of emotional intensity, (4) total duration of response, and, (5) duration and rate of return to euthymic baseline. In addition to these features, the total response time from emotion onset to emotion offset is also of importance. Despite its potential utility for understanding emotion experience and expression throughout the lifespan, Thompson's (1994) model of emotion dynamics has primarily been tested only in specialized infant populations to date (e.g., Frodi & Thompson, 1985; Thompson, Cicchetti, Lamb, & Malkin, 1985). We propose that several features of Thompson's emotion dynamics model, and its quantitative emotion dynamic parameters, could be useful to distinguish the emotional features of "optimally adaptive" and maladaptive emotional reactivity, potentially shedding light on normative variation in emotional response, as well as identifying, defining, and quantifying the emotional characteristics of early-onset affective disorders.

Toward this end, application and integration of an emotional competence model described by Saarni (1999) in conjunction with Thompson's (1994) emotion dynamics model is also of interest. "Emotional competence," defined by the characteristics of healthy or "optimal" emotional development has been described by Saarni (1999), who proposes that the capacity to experience a broad range of discrete emotions at sufficient intensity for reasonable duration is optimal and inherent in achieving emotional maturity or competence. These capacities for a broad range, repertoire, and ability to experience and regulate emotional responses, both positive and negative, may be seen as adaptive, because they are key to meaningful and satisfying interpersonal and intrapsychic functioning. Notably, this principle is also central to many psychodynamic models of mental health.

By integrating and extending upon Thompson's (1991, 1994) emotion dynamics model and Saarni's (1999) emotional competence model, we propose a novel model applying the concept of "optimal emotional reactivity curves" to defining mood disorders and associated risk states in young children. An "optimal" reactivity curve (see Figure 10.2) is characterized by an individual who is able to react spontaneously to an emotionally evocative incentive event (either external or internal) in a timely manner, experience an emotional peak of sufficient intensity, and then, within a reasonable time, return to a euthymic baseline.

Relative to the "optimal" reactivity, we hypothesize that depression

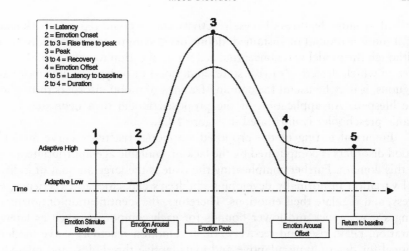

FIGURE 10.2. Proposed model of emotion reactivity curves.

could manifest as a diminution in the intensity or duration of joyful responses and/or as an amplification in the intensity or duration of sad reactions. Latencies of such responses, as well as abilities to return to a euthymic baseline, are all elements of response characteristics that may be key to defining risk states and overt mood disorders. In other words, depressed children may become sad quickly and may also remain sad for extended periods. In addition, it may also take depressed children extended periods of time to react with joy, and they may remain joyful for a very short period of time. In keeping with this model, we have previously reported that preschoolers' inability to experience pleasure in daily activities and play, a well-known phenomenon in older depressed children and adults called "anhedonia," was a highly specific marker of depression among preschool children (Luby, Mrakotsky, et al., 2004). Thus, one might hypothesize that anhedonic depressed children would have an inability to sustain joy, leading to shorter durations, lower peaks, and a quick return to their baseline. Accordingly, data from the same sample have shown that preschoolers defined as depressed, based on DSM-IV criteria according to parent report, were also objectively observed to display less enthusiasm and more negativity than nondepressed preschoolers during mildly stressful and semistructured parent–child interaction tasks (Luby et al., 2006). Such findings indicate the potential importance of investigating children's emotional reactivity within various contexts, relationships, and events in relation to specific emotions known to be associated with early-onset mood disorders.

Conversely, a manic state could be characterized by an excessively sustained positive emotion (e.g., "elation"), an inability to return to a euthymic baseline, as well as insufficient appropriate negative emotion in response to sad or negative events. We propose that deviations in any or all of the described dynamic features of these reactivity curves could represent risk states or, if more profound or sustained, define overt symptoms of mood disorders. Although the model was conceptualized for application to young children, an area in which detection of risk states and mood disorders remains more ambiguous, it may be useful for defining features of mood disorders throughout the lifespan. An application of the proposed model to a depressed and a manic preschooler is illustrated in Figure 10.3.

Empirical testing of the proposed emotional reactivity curve model in mood disorders is complicated by the lack of available age-appropriate norms in this domain. Further complicating the issue is the large amount of individual variation in normally developing children's capacities to experience, express, and regulate their emotions. Therefore, the identification of normative ranges (e.g., upper and lower bounds for each component, such as latency, duration, peak, rise, and recovery) of the emotion reactivity curve model is critical for determining adaptive and maladaptive thresholds, and related to this, defining the parameters of mood disorders. Mapping the core components of emotion reactivity curves in a population of normative and clinical preschoolers could provide unprecedented measurable clinical thresholds.

As others have suggested (e.g., Belden & Luby, 2004; Thompson, 1994), we speculate that the proposed emotion reactivity curves will vary in relation to a child's internal characteristics such as temperamental disposition, external characteristics such as psychosocial environment, as well as caregivers' approach to the socialization of emotion during interactions with their preschoolers. "Optimally adaptive" emotional reactivity may also vary with cultural environment and social expectation. Another important consideration is that characteristics of emotion reactivity curves might be emotion-specific. For example, a child may be able to effectively control his or her feelings of sadness but at the same time have chronic and uncontrollable feelings of guilt and shame. Thus, it may be important to examine emotion dynamics not only

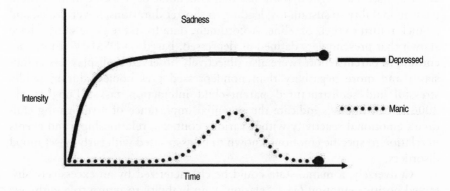

FIGURE 10.3. Depressed and manic preschoolers' responses to a sadness-inducing event: Hypothesized emotion reactivity curves.

in relation to positive or negative emotion valences in general but also for specific key emotions within those valences. As previously discussed, in relation to preschool depression, it may be just as important to assess children's inability to sustain the arousal of joy and pleasure as it is to examine their reactivity while experiencing sadness.

Emotion Dynamic Features: Application to the Identification, Prevention, and Treatment of Mood Disorders

Positive and/or negative emotion arousal (e.g., joy and sadness) at appropriate or inappropriate times, are thought to promote or undermine adaptive functioning beginning in infancy and continuing throughout the lifespan. When an individual experiences extremes of either joy or sadness, or inappropriate joy in response to a sad event, this undermines social functioning. We propose that mapping the dynamic trajectories of a young child's impaired emotional response gives us a novel tool to identify, quantify, and measure what may be the specific features of an individual child's emotion dysregulation leading to risk states or manifest mood disorders. Most importantly, this method could be particularly useful for the design of more targeted prevention and/or intervention strategies. Furthermore, if in fact the conceptualization of this model can be operationalized, empirically tested, and validated, then emotion reactivity curves could potentially provide clinicians with a useful tool for understanding and assessing the unique individual features (e.g., reactivity characteristics) of mood disorder manifestations in individual children.

CONCLUSION

Large bodies of developmental research have provided evidence for early alterations in neurobiology and affect development in infants and preschoolers at high risk for depression, setting the stage for studies of clinical depressive disorders in young children. Subsequently, Luby and colleagues have provided evidence that children as young as 3 years, 6 months of age can display a valid clinical depressive syndrome (Luby et al., 2002, 2003b). These data suggest that the current DSM-IV criteria can be applied to preschool children when the assessment is modified to account for age-adjusted manifestations of the symptom states. Discriminant validity, as well as convergent validity based on biological and neuropsychological markers also supports the existence of a valid preschool depressive syndrome (Luby et al., 2003a; Mrakotsky, 2001). Furthermore, observational findings that demonstrate decreases in positive emotions and increases in negative emotions during dyadic interactions with the caregiver lend further support to this construct (Luby et al., 2006). In addition, preliminary evidence also suggests that there are alterations in specific aspects of emotion development, such as depressed young children's decreased ability to recognize and label the facial affect of others (Mrakotsky, 2001). Validation of these findings in independent study samples is now warranted.

Age-appropriate tools are now available for the assessment of mood disorders in young children (e.g., Preschool Age Psychiatric Assessment [PAPA]; Egger, Ascher, & Angold, 1999). These include developmentally modified parental interviews, age-appropriate direct interviews of the child using puppets (Berkeley Puppet Interview), and observational measures of emotional reactivity and parent–child relationship quality (Egeland & Hiester, 1995; Goldsmith, Reilly, & Lemery, 1995). A novel measure of affect recognition and labeling, as well as other cognitive and neuropsychological measures, may also be a useful component of a comprehensive assessment of affective disorders in young children (Mrakotsky & Luby, 2000, unpublished measure).

We have proposed a novel developmental model that integrates principles of emotion dynamics and emotional competence to define the features of adaptive and maladaptive emotional reactivity curves during early childhood. We have proposed that the quantification and analyses of such emotional reactivity curves could inform investigations of normative emotional development, as well as our understanding of the developmental psychopathology of mood disorders. We also suggest that quantitative analyses of such response characteristics might be useful for the design of targeted prevention and intervention efforts.

Whereas this data will be useful to advance the identification and assessment of risk states and clinical depressive syndromes in very young children, there is much smaller body of data to inform the recognition and assessment of manic episodes and therefore bipolar disorders in young children. There have been exciting new data on the nosology and longitudinal course of bipolar disorders in school-age children and adolescents (Biederman et al., 2000; Geller et al., 1998, 2001; Geller, Tillman, Craney, & Bolhofner, 2004). To date there is only one published large-scale investigation describing the phenomenology of bipolar disorders arising in the preschool period (Luby & Beldin, in press). This investigation provides evidence for a specific mania symptom constellation that is associated with impairment and shows discriminant validity from other disruptive behavioral disorders (Luby & Beldin, in press). The symptoms of grandiosity and elation emerged as highly specific markers of the disorder in preschoolers. Further replication in independent study samples is now warranted.

Two case studies are described (and numerous others have been observed) that lend support to and describe characteristics bipolar disorders arising in the preschool period of development. The increasing frequency of clinically observed putative bipolar symptoms among preschool children by the authors, as well as other clinicians, also supports this hypothesis. A number of the measurement strategies we have described, as well the emotion dynamic model, would theoretically also be applicable to the assessment of early-onset bipolar disorders inasmuch as they target the assessment of mood and affect, and emotional reactivity. However, the use of these measures and strategies for capturing the early manifestations of mania or hypomania have just been initiated and will undoubtedly be the focus of future study.

REFERENCES

American Psychiatric Association. (1980). *Diagnostic and statistical manual of mental disorders* (3rd ed.). Washington, DC: Author.

Asarnow, J. R., Jaycox, L. H., Duan, N., LaBorde, A. P., Rea, M. M., Murray, P., et al. (2005). Effectiveness of a quality improvement intervention for adolescent depression in primary care clinics: A randomized controlled trial. *Journal of the American Medical Association, 293*(3), 311–319.

Belden, A., & Luby, J. (2006). Preschoolers' depression severity and behaviors during dyadic interactions: The mediating role of parental support. *Journal of the American Academy of Child and Adolescent Psychiatry, 45*(2), 213–222.

Biederman, J., Mick, E., Faraone, S., Spencer, T., Wilens, T., & Wozniak, J. (2000). Pediatric mania: A developmental subtype of bipolar disorder? *Biological Psychiatry, 48*, 458–466.

Bowlby, J. (1980). *Attachment and loss: Vol. 3. Loss, sadness, and depression.* New York: Basic Books.

Campos, J. J., Campos, R. G., & Barrett, K. C. (1989). Emergent themes in the study of emotional development and emotion regulation. *Developmental Psychology, 25*, 394–402.

Campos, J., Mumme, D., Kermoian, R., & Campos, R. (1994). A functionalist perspective on the nature of emotion. *Monographs of the Society for Research in Child Development, 59*(1–2, Serial No. 240), 284–303.

Carlson, G. A., & Cantwell, D. P. (1980). Unmasking masked depression from childhood through adulthood: Analysis of three studies. *American Journal of Psychiatry, 145*, 1222–1225.

Cicchetti, D., Ackerman, B., & Izard, C. (1995). Emotions and emotion regulation in developmental psychology. *Developmental Psychopathology, 7*, 1–10.

Cicchetti, D., & Toth, S. (1998). The development of depression in children and adolescents. *American Psychologist, 53*(2), 221–241.

Denham, S. A. (1998). *Emotional development in young children.* New York: Guilford Press.

Denham, S., & Zoller, D. (1991). "When my hamster died, I cried": Preschooler's attributions of the causes of emotions. *Journal of Genetic Psychology, 152*, 371–373.

Egeland, B., & Hiester, M. (1995). The long-term consequences of day-care and mother–infant attachment. *Child Development, 66*(2), 474–485.

Egger, H. L., Ascher, & Angold, A. (1999). *Preschool Age Psychiatric Assessment.* Duke University Medical Center, Durham, NC.

Fridja, N. (1986). *The emotions.* New York/Paris, France: Cambridge University Press/Editions de La Maison des Sciences de L'Homme.

Frodi, A., & Thompson, R. (1985). Infants' affective responses in the Strange Situation: Effects of prematurity and of quality of attachment. *Child Development, 56*, 1280–1290.

Geller, B., Hoog, S., Heiligenstein, J., Ricardi, R., Tamura, R., & Kluszynski, S. (2001). Fluoxetine treatment for obsessive–compulsive disorder in children and adolescents: A placebo-controlled clinical trial. *Journal of the American Academy of Child and Adolescent Psychiatry, 40*(7), 773–779.

Geller, B., Tillman, R., Craney, J. L., & Bolhofner, K. (2004). Four-year prospective outcome and natural history of mania in children with a prepubertal and early adolescent bipolar disorder phenotype. *Archives of General Psychiatry, 61*, 459–67.

Geller, B., Williams, M., Zimmerman, B., Frazier, J., Beringer, L., & Warner, K. (1998).

Prepubertal and early adolescent bipolarity differentiate from ADHD by manic symptoms, grandiose delusions, ultra-rapid or ultradian cycling. *Journal of Affective Disorders, 51*, 81–91.

Goldsmith, H. H., Reilly, J., & Lemery, K. S. (1995). *Laboratory Temperament Assessment Battery: Preschool Version.* University of Wisconsin, Madison, WI.

Izard, C. E., Fantauzzo, C., Castle, J., Haynes O., Rayais, M., & Putnam, P. (1995). The ontogeny and significance of infants' facial expression in the first 9 months of life. *Developmental Psychology, 31*, 997–1013.

Izard, C., Hembree, E., & Huebner, R. (1987). Infants' emotional expressions to acute pain: Developmental change and stability of individual differences. *Developmental Psychology, 23*, 105–113.

Kagan, J., Lapidus, D., & Moore, M. (1978). Infant antecedents of cognitive functioning: A longitudinal study. *Child Development, 49*, 1005–1023.

Kashani, J. H. (1982). Depression in the preschool child. *Journal of Children in Contemporary Society, 15*, 11–17.

Kashani, J. H., & Carlson, G. A. (1985). Major depressive disorder in a preschooler. *Journal of the American Academy of Child and Adolescent Psychiatry, 24*(4), 490–494.

Kashani, J. H., Holcomb, W. R., & Orvaschel, H. (1986). Depression and depressive symptoms in preschool children from the general population. *American Journal of Psychiatry, 143*(9), 1138–1143.

Kashani, J. H., & Ray, J. S. (1983). Depressive related symptoms among preschool-age children. *Child Psychiatry and Human Development, 13*, 233–238.

Kashani, J. H., Ray, J. S., & Carlson, G. A. (1984). Depression and depressive-like states in preschool-age children in a child development unit. *American Journal of Psychiatry, 141*(11), 1397–1402.

Klein, D. F. (1974). Endogenomorphic depression. *Archives of General Psychiatry, 31*, 447–454.

Kochanska, G., Gross, J., Lin, M., & Nichols, K. (2002). Guilt in young children: Development, determinants, and relations with a broader system of standards. *Child Development, 72*, 461–482.

Kovacs, M., Devlin, B., Pollock, M., Richards, C., & Mukerji, P. (1997). A controlled family history study of childhood-onset depressive disorder. *Archives of General Psychiatry, 54*(7), 613–623.

Lemery, K. S., Essex, M. J., & Snider, N. A. (2002). Revealing the relation between temperament and behavior problem symptoms by eliminating measurement confounding: Expert ratings and factor analyses. *Child Development, 73*, 867–882.

Lengua, L. J. (2002). The contribution of emotionality and self-regulation to the understanding of children's response to multiple risk. *Child Development, 73*, 144–61.

Lewis, M., Alessandri, S., & Sullivan, M. (1990). Violation of expectancy, loss of control, and anger expressions in young infants. *Developmental Psychology, 26*, 745–751.

Luby, J., & Belden, A. (in press). Defining and validating bipolar disorder in the preschool period. *Development and Psychopathology.*

Luby, J., Heffelfinger, A., Koenig-McNaught, A., Brown, K., & Spitznagel, E. (2004). The Preschool Feelings Checklist: A brief and sensitive screening measure for depression in young children. *Journal of the American Academy of Child and Adolescent Psychiatry, 43*(6), 708–717.

Luby, J. L., Heffelfinger, A., Mrakotsky, C., Brown, K., Hessler, M., & Spitznagel, E. (2003a). Alterations in stress cortisol reactivity in depressed preschoolers relative to psychiatric and no-disorder comparison groups. *Archives of General Psychiatry, 60*(12), 1248–1255.

Luby, J. L., Heffelfinger, A. K., Mrakotsky, C., Brown, K. M., Hessler, M. J., Wallis, J. M., et al. (2003b). The clinical picture of depression in preschool children. *Journal of the American Academy of Child and Adolescent Psychiatry, 42*(3), 340–348.

Luby, J., Heffelfinger, A., Mrakotsky, C., Hessler, M., Brown, K., & Hildebrand, T. (2002).

Preschool major depressive disorder: Preliminary validation for developmentally modified DSM-IV criteria. *Journal of the American Academy of Child and Adolescent Psychiatry, 41*(8), 928–937.

Luby, J., Heffelfinger, A., Mrakotsky, C., & Hildebrand, T. (1999). *Preschool Feelings Checklist*. St. Louis, MO: Washington University.

Luby, J., Mrakotsky, C., Heffelfinger, A., Brown, K., & Spitznagel, E. (2004). Characteristics of depressed preschoolers with and without anhedonia: Evidence for a melancholic depressive subtype in young children. *American Journal of Psychiatry, 161*, 1998–2004.

Luby, J., Sullivan, J., Belden, A., Stalets, M., Blankenship, S., & Spitznagel, E. (2006). An observational analysis of behavior in depressed preschoolers: Further validation of early onset depression. *Journal of the American Academy of Child and Adolescent Psychiatry, 45*(2), 203–212.

McCoy, C., & Masters, J. (1985). The development of children's strategies for the social control of emotion. *Child Development, 56*, 1214–1222.

Mota-Castillo, M., Torruella, A., Engels, B., Perez, J., Dedrick, C., & Gluckman, M. (2001). Valproate in very young children: An open case series with a brief follow-up. *Journal of Affective Disorders, 67*, 193–197.

Mrakotsky, C. (2001). *Visual perception, spatial cognition and affect recognition in preschool depressive syndromes*. Vienna/St. Louis, MO: University of Vienna/Washington University.

Mrakotsky, C., & Luby, J. (2000). *The Facial Affect Comprehension Evaluation (FACE): A test for emotion perception and emotion recognition in the preschool age* [Unpublished measure]. Vienna/St. Louis, MO: University of Vienna/Washington University.

Nottelmann, E., Biederman, J., Birmaher, B., Carlson, G. A., Chang, K., Fenton, W., et al. (2001). National Institute of Mental Health Research Roundtable on prepubertal bipolar disorder. *Journal of the American Academy of Child and Adolescent Psychiatry, 40*(8), 871–878.

Poznanski, E. O., Grossman, J. A., Buchsbaum, Y., Banegas, M., Freeman, L., & Gibbons, R. (1984). Preliminary studies of the reliability and validity of the children's depression rating scale. *Journal of the American Academy of Child and Adolescent Psychiatry, 23*, 191–197.

Poznanski, E., & Zrull, J. P. (1970). Childhood depression: Clinical characteristics of overtly depressed children. *Archives of General Psychiatry, 23*(1), 8–15.

Robins, C., & Block, P. (1988). Personal vulnerability, life events, and depressive symptoms: A test of a specific interaction model. *Journal of Personality and Social Psychology, 54*, 847–852.

Rotenberg, K., Mars, K., & Crick, N. R. (1987). Development of children's sadness. *Psychology and Human Development, 2*(1), 13–25.

Saarni, C. (1999). *The development of emotional competence*. New York: Guilford Press.

Scheffer, R. E., Niskala, & Apps, J. A. (2004). The diagnosis of preschool bipolar disorder presenting with mania: Open pharmacological treatment. *Journal of Affective Disorders, 82*(Suppl. 1), S25–S34.

Spitz, R. (1945). Hospitalism: An inquiry into the genesis of psychiatric conditions in early childhood. *Psychoanalytic Study of the Child, 1*, 53–74.

Spitz, R. (1946). Anaclitic depression: An inquiry into the genesis of psychiatric conditions in early childhood. *Psychoanalytic Study of the Child, 1*, 47–53.

Spitz, R. (1949). Motherless infants. *Child Development, 20*, 145–155.

Sroufe, L. (1979). Socioemotional development. In J. Osofsky (Ed.), *The handbook of infant development* (pp. 462–516). New York: Wiley.

Sroufe, L. (1995). *Emotional development: The organization of emotional life in the early years*. Cambridge, UK: Cambridge University Press.

Tangney, J., Wagner, P., & Gramzow, R. (1992). Proneness to shame, proneness to guilt, and psychopathology. *Journal of Abnormal Psychology, 101*(3), 469–478.

Thompson, R. A. (1990). Emotion and self-regulation. In R. A. Thompson (Ed.), *Nebraska*

Symposium on Motivation, 1988: Socioemotional development: Current theory and research in motivation (Vol. 36, pp. 367–467). Lincoln: University of Nebraska Press.

Thompson, R. A. (1991). Emotional regulation and emotional development. *Educational Psychology Review, 3,* 269–307.

Thompson, R. A. (1994). Emotion regulations: A theme in search of definition. In N. A. Fox (Ed.), *The development of emotion regulation: Biological and behavioral considerations* (pp. 25–166). Chicago: University of Chicago Press.

Thompson, R. A., & Calkins, S. D. (1996). The double-edged sword: Emotional regulation for children at risk. *Developmental Psychopathology, 8,* 163–182.

Thompson, R., Cicchetti, D., Lamb, M. E., & Malkin, C. (1985). Emotional responses of Down syndrome and normal infants in the Strange Situation: The organization of affective behavior in infants. *Developmental Psychology, 21,* 828–841.

Tumuluru, R. V., Weller, E. B., Fristad, M. A., & Weller, R. A. (2003). Mania in six preschool children. *Journal of Child and Adolescent Psychopharmacology, 13*(4), 489–494.

Tuzun, U., Zoroglu, S. S., & Savas, H. A. (2002). A 5-year-old boy with recurrent mania successfully treated with carbamazepine. *Psychiatry and Clinical Neurosciences, 56*(5), 589–591.

Weissman, M. M., Prusoff, B., Gammon, D., Merikangas, K., Leckman, J., & Kidd, K. (1984). Psychopathology in the children (ages 6–18) of depressed and normal parents. *Journal of the American Academy of Child and Adolescent Psychiatry, 23*(1), 78–84.

White, B. L. (1985). *The first three years of life.* New York: Prentice-Hall.

Zahn-Waxler, C., Cole, P., & Barrett, K. (1991). Guilt and empathy: Sex differences and implications for the development of depression. In J. Garber & K. A. Dodge (Eds.), *The development of emotion regulation and dysregulation* (pp. 243–272). New York: Cambridge University Press.

Zahn-Waxler, C., & Robinson, J. (1995). Empathy and guilt: Early origins of feelings of responsibility. In J. P. Tangney & K. W. Fischer (Eds.), *Self-conscious emotions: The psychology of shame, guilt, embarrassment, and pride* (pp. 143–173). New York: Guilford Press.

Zeman, J., Shipman, K., & Suveg, C. (2002). Anger and sadness regulations: predictions to internalizing and externalizing symptoms in children. *Journal of Clinical Child and Adolescent Psychology, 31*(3), 393–398.

Zito, J., Safer, D., dosReis, S., Gardner, J., Boles, M., & Lynch, F. (2000). Trends in the prescribing of psychotropic medications to preschoolers. *Journal of the American Medical Association, 283,* 1025–1030.

11

Attachment Disorders

BRIAN S. STAFFORD and CHARLES H. ZEANAH

Although attachment-disordered behavior has been described in the literature for more than 50 years, there was almost no research on attachment disorders until the mid-1990s. The delay has led to much confusion in the lay, social care, and professional circles regarding terminology, focus, breadth, and significance of attachment-disordered behavior. Some of the confusion comes from the disparity between clinical research into attachment-disordered behavior and the exponential expansion of developmental research on attachment theory in typical and atypical populations. Also contributing to this confusion is the lack of empirically sound treatments for attachment disordered and other socially disordered behavior.

In this chapter, we first review a developmental perspective on attachment, with special attention to the preschool period and attachment behavioral strategies and internal representations of attachment in preschool children. Next, we review the phenomenology of the reactive attachment disorder (RAD) construct, including what is known about signs of disordered attachment in children within institutions, children adopted out of institutions, and abused/neglected children in foster care. We also review what is known and unknown regarding prevalence and longitudinal course of RAD. Finally, we offer guidelines for assessment and treatment of preschool children with these disorders, including treatments to be avoided.

DEVELOPMENT OF ATTACHMENT

The fundamental goal of the attachment system is to ensure survival of offspring by promoting mutual proximity of infants and caregivers, thereby providing protection from danger. To ensure proximity-seeking behavior, infants

231

must have the ability to reference and respond to their caregivers' signals and to signal their caregivers. Although the evolutionary goal of this motivational system is proximity seeking, another function of this system is to regulate the infant's developing emotional states. The attachment system also motivates young children to seek comfort, support, nurturance, and protection from discriminated attachment figures.

Since children are not born attached to their caregivers, they must learn through their experiences to develop a preference for an attachment figure who will meet their needs (Ainsworth, 1967; Bowlby, 1982). Human infants appear to develop the capacity to form a preferred attachment to a caregiver by the latter part of the first year of life under species-typical circumstances. Infants become attached to caregivers with whom they have had significant social interaction through an unfolding developmental process. At birth the infant shows *undiscriminating responsiveness* to people through behavioral signaling (Stage I). From age 2–3 months the infant demonstrates continuing responsiveness to other people but begins to show *differential responsiveness* to its mother and other primary caregivers (Stage II). Important changes in cognitive, emotional, communicative, and memory development occur at around 6 to 7 months. The onset of locomotion (crawling and walking) allows children to display new attachment behaviors (following, establishing a secure base, refueling, *proximity maintenance* [Stage III], returning to a safe haven, and burying their face in the mother's lap, and, finally, differential clinging to mother when distressed [Ainsworth, 1967]. Elaboration of cognitive skills and memory allows for the development of a rudimentary "internal working model" that allows the infant to achieve an end goal of "proximity" and to select behaviors that will help to accomplish this. Expansion of communicative skills allows for further visual and vocal engagement, and signaling with others. Finally, in the preschool years, further cognitive, communicative, and emotional development allow for the formation of the *goal-corrected partnership* seen in the toddler and preschool years (Stage IV).

The attachment system is complemented by other important behavioral systems, including the *exploratory system,* the *wariness system*, and the *sociable/affiliative system*. The exploratory system, fueled by the newfound skills of locomotion, enhances the infant's ability to learn and interact with the physical and social environment. The attachment and exploratory systems frequently act in concert. When the child feels comfortable with a caregiver's availability, attachment is readily deactivated and the child will likely explore the immediate environment. However, if the attachment system is activated by fear or distress, exploration ceases, seeking proximity to the caregiver becomes primary, and the motivation to explore diminishes. The sociable/affiliative system motivates the young child to engage socially with others. Wariness in novel situations has obvious survival value. The behaviors associated with these systems are coordinated in such a manner that they inhibit or potentiate one another.

What is observed between 6 and 12 months is that the infant begins to define sharply an attachment to its mother, with a striking decline in friendliness to others, and "maintenance of proximity to a discriminated figure by means of locomotion as well as signals" (Bowlby, 1969, p. 267). Protests at the mother's departure also develop. Ainsworth interpreted this as indicating that the infant had formed a "mental representation" of the mother. The attachment figure also serves as a "secure base" from which the child may explore the environment and as a "safe haven" to whom the child returns when stressed. In addition, from ages 12–14 months, the infant begins to show developing attachments to figures other than the primary caregiver and may develop a hierarchy of attachment figures.

The Strange Situation procedure (SSP; Ainsworth et al., 1978) is a laboratory procedure designed to evaluate the organization of child behaviors at a time of low and high attachment stress to reveal patterns of balancing the motivation to explore the environment and the motivation to seek comfort from a discriminated attachment figure. The SSP consists of eight discrete episodes designed to increasingly activate the infant's attachment system through interactions with an attachment figure and a stranger. Much of the behavior observed during the SSP is a balance between the infant's wariness, exploratory, and sociable behavioral systems, and the attachment system. Patterns of attachment in the SSP are derived from the organization of behaviors the infant displays toward familiar and unfamiliar adults during a series of brief, controlled separations and reunions when the infant is between 12 and 20 months of age.

Secure, avoidant, and ambivalent attachments are "organized" patterns, whereas avoidant and ambivalent patterns are also known as insecure strategies, and a disorganized attachment is considered nonorganized (Table 11.1). A secure attachment demonstrates a comfortable balance between infants' attachment and exploratory systems. *Securely attached* infants use the caregiver as a *secure base* from which to explore. *Insecure–avoidant* infants seem to be preoccupied with exploration, though aware of the caregiver. *Insecure–resistant* infants are reluctant to leave the caregiver to explore and may become fretful

TABLE 11.1. Classifications of Attachment in Toddlers and Preschoolers

Author (year)	Secure strategies	Insecure strategies			
Ainsworth, Blehar, Waters, & Wall (1978)	Secure	Avoidant	Resistant	Disorganized	Unclassifiable
Cassidy & Marvin (1987)	Secure	Avoidant	Dependent	Controlling/ disorganized	Insecure/other
Crittenden (2000)	Balanced	Defended	Coercive	Defended/ coercive	Anxious/ depressed	Insecure /other
	Organized strategies			Not organized strategies	

even before her departure. They are extremely distressed by her departure, but greet her return with a mixture of contact seeking and rejection (resistance to comfort or contact). Infants with *disorganized* attachments demonstrate atypical reunion behaviors, such as dissociative or disoriented episodes, as well as a combination of secure, avoidant, and ambivalent behaviors that are poorly integrated (Main & Solomon, 1986).

These patterns have been correlated with observations of parental care preceding the SSP evaluation. Infants who demonstrated a secure attachment in the SSP have caregivers that are observed to be emotionally responsive to their infants' distress and bids for comfort. Infants with insecure–avoidant attachments have caregivers that are striking in their aversion to providing physical comfort and that express little emotion to their infants. Finally, caregivers of insecure–resistant/ambivalent infants respond inconsistently to their infant's bids. Disorganized attachments are associated with high-risk environments and are supposed to be attachment sequelae of threatening, frightening or dissociated caregiving (Main & Hesse, 1990). This pattern is thought to represent the simultaneous activation of the attachment system and the fear/wariness system. This yoking presents the infant with an inherent conflict. Fear of the parent activates the attachment system and the drive for proximity; however, as proximity increases, the fear does as well, which may lead to contradictory approaches. In these scenarios, the attachment figure is both the *solution* and the *source* of the attachment alarm.

To summarize, infants develop attachments to caregivers with whom they have had significant social interaction. The Strange Situation attachment "classification" that they develop is a laboratory pattern of behaviors representing the balance of their exploratory, sociable, wariness, and attachment systems, and that has been validated against naturalistic patterns of interaction in the home.

Attachment in Preschoolers

As children enter the preschool period, they make increasing excursions into other physical and social environments. Although separation distress becomes less evident and refueling periods become briefer as the child develops, attachment is no less important. Rather, gradually less physical contact with the attachment figure in times of distress is required as attachment becomes less directly tied to observable behavior. Further development of motor locomotion, communicative ability, and cognitive processing lead to significant changes in the behaviors and internal working models associated with attachment behaviors. Marvin and Greenberg (1982) suggested that there is a developmental coupling of the wariness and sociable systems and a decoupling of the attachment and sociable systems. This allows preschoolers the increased ability to deal with strangers on their own. In addition, preschoolers' expanding cognitive and emotional capacities allow them to develop an early understanding of the parents' own feelings and motives. These factors usher in what Bowlby (1982) described as a "goal-corrected partnership" with their caregiver.

Expectations regarding availability of attachment figures and their response to bids for proximity are largely settled by the preschool years. These include the strategies for managing the need for proximity and feelings of anger, fear, and desire for comfort. At this time the preschooler has developed an internal working model of how emotional regulation of the self is best achieved through interaction with the caregiver. This includes aspects of warmth, empathy, and nurturance, and trust and security. Other developmentally salient tasks of the preschool period that are pertinent to attachment include physical and psychological protection and vigilance/self-protection.

Preschool children, whose cognitive and linguistic skills are substantially more advanced than those of infants in the second year of life, seek opportunities to communicate with their attachment figures regarding their mutual access to one another. Without such communication, even children who expect, based upon past experiences, that their attachment figures will be available, if needed, may feel both anxiety and anger. Preschoolers increasingly organize their interactions with attachment figures on the basis of physical orientation, eye contact, nonverbal expressions, affect, and conversations about separations, reunions, feelings, shared activities, and plans.

Thus, although the SSP is typically implemented in preschool-age children identically to the way Ainsworth et al. (1978) originally described, behaviors salient for coding patterns of attachment are different. As shown in Table 11.1, there are two systems of classifying attachment in preschoolers. The Cassidy–Marvin system (Cassidy & Marvin, 1987) follows conceptually and practically as a developmental elaboration of the Ainsworth system for infants. The Crittenden (2000) dynamic–maturational approach to preschool attachment, on the other hand, represents a substantial departure from the traditional approach. This approach derives from Crittenden's assertion that, in the preschool period, there occurs a developmental reorganization of the child's processes for generating self-relevant meanings and for organizing strategic behaviors. In her system, the manner in which cognition (temporal ordering) and affect (display of emotion) are combined create the patterns of attachment seen in the SSP.

In both systems, attachment groups are distinguished by identifying the communicative or defensive goals that underlie attachment patterns. Rather than a correspondence of behavior to pattern of attachment, as was found in infancy, the behavior of children in the preschool years is considered in terms of its function for each child in the context of the dyadic relationship. Strategy, in other words, becomes the defining feature of pattern of attachment in the preschool years. As shown in Table 11.1, these strategies may be dichotomized as secure–insecure or as organized–not organized.

Attachment classifications, therefore, during this period take into account the child's ability to maintain protective proximity and the attachment figure's contribution to the interaction with the child. Because the attachment strategy is constructed interpersonally, it is considered a dyadic characteristic, not an individual feature. Unfortunately, preliminary findings suggest that the two systems share little agreement about how to classify attachment, although much more work is needed in this area to address this question.

Developmental research in attachment continues to grow exponentially. Ironically, however, clinical disorders of attachment have only recently received attention. For example, in Cassidy and Shaver's encyclopedic *Handbook of Attachment* (1999), there are over 2,000 references cited about attachment, but not a single reference to attachment disorders. This disparity points to the need for more attention to clinical disorders of attachment.

CLINICAL PERSPECTIVES ON DISTURBED ATTACHMENT: REACTIVE ATTACHMENT DISORDER

Concern about social behavior in maltreated and institutionalized children has been apparent from the early part of the 20th century. Nevertheless, RAD did not appear in formal nosologies until the third edition of the *Diagnostic and Statistic Manual of Mental Disorders* (DSM-III) was published (American Psychiatric Association, 1980). Even then, despite its potential importance, there were no published studies addressing its validity until 15 years later.

In the current DSM-IV-TR conceptualization, the disorder is defined by aberrant social behaviors that appear in early childhood and are evident across social contexts. Two unique patterns are defined: an emotionally withdrawn/inhibited pattern and an indiscriminately social/disinhibited pattern. DSM-IV-TR (American Psychiatric Association, 2000) defines RAD as a markedly disturbed and developmentally inappropriate social relatedness in most contexts, beginning before age 5 years, as evidenced by either restricted or indiscriminate social interaction. Developmental delay or autism cannot strictly account for the abnormal social relatedness. In addition, evidence of pathogenic care such as institutionalization, emotional or physical neglect, or multiple changes in primary caregivers, must be the basis for the behavioral abnormalities; that is, the described social abnormalities must be the result of "pathogenic care."

In keeping with the DSM-IV definition of psychopathology as located within the individual, RAD is not conceptualized as a relationship-specific disorder; rather, it is a disorder of social relatedness within the child, expressed across different relationships. An emotionally withdrawn/inhibited type and an indiscriminately social/disinhibited type have been described.

Emotionally Withdrawn/Inhibited RAD

The inhibited type is marked by the child's emotional withdrawal, failure of social and emotional reciprocity, and lack of seeking or responding to comfort when distressed. The child exhibits an absence of the expected tendency to initiate or respond appropriately to social interactions, exhibiting instead excessively inhibited, hypervigilant, or highly ambivalent reactions.

Attachment behaviors, such as seeking and accepting comfort, showing and responding to affection, relying on caregivers for help, and cooperating with caregivers, are absent or markedly restricted. In addition, exploratory behavior is frequently limited due to the absence of a preferred attachment figure. Children with this disorder may also demonstrate problems of emotion regulation that range from affective blunting to withdrawal, to "frozen watchfulness" (American Psychiatric Association, 2000, p. 127). This type has been described both in institutionalized children (Tizard & Rees, 1975; Zeanah et al., 2004) and in abused and neglected children (Boris et al., 2004; Zeanah et al., 2004). Notably, this type has not been identified in young children adopted out of institutions (see Chisholm, 1998; O'Connor & Rutter, 2000), perhaps because, once adopted, as young children form attachments, signs of the inhibited type disappear. There does not appear to be any critical or sensitive period for this finding. It is more likely an indicator that the emotional environment is markedly insufficient. Zeanah, Smyke, and Dumitrescu (2002) have suggested that the inhibited type of RAD is equivalent to the absence of a discriminated attachment in children who are cognitively capable of forming attachments. This explains their failure to seek or respond to comforting when distressed and their lack of differentiation among caregivers.

In keeping with this hypothesis, Smyke, Dumitrescu, and Zeanah (2002) reported that a substantial minority of institutionalized young children (13%) in Romania had signs of the emotionally withdrawn/inhibited type compared with very few signs in a never-institutionalized group of children. Furthermore, the frequency of the emotionally withdrawn/inhibited type of disorder was significantly lower (7%) in a unit that had fewer caregivers (four as opposed to 17 on typical units) regularly assigned to care for the children in a particular group. This provided these children with a greater opportunity to develop a focused attachment. It appears that emotionally withdrawn/inhibited attachment disorder in abused and neglected children may also be transient. Zeanah et al. (2004) found that symptoms of inhibition were reliably present 3 months after foster care, but other studies of ex-institutionalized infants did not reliably find these symptoms after a year in care (O'Connor, Brendenkamp, & Rutter, 1999; O'Connor & Rutter, 2000). According to a recent descriptive study, children may begin to organize attachments to new caregivers within days of placement (Stovall & Dozier, 2000). Behavioral symptoms of inhibition may eventually disappear, but it is not known whether these symptoms have developmental sequelae, such as social cognition, emotion regulation, or internal working models of close relationships.

Indiscriminately Social/Disinhibited RAD

This pattern is characterized by more child interaction with caregivers than that in the emotionally withdrawn/inhibited pattern but failure to demonstrate selectivity in interacting with others. Specifically, these young children will seek comfort, support and nurturance indiscriminately. Stranger wariness, which appears as early as 7 months of age and remains apparent for several years, is absent. Children exhibiting this type of RAD may approach strangers without appropriate social wariness and/or may seem overly familiar and overly comfortable with them. They may readily seek comfort or help from a stranger, and may demonstrate a variety of social relatedness problems that depend upon accurately reading social cues and understanding interpersonal boundaries.

This pattern of RAD has been observed in maltreated children soon after they are placed in foster care (Zeanah et al., 2004). It also has been observed in institutionalized young children (Zeanah et al., 2002), as well as in children adopted out of institutions (O'Connor & Rutter, 2000). Chisholm, Carter, Ames, and Morison (1995), for example, found greater rates of this socially abnormal behavior in children who had spent at least 8 months in an institution. These behaviors persisted over time, as they were evident at both 11 and 39 months postadoption. O'Connor, Bredenkamp, and Rutter (1999) also found high rates of disinhibited social behavior in previously institutionalized children adopted into English homes. Furthermore, a linear relationship was found that between the duration of early deprivation and the number of signs of indiscriminate behavior at ages 4 and 6 years. Along these lines, O'Connor and Rutter (2000) found that children exhibiting indiscriminate behavior at age 6 had experienced deprivation for twice as long (22 months) as children exhibiting no signs of indiscriminate behavior (11 months). Interestingly, even after children have developed a selective attachment to their adoptive parents they may continue to exhibit indiscriminate behavior (Chisholm, 1998; O'Connor, Marvin, Rutter, Olrick, & Brittner, 2002).

Importantly, in both maltreated and institutionalized children, signs of indiscriminately social/disinhibited RAD frequently co-occurred with signs of emotionally withdrawn/inhibited behavior (Zeanah et al., 2002, 2004). This led to criteria describing a mixed-type RAD in the recently described Research Diagnostic Criteria for Preschool Age (RDC-PA; American Academy of Child and Adolescent Psychiatry, 2004).

A Clinical/Developmental Divergence: RAD and Classifications of Attachment

To address the question of how Strange Situation classifications of attachment mapped onto clinical disorders of attachment, Boris and Zeanah (1999) proposed a spectrum of attachment disturbances, ranging from secure attachment (completely nondisturbed) to insecure, to disorganized, to secure base distortions, to reactive attachment disorder (completely disturbed). Until recently, there was no empirical testing of this proposed classification system. Results from several different samples have failed to support the spectrum, however, suggesting instead that the situation may be more complicated.

In her study of adopted Romanian infants, for example, Chisholm (1998) found no differences in indiscriminate friendliness between preschoolers classified as securely attached and as insecurely attached at 39 months of age. She also found that rates of secure attachment, as assessed by parental report, increased from 11 to 39 months in children who were institutionalized for at least 8 months, although indiscriminate friendliness did not diminish during this time. Likewise, O'Connor et al. (2000) found that a number of children classified as securely attached in a home-based SSP also exhibited indiscriminate behavior.

Further evidence also suggests that measures of attachment-disordered behavior diverge from laboratory measures of attachment behavior in institutions. Zeanah, Smyke, Koga, and Carlson (2003) compared a normative community preschool sample with an institutionalized group of Romanian children ages (11–31 months) with a battery of assessments of attachment and attachment-disordered behavior. They studied the children's relationship with their favorite caregiver—as reported by the caregivers—during the SSP, and also elicited from the caregiver signs of emotionally withdrawn/inhibited and indiscriminately social/disinhibited RAD, and objectively coded inhibited and disinhibited behavior observed in the SSP. They found that very few preschoolers (22%) in the institutions had organized an attachment to their favorite caregivers, whereas 78% of children living with their parents had organized attachments to their mothers. A significantly higher percentage of the institutionalized children (67.4%) than the home-reared children (22%) were classified as having disorganized attachments. In addition, 11% of the institutionalized group had so little attachment behavior that they could not even be classified disorganized, and instead received a designation of "unclassifiable." Surprisingly, having an organized attachment was not significantly related to caregiver ratings of signs of either emotionally withdrawn/inhibited RAD or indiscriminately social/disinhibited RAD.

In fact, the attachments among institutionalized children were so different that the investigators developed a new rating that assessed the degree to which a child had even formed an attachment to the caregiver. This was needed because many of the behaviors were so incompletely organized. A 5-point Likert scale was developed to identify fully formed attachments (5), developing attachments (2–4), and lack of attachment (1). Using this new approach, they found that only 3 of 95 institutionalized children were blindly rated as having fully formed attachments (scored as a 5), whereas all of the never-institutionalized children were rated as having fully formed attachments (Zeanah et al., 2003). Interestingly, in this sample, ratings of emotionally withdrawn/inhibited RAD were moderately intercorrelated ($r = .44$) with degree of attachment formation on the Likert scale, whereas ratings of indiscriminately social/disinhibited attachment were unrelated to degree of attachment formation. Taken together, these results suggest that clinical disturbances as reflected in signs of RAD are related to how fully developed and expressed attachment behaviors are, but not necessarily to the organization of any particular pattern of attachment.

Prevalence of RAD

The prevalence of RAD is unknown, but it is believed to be a rare condition. The number of children who are "at risk" for the disorder based upon "pathogenic care" is alarmingly high. In the United States, the number of children validated as having been maltreated by Child Protective Services approaches 2 million annually. Controversies regarding the definition and measurement challenges remain obstacles to assessing prevalence accurately.

Course of RAD

As noted, studies of young children adopted out of institutions after age 6 months have demonstrated that signs of indiscriminately social/disinhibited RAD tend to persist even after the dramatic environmental improvements that adoption is believed to entail (Chisholm, 1998; O'Connor and Rutter, 2000). Nevertheless, in the longest follow-up of children adopted out of institutions, signs of indiscriminate behavior persisted as long as 4 years in some children assessed at the age of 8 years (Tizard & Hodges, 1978). When these children were 16 years old, indiscriminate behavior was not as readily identified, but superficial and indiscriminate peer relations were evident in those children who had previously shown indiscriminate behavior with caregivers (Hodges & Tizard, 1989). These findings are important in suggesting that heterotypical continuity or developmental transformation of children with the disorder, or with the core signs of indiscriminate sociability, may occur. The developmental transformation of core symptom manifestation must be considered as more longitudinal studies of children previously diagnosed with RAD appear and define the course of the disorder more accurately.

The course of the emotionally withdrawn/inhibited pattern of RAD appears to be quite different; that is, this form of disorder is readily identifiable in young children who are institutionalized (Smyke et al., 2002) but is not described in children adopted out of institutions (O'Connor & Rutter, 2000; Chisholm, 1998). These findings suggest that the disorder resolves once a child is placed in a stable and nurturing environment.

The sequelae of either subtype of the disorder are understudied; however, all three studies examining patterns of attachment have found more than 40% of children exhibit atypical insecure patterns several years after adoption (Chisholm, 1998; Marcovitch et al., 1997; O'Connor, et al., 2002). Importantly, the consequences of these aberrant attachment patterns for children's subsequent psychological and social adjustment remains unclear.

ASSESSMENT OF RAD

No established protocol exists for diagnosing RAD. There is, however, promising support for the utility of structured observations and interviews (Boris et al., 2004). Since clinical observations of inhibited and disinhibited behavior are central to the diagnosis, they serve as a natural starting point (O'Connor & Zeanah, 2003). Observations of infants' responses toward caregivers and toward strangers are essential. In addition, structured episodes that activate the wariness system, as in the SSP separations, allow clinicians to observe attachment behaviors upon reunion and to contrast behavior toward an attachment figure and a stranger. Unfortunately, at this point, there is no "gold standard" procedure that definitively diagnoses or classifies either the emotionally withdrawn/inhibited pattern or the indiscriminately social/disinhibited pattern. The SSP is limited in its ability to elicit current RAD criteria (Boris, Fueyo, & Zeanah, 1997), although separation and reunion responses are indeed clinically relevant in cases of disorganization/disorientation, role reversal, and controlling behaviors. Although observational research paradigms show promise (Boris et al., 2004), a clinical assessment should include observation of free-play with caregivers and arousal of the attachment system by separations and reunions with caregivers and strangers, and/or the introduction of a potentially arousing novel object to sense whether the child (1) becomes distressed, (2) uses others for comfort, and (3) has a preference for the caregiver.

Likewise, although there is no "gold standard" interview, several groups have demonstrated the adequacy of semistructured clinical interviews in the identification of disordered attachment behaviors (Smyke, Dumitrescu, & Zeanah, 2002; O'Connor & Rutter, 2000). The interview should cover all of the possible symptoms associated with all descriptions of RAD and explore the contextual determinants of the behavior, as well as the course of these behaviors. The use of parent-based questionnaires has inherent difficulties that should be considered. Since clinicians have difficulty agreeing upon diagnostic criteria, it is likely that parents will have different understandings of such 169attachment disorder," " indiscriminate sociability," and so forth.

At present, we recommend detailed observations in naturalistic and clinical settings, as well as obtaining multiple focused reports from caregivers. This approach must suffice until further empirical clarifications of the diagnostic features are available. At this point, it is most important to observe general social relatedness, as well as specific attachment behaviors, between the preschoolers and the primary caregivers.

Comorbidity/Differential Diagnosis

Mental Retardation/Cognitive Delays

Infants do not form selective attachments until they are 7 to 9 months of age. Consequently, it does not make sense to diagnose an attachment disorder in children who have not yet attained a cognitive age of 9 or 10 months. Because psychosocial neglect is often associated with cognitive delays and RAD, young children with RAD often present with comorbid developmental delays, though exact rates of comorbidity are not yet available (O'Connor et al., 1999, Zeanah, 2000). Thus, from a clinical perspective, it is important to ascertain a young child's developmental or cognitive age, if RAD is suspected, to determine whether the child is capable of having formed selective attachments and to determine whether cognitive delays are present and should also be targeted for treatment.

Autism Spectrum Disorders

DSM-IV-TR criteria specify that children diagnosed with pervasive developmental disorder (PDD) may not also be diagnosed with RAD, though this requirement has been criticized on empirical and logical grounds (Zeanah, 1996).

Distinguishing between PDD and RAD may be a diagnostic challenge. There are similarities in the clinical pictures between children with autism spectrum disorders (ASDs) and children with emotionally withdrawn/inhibited type RAD that require careful assessment, and in some children, distinguishing between the two disorders is complicated. Preschoolers diagnosed with ASDs as well as those with RAD, emotionally withdrawn/inhibited type, demonstrate deficits in reciprocal social interaction, as well as deviant emotional regulation. Also complicating the picture is that children with ASDs frequently have cognitive delays and stereotypies, conditions that are also frequently observed with institutionalization or profound neglect, and are therefore frequently seen in young children with RAD.

One obvious distinguishing feature is that ASDs most often occur in the absence of extreme psychosocial deprivation. Because severe deprivation is associated with "quasi-autistic" syndromes (Rutter et al., 1999), one can definitely rule out RAD if there is no history of severe deprivation, but one cannot rule out either disorder in the presence of a history severe deprivation.

Deficits in joint attention, language abnormalities, and selective impairment in symbolic play are characteristic of ASDs, but in children with emotionally withdrawn/inhibited type RAD, there is no reason to expect these developmental functions to be impaired in the absence of cognitive delay above the 18-month age level.

There are also important differences in social behavior. Children with RAD should not manifest the restricted and peculiar interests of children with PDD. Furthermore, children with PDD spectrum disorders do form selective attachments, although their attachment behaviors may be unusual, including stereotypies that normally lead to a disorganized classification (Capps, Sigman, & Mundy, 1994).

Posttraumatic Stress Disorder

Children who have been abused, or who have witnessed violence, may show fear, clinging, or withdrawal from caregivers (Hinshaw-Fuselier, Boris, & Zeanah, 1999). These signs are consistent not only with the hyperarousal and avoidant clusters of a preschooler's posttraumatic symptomatology (Scheeringa,

Peebles, Cook, & Zeanah, 2001) but also the inhibited, hypervigilant, or highly ambivalent and contradictory responses described in DSM-IV-TR RAD criteria. Clearly, abuse and exposure to domestic violence qualify as "pathogenic care," but it is uncertain whether these symptoms should primarily be considered as posttraumatic stress disorder (PTSD) or RAD, emotionally withdrawn/inhibited type. Surprisingly, few data are available to clarify this clinical distinction; no studies to date have assessed abused and neglected children for both PTSD and RAD. Scheeringa, Zeanah, Drele, and Larrieu (1995) reported that children who had experienced chronic, enduring traumas rather than discrete, "single-blow" traumas were more likely to demonstrate numbing of responsiveness, and this is reminiscent of the emotional blunting that characterizes RAD, emotionally withdrawn/inhibited type. At this point, we recommend systematic assessment and careful consideration of both disorders in children with histories of significant maltreatment.

Conduct Disorder

There has been much confusion with regard to older children and adolescents about RAD and psychopathy (Zeanah, 2000; International Classification of Diseases [ICD-10]); that is, some have asserted that children exhibiting aggression, victimization of others, stealing, lying, defiance, bossiness, cruelty to animals, destruction of property or self, defiance, intense displays of anger or rages, and a grandiose sense of self have attachment disorders. These so-called "signs and symptoms" of RAD are behaviors and problems commonly found in symptomatic maltreated children, but are not appropriately classified using conventional definitions of RAD.

In fact, there are no well-validated means of measuring attachment in school-age children, and as such, there are few reliable indicators of attachment disordered behavior in this age group. RAD, emotionally withdrawn/inhibited type, has not been described in school-age children, although indiscriminate sociability has been described (O'Connor et al., 2002; Tizard & Hodges, 1978).

Although it appears that institutional care and abuse/neglect may be associated with externalizing behavior disorders (Egger, Smyke, Koga, & Zeanah, 2005; Reams, 1999), conduct disorder in young children has not been formally assessed. The relation between these externalizing problems and signs of attachment disorder appears to be limited, however (O'Connor & Zeanah, 2003). From a clinical perspective, however, it seems prudent to assess children with histories of maltreatment or institutional care for both RAD, indiscriminately social/disinibited type, and conduct disorder, because they may co-occur.

Attention-Deficit/Hyperactivity Disorder

Young children with RAD, disinhibited type, demonstrate a persistent pattern of socially impulsive behavior. These behaviors must be distinguished from the impulsivity that characterizes attention-deficit/hyperactivity disorder (ADHD). Complicating the distinction is evidence that a syndrome of inattention and overactivity may develop in the context of institutionalization (Kreppner et al., 2001; Roy, Rutter, & Pickles, 2004). Signs of inattention–overactivity are correlated with duration of deprivation among institutionalized children and may constitute an institutional–deprivation syndrome. What remains to be determined is the similarity of this syndrome to more typical ADHD (Kreppner et al., 2001). Although ADHD and the disinhibited type of RAD may be associated with social impulsivity, there is no reason to expect children with indiscriminately social/disinhibited RAD to manifest inattention or hyperactivity. If, on the other hand, the child meets criteria for both disorders, both diagnoses should be assigned.

INTERVENTION FOR RAD

By definition, attachment disorders are encountered in children who have not experienced an opportunity to form lasting and supportive relationships. Common scenarios include children raised in institutions, placed in multiple foster care homes, or those who have had extremely adverse experiences with caregivers. Intervention, therefore, should take into account the developmental needs of preschoolers and their caregivers, as well as children's previous relationship experiences, current placement, and other significant relationships.

An assessment of parental fitness may be warranted if the child currently resides in a dangerous or destructive caregiving environment. If the child's safety cannot be ensured, removal of the child is mandated by law in all 50 states. Although placement in foster care necessarily disrupts the child's relationship with the primary caregiver, safety must be established as the first priority.

If children lack an attachment figure, providing them with one should be the next priority. Smyke, Wajda-Johnston, and Zeanah (2004), Zeanah and Smyke (2005) and others (e.g., Dozier, Lindhiem, & Ackerman, 2005) have outlined approaches designed to facilitate attachment between young maltreated children and their foster parents. Clearly, the younger the child at placement, the less likely clinical signs of disturbed attachment are to develop. In addition, what appears to be most crucial is an appropriate parental figure who can provide sustenance, stimulation, support, structure, and surveillance. In addition to these functions, clinicians and researchers have identified caregiver characteristics of attachment figures that are more likely to foster secure attachments in their children. Along these lines, Dozier, Stovall, Albus, and Bates (2001) found that foster parents who have autonomous narratives, as assessed by the Adult Attachment Interview (AAI), about their own experiences of receiving care from their parents were more likely to develop secure attachments with their foster children. Another interview, the Working Model of the Child Interview (WMCI; Zeanah & Benoit, 1995), assesses a caregiver's representation of a specific child and his or her relationship with that child. *Balanced* narratives produced from this measure are similarly associated with security of attachment. These interviews assess the caregiver's ability to discuss and reflect upon caregiving experiences (AAI), and to take an emotional perspective about this child's experiences, circumstances, personality, and his or her own relationship with the child (WMCI).

Children with RAD and their caregivers typically come from impoverished settings and may require numerous social agencies to address their significant physical needs. As a result, their needs may be best approached through an organized community system of care (Marx, Benoit, & Kamradt, 2003; Klaehn & Martner, 2003). A template of treatment typically includes referral and case management from social service and developmental agencies, education regarding the child's developmentally appropriate individual needs, and further assessments of the child and the caregiving relationship to determine the appropriate therapeutic approach. More affluent families that foster or adopt toddlers with attachment disturbances may not require the system of care approach, but they also benefit from educational, development, and therapeutic environs. In addition, in cases of foster parenting or adoption, it is important to identify the caregiver's motivation to become the caregiver of a nonbiological child.

After placement in care, determining whether reunification is possible, or whether the child should be freed for adoption should be implemented immediately. Clinical approaches designed to minimize harm to the child in the context of disrupted relationships have been advocated (Smyke et al., 2004; Zeanah & Smyke, 2005). These approaches emphasize building new attachment relationships and helping the child gradually transition from one setting to the next. Disruptions in placement can be very disturbing to young children and should be kept to a minimum; however, certain circumstances may necessitate a disruption. Throughout, it is necessary to maintain a focus on the child's best interests while determining whether reunification or termination of parental rights and adoption is indicated.

Some significant and common caregiver barriers to intervention include depression, substance abuse, unresolved trauma/loss, and domestic violence. Immediate referral to address these concerns is warranted. Clinicians commonly identify disordered attachment behaviors by the child as a barrier to a successful relationship. Caregivers frequently highlight disordered sleep and feeding behaviors, as well as excessive tantrum and aggressive behaviors, as barriers to mutually rewarding relationships.

Although no studies to date have evaluated specific psychotherapeutic approaches to young children with RAD, it stands to reason that the treatment should be relationship-focused, aimed at enhancing–building–reconstructing the caregiver–child relationship. A number of attachment-based interventions (see Lieberman & Zeanah, 1999, for a review) have been applied and shown to be effective for parent–infant dyads at high risk for insecurity.

Nevertheless, no studies have compared attachment-based interventions with alternative interventions, and the mechanisms underlying treatment response are unclear.

Child–parent dyadic psychotherapy is a multifaceted intervention that combines insight-oriented psychotherapy, unstructured developmental guidance, emotional support, and concrete assistance to caregivers and their toddlers (see Van Horn & Lieberman, Chapter 16, this volume). This method uses joint or "dyadic" work with the caregivers and toddlers, with the ultimate goal of improving parent–toddler relationships and the child's socioemotional functioning by providing a therapeutic relationship characterized by flexibility and receptiveness to the parent's and the child's needs. Interactions between dyads are observed and serve as a catalyst to the caregiver's affective experience, as well as a link to her own relationship experiences both in the past and the present. Enduring changes in the parent's and child's experiences of one another occur through the corrective emotional experience with the therapist and with each other during sessions.

Interaction guidance (McDonough, 2004) is a dyadic therapy designed to meet the needs of families who have not previously been successfully engaged in treatment and may be overburdened by poverty, lack of education, large family size, substance abuse, inadequate housing, and lack of social support. The interaction guidance approach assists family members in gaining enjoyment from their relationships with their child and in developing an understanding of their child's behavior through an experience of interactive play. Through immediate and reflective viewing of videotaped play interactions, the caregiver is praised for his or her appropriate interactive strengths. Parent-initiated discussions of more troublesome interactions may also become a focus of treatment.

Another treatment informed by attachment theory is the novel group therapy known as the Circle of Security (Marvin, Cooper, Hoffman, & Powell, 2002). The group protocol consists of a 20-week parent education and psychotherapy intervention designed to shift patterns of attachment–caregiving interactions in high-risk caregiver–child dyads to a more appropriate developmental pathway. With the use of edited videotapes of their interactions with their children, caregivers are encouraged to increase their sensitivity and appropriate responsiveness to their children's signals relevant to moving away from the caregiver to explore, and moving back for comfort and soothing. The treatment also focuses on increasing caregivers' ability to reflect on their own and their child's behavior, thoughts, and feelings regarding their attachment–caregiving interactions; and to reflect on experiences in their own histories that affect their current caregiving patterns.

Treatments to Be Avoided

Although the empirical evidence base for treatment of RAD remains thin, there is a group of treatments that we believe should be avoided. These treatments are known as "attachment therapy," "holding therapy," "rage reduction therapy," and "rebirthing therapy," among other names, but they all share certain core features. First, this group of treatments describes children with RAD as having suppressed rage that results from an early trauma and leads to behavioral problems, shallow emotions, and manipulative and insincere relations with others. Treating this form of RAD, supposedly an early manifestation of later antisocial behavior, in which the child actively resists attachment to others, requires that the resistance be "broken." The treatment for this disorder include various coercive methods to enrage the child, in order to have him or her express the suppressed rage, and to demonstrate that the parent is in charge.

These therapies have been severely criticized for lacking a coherent rationale and any meaningful empirical support (Mercer, 2002, 2003). Although establishing parental control may be an important part of therapy, the coercive techniques employed in holding therapy are unnecessary to achieve it and are inconsistent with both attachment theory and research (Lieberman & Zeanah, 1999). Second, these empirically unsupported treatments are also unacceptably dangerous: Six deaths have been attributed either to the therapeutic approaches themselves, or to parenting practices associated with them. Further contraindications are that obtaining compliance through coercive means runs the risk of retraumatizing already traumatized children and could therefore be psychologically harmful. Third, there is little support for the notion that anger and catharsis can be therapeutic. In fact, there is a strong clinical consensus that expressing anger over previous maltreatment is, in and of itself, unlikely to be therapeutic. Fourth, the emphasis on the linear connection between disturbed attachments and psychopathy is unsupported and lends itself to inaccurate scare tactics with vulnerable families. Furthermore, the emphasis on individual psychopathology in the child may lead to an unnecessary and unwise preoccupation with power, control, and dominance; may serve as a distraction from the relational nature of attachments; and may lead away from issues of the parent tracking and responding to the child's needs. For all of these reasons, many professional groups have denounced "attachment therapies" or "holding therapies" in official statements (see Boris & Zeanah, 2005; Chaffin et al., 2006).

CONCLUSIONS

RAD is a disorder of attachment and social relatedness affecting young children who have been severely neglected early in life. Though not well studied until the past decade, the disorder has been recognized for some time in young children who have been maltreated or raised in institutions. Many questions about the disorder remain unanswered, especially regarding why similar conditions of risk (i.e., neglect) give rise to such phenomenologically distinct forms of the disorder: an emotionally withdrawn/inhibited type and an indiscriminately social/disinhibited type. Furthermore, the long-term consequences of these disorders of early childhood are unclear, although increased risk for aberrant patterns of attachment even years after adoption suggest that early adverse experiences may not be completely remediated.

REFERENCES

Ainsworth, M. D. S. (1964). Patterns of attachment behavior shown by the infant in interaction with his mother. *Merrill–Palmer Quarterly, 1,* 51–58.

American Academy of Child and Adolescent Psychiatry. (2003). *Policy statement: Coercive interventions for reactive attachment disorder.* Washington, DC: Author.

American Academy of Child and Adolescent Psychiatry Task Force on Research Diagnostic Criteria: Infancy and Preschool. (2003). Research diagnostic criteria for preschool children: The process and empirical support. *Journal of the American Academy of Child and Adolescent Psychiatry, 42,* 1504–1512.

Ainsworth, M. D. S. (1967). *Infancy in Uganda: Infant care and the growth of love.* Baltimore: Johns Hopkins University Press.

Ainsworth, M. D. S., Blehar, M., Waters, E., & Wall, S. (1978). *Patterns of attachment: A psychological study of the Strange Situation.* Hillside, NJ: Erlbaum.

American Professional Society on the Abuse of Children. (2005). *Report of the APSAC task force on attachment therapy, reactive attachment disorder, and attachment problems.*

American Psychiatric Association. (1980) *Diagnostic and statistic manual of mental disorders* (3rd ed., rev.). Washington, DC: Author.

American Psychiatric Association. (2000) *Diagnostic and statistic manual of mental disorders* (4th ed., text rev.). Washington, DC: Author.

American Psychiatric Association. (2002). *Position statement: Reactive attachment disorder.* Washington, DC: Author.

Boris, N. W., Fueyo, M., & Zeanah, C. H. (1997). The clinical assessment of attachment in children under five. *Journal of the American Academy of Child and Adolescent Psychiatry, 36,* 291–293.

Boris, N. W., Hinshaw-Fuselier, S. S., Smyke, A. T., Scheeringa, M., Heller, S. S., & Zeanah, C. H. (2004). Comparing criteria for attachment disorders: Establishing reliability and validity in high-risk samples. *Journal of the American Academy of Child and Adolescent Psychiatry, 43,* 568–577.

Boris, N. W., & Zeanah, C. H. (1999). Disturbances and disorders of attachment in infancy: An overview. *Infant Mental Health Journal, 20,* 1–9.

Boris, N. W., & Zeanah, C. H. (2005). Practice parameters for the assessment and treatment of children and adolescents with Reactive Attachment Disorder of Infancy and Early Childhood. *Journal of the American Academy of Child and Adolescent Psychiatry,* 44(11), 1206–1219.

Bowlby, J. (1969). *Attachment and loss. Volume 1.* New York: Basic Books.

Bowlby, J. (1982). Attachment and loss: Retrospect and prospect. *American Journal of Orthopsychiatry, 52*(4), 664–678.

Capps, L., Sigman, M., & Mundy, P. (1994). Attachment security in children with autism. *Development and Psychopathology, 6,* 249–262.

Cassidy, J., & Marvin. R. S. (1987). *Attachment organization in preschool children: Coding guideline.* Unpublished coding manual. Seattle: Mac Arthur Working Group on Attachment.

Cassidy, J., & Shaver, P. (Eds.). (2000). *Handbook of attachment.* New York: Guilford Press.

Chaffin, M., Hanson, R., Saunders, B. E., Nichols, T., Barnett, D., Zeanah, C., et al. (2006). Report of the APSAC Task Force on Attachment Therapy, Reactive Attachment Disorder, and Attachment Problems. *Child Maltreatment, 11*(1), 76–89.

Chisholm, K. (1998). A three year follow-up of attachment and indiscriminate friendliness in children adopted from Romanian orphanages. *Child Development, 69*(4), 1092–1106.

Chisholm, K., Carter, M. C., Ames, E. W., & Morison, S. J. (1995). Attachment security and indiscriminately friendly behavior in children adopted from Romanian orphanages. *Development and Psychopathology, 7*(2), 283–294.

Crittenden, P. M. (2000). A dynamic–maturational exploration of the meaning of security and adaptation: Empirical, cultural and theoretical considerations. In P. M. Crittenden & A. H. Claussen (Eds.), *The organization of attachment relationships: Maturation, culture, and context* (pp. 358–383). New York: Cambridge University Press.

Dozier, M., Lindhiem, O., & Ackerman, J. P. (2005). Attachment and biobehavioral catch-up: An intervention targeting specific identified needs of foster infants. In L. Berlin, Y. Ziv, L. Amaya-Jackson, & M. Greenberg (Eds.), *Enhancing early attachments: Theory, research, intervention, and policy.* New York: Guilford Press.

Dozier, M., Stovall, K. C., Albus, K., & Bates, B. (2001). Attachment for infants in foster care: The role of caregiver state of mind. *Child Development, 72*, 1467–1477.

Egger, H., Smyke, A. T., Koga, S., & Zeanah, C. H. (2005, April). *Psychiatric disorders in institutionalized children: Results of a randomized controlled trial.* Paper presented at the biennial meeting of Society for Research in Child Development, Atlanta, GA.

Hinshaw-Fuselier, S., Boris, N., & Zeanah, C. H. (1999). Reactive attachment disorder in maltreated twins. *Infant Mental Health Journal, 20*, 42–59.

Hodges, J., & Tizard, B. (1989). Social and family relationships of ex-institutional adolescents. *Journal of Child Psychology, Psychiatry, and Allied Disciplines, 30*, 77–97.

Klaehn, R., & Martner, J. (2003). A conceptual framework for an early childhood system of care. In A. J. Pumariega & N. C. Winters (Eds.), *The handbook of child and adolescent systems of care* (pp. 203–223). Hoboken, NJ: Wiley.

Kreppner, J. M., O'Connor, T., Rutter, M., & the English and Romanian Adoptees Study Team. (2003). Can inattention/overactivity be an institutional deprivation syndrome? *Journal of Abnormal Child Psychology, 29*, 513–528.

Lieberman, A. (2004). Child–parent psychotherapy. In A. Sameroff, S. McDonough, & K. Rosenblum (Eds.), *Treatment of infant–parent relationship disturbances.* New York: Guilford Press.

Lieberman, A., & Zeanah, C. H. (1999). Contributions of attachment theory to infant–parent psychotherapy and other interventions with infants and young children. In J. Cassidy & P. Shaver (Eds.), *Handbook of attachment* (pp. 555–574). New York: Guilford Press.

Main, M., & Hesse, E. (1990). Parent's unresolved traumatic experiences are related to infant disorganized attachment status: Is frightened and/or frightening parental behavior the linking mechanism? In M. T. Greenberg, D. Cicchetti, & E. M. Cummings (Eds.), *Attachment in the preschool years: Theory, research, and intervention* (pp. 161–182). Chicago: University of Chicago Press.

Main, M., & Solomon, J. (1986). Discovery of an insecure–disorganized/disoriented attachment pattern. In T. B. Brazelton & M. W. Yogman (Eds.), *Affective development in infancy* (pp. 95–124). Norwood, NJ: Ablex.

Marcovitch, S., Goldberg, S., Gold, A., Washington, J., Wasson, C., Krekewich, K., et al. (1997). Determinants of behavioural problems in Romanian Children Adopted in Ontario. *International Journal of Behavioral Development, 1*, 17–31.

Marvin, R., Cooper, G., Hoffman, K, & Powell, B. (2002). The circle of security project: Attachment-based intervention with caregiver-preschool child dyads. *Attachment and Human Development, 4*, 107–124.

Marvin, R., & Greenberg, M. (1982). Preschoolers changing conceptions of their mothers: A social cognitive study of mother–child attachment. In D. Forbes & M. T. Greenberg (Eds.), *New directions for child development: No. 18. Children's planning strategies* (pp. 47–60). San Francisco: Jossey-Bass.

Marx, L., Benoit, M., & Kamradt, B. (2003). Foster children in the child welfare system. In A.

J. Pumariega & N. C. Winters (Eds.), *The handbook of child and adolescent systems of care* (pp. 332–352). Hoboken, NJ: Wiley.

McDonough, S. (2004). Interaction guidance. In A. Sameroff, S. McDonough, & K. Rosenblum (Eds.), *Treatment of infant–parent relationship disturbances* (pp. 79–96). New York: Guilford Press.

Mercer, J. (2002). Attachment therapy: A treatment without empirical support. *Scientific Review of Medical Practice, 2,* 105–112.

Mercer, J. (2003). Violent therapies: The rationale behind a potentially harmful child psychotherapy. *The Scientific Review of Medical Practice, 3,* 27–37.

O'Connor, T. G., Bredenkamp, D., Rutter, M., & the English and Romanian Adoptees Study Team. (1999). Attachment disturbances and disorders in children exposed to early severe deprivation. *Infant Mental Health Journal, 20,* 10–29.

O'Connor, T. G., Marvin, R. S., Rutter, M., Olrick, T., & Brittner, P. A. (2002). Child–parent attachment following early institutional deprivation. *Development and Psychopathology, 15*(1), 19–38.

O'Connor, T. G., & Rutter, M. (2000). Attachment disorder behavior following early severe deprivation: Extension and longitudinal follow-up. *Journal of the American Academy of Child and Adolescent Psychiatry, 39,* 703–712.

O'Connor, T. G., & Zeanah, C. H. (2003). Attachment disorders: Assessment strategies and treatment approaches. *Attachment and Human Development, 5,* 223–244.

Reams, R. (1999). Children birth to three entering the state's custody. *Infant Mental Health Journal, 20,* 166–174.

Roy, P., Rutter, M., & Pickles, A. (2004). Institutional care: Associations between overactivity and lack of selectivity in social relationships. *Journal of Child Psychology, Psychiatry and Allied Disciplines, 45*(4), 866–873.

Rutter, M., Andersen-Wood, L., Beckett, C., Bredenkamp, D., Castle, J., Groothues, C., et al. (1999). Quasi-autistic patterns following severe early global privation. English and Romanian Adoptees (ERA) Study Team. *Journal of Child Psychology and Psychiatry, 40*(4), 537–549.

Scheeringa, M., Peebles, C., Cook, C., & Zeanah, C. H. (2001). Towards establishing the procedural, criterion, and discriminant validity of PTSD in early childhood. *Journal of the American Academy of Child and Adolescent Psychiatry, 40,* 52–60.

Scheeringa, M., Zeanah, C. H., Drell, M., & Larrieu, J. (1995). Two approaches to the diagnosis of post-traumatic stress disorder in infancy and early childhood. *Journal of the American Academy of Child and Adolescent Psychiatry, 34,* 191–200.

Smyke, A. T., Dumitrescu, A., & Zeanah, C. H. (2002). Disturbances of attachment in young children: I. The continuum of caretaking casualty. *Journal of the American Academy of Child and Adolescent Psychiatry, 41,* 972–982.

Smyke, A. T., Wajda-Johnston, V., & Zeanah, C. H. (2004). Working with young children in foster care. In J. D. Osofsky (Ed.), *Young children and trauma* (pp. 260–284). New York: Wiley.

Stovall, K. C., & Dozier, M. (2000). The development of attachment in new relationships: Single subject analyses for 10 foster infants. *Development and Psychopathology, 12,* 133–156.

Tizard, B., & Hodges, J. (1978). The effect of early institutional rearing on the development of eight-year old children. *Journal of Child Psychology and Psychiatry, 19,* 99–118.

Tizard, B., & Rees, J. (1975). The effect of early institutional rearing on the behavioral problems and affectional relationships of four-year-old children. *Journal of Child Psychology and Psychiatry, 27,* 61–73.

World Health Organization. (1992). *The ICD-IO classification of mental and behavioral disorders: Clinical descriptions and diagnostic guidelines.* Geneva: Author.

Zeanah, C. H. (1996). Beyond insecurity: A re-conceptualization of attachment disorders of infancy. *Journal of Consulting and Clinical Psychology, 64,* 42–52.

Zeanah, C. H. (2000). Disturbances of attachment in young children adopted from institutions. *Journal of Developmental and Behavioral Pediatrics, 21,* 230–236.

Zeanah, C. H., & Benoit, D. (1995). Clinical applications of a parent perception interview in infant mental health. *Child and Adolescent Psychiatry Clinics of North America, 4,* 539–554.

Zeanah, C. H., Scheeringa, M. S., Boris, N. W., Heller, S. S., Smyke, A. T., & Trapani, J. (2004). Reactive attachment disorder in maltreated toddlers. *Child Abuse and Neglect: The International Journal, 28,* 877–888.

Zeanah, C. H., & Smyke, A. T. S. (2005). Building attachment relationships following maltreatment and severe deprivation. In L. Berlin, Y. Ziv, L. Amaya-Jackson, & M. Greenberg (Eds.), *Enhancing early attachments* (pp. 195–216). New York: Guilford Press.

Zeanah, C. H., Smyke, A. T., & Dumitrescu, A. (2002). Disturbances of attachment in young children: II. Indiscriminate behavior and institutional care. *Journal of the American Academy of Child and Adolescent Psychiatry, 41,* 983–989.

Zeanah, C. H., Smyke, A., Koga, A., & Carlson, E. (2003, May). *Attachment in institutionalized children.* Paper presented at the biennial meeting of the Society for Research in Child Development, Tampa, FL.

12

Autism Spectrum Disorders

SOMER L. BISHOP and CATHERINE LORD

Autism, a neurodevelopmental disorder that emerges in early childhood and persists throughout the lifespan, is one of a spectrum of disorders, which includes Asperger syndrome, pervasive developmental disorder not otherwise specified (PDD NOS), childhood disintegrative disorder (CDD), and Rett syndrome. These disorders are currently classified under the umbrella term of pervasive developmental disorder (PDD) in both the fourth edition of the *Diagnostic and Statistical Manual of Mental Disorders* (DSM-IV; American Psychiatric Association, 1994) and the *International Classification of Diseases* (ICD-10; World Health Organization, 1992), but the term autism spectrum disorder (ASD) is now more commonly used. Given our current state of knowledge, ASD may be a more useful description, because it specifies autism as the prototype and includes other disorders in the spectrum based on their symptom overlap with autism. This better reflects current research suggesting that at least some of the disorders classified as PDD in the major diagnostic frameworks are differentiated from autism primarily by the severity, trajectory, or breadth of symptoms (e.g., atypical autism, PDD NOS, Asperger syndrome), whereas they are presumably differentiated from non-ASDs by a number of qualitative, developmental, and possibly biological factors. We discuss briefly the question of whether to include disorders with known etiologies (e.g., fragile X syndrome, tuberous sclerosis) that often have symptom overlap with autism.

According to DSM-IV and ICD-10, autism is characterized both by deficits in social reciprocity and communication, and by the presence of restricted and repetitive behaviors and/or interests. A diagnosis of autism is based on both the presence of abnormal behaviors and the absence of typical development. To receive a diagnosis of autism, a child must show abnormalities in so-

252

cial interaction and language, as used in social communication or symbolic/ imaginative play before the age of 3 years.

These onset criteria are notable for two reasons. First, they include children who do not yet have difficulties in all three of the areas that define autism. Thus, a child who has a language delay and speaks very rarely at age 2, but does not have any unusual repetitive behaviors at that time, could meet criteria for autism at age 3 in the event that he or she developed more obvious social difficulties and repetitive behaviors later in preschool years.

Second, children who, often retrospectively, are reported not to have shown any abnormalities or delays prior to age 3 are excluded from the autism classification, though they can receive other ASD diagnoses (PDD NOS, Asperger syndrome, CDD, or atypical autism) in DSM-IV and ICD-10. This aspect of the criteria is more controversial. A number of studies have indicated that classifying children with ASD on the basis of gross language measures, such as saying single words by 24 months or simple phrases by 36 months, is not predictive of later differences (Eisenmajer et al., 1998). The original distinction in ICD-10 and DSM-IV regarding onset was made to clarify the differences between autism and early-onset schizophrenia, which rarely occurs before adolescence (Kolvin, Ounsted, Richardson, & Garside, 1971). Because there is now a much better understanding of the differences between ASD and schizophrenia, specifying an onset criterion to make this distinction may be less necessary.

EARLY MANIFESTATIONS

The most common symptom first reported by parents is language delay, which is related to many other disorders that are more prevalent than ASDs. Recent studies suggest that there are often other signs of ASD before the end of the first year of life (Baranek, 1999; Werner, Osterling, & Dawson, 2000), some of which may be specific to ASD (e.g., unusual eye contact), but others which are not (e.g., regulatory problems in children at 6 months).

Many parents first suspect that something is not quite right with their child's development when they notice that he or she is "not yet talking." "Not yet talking" has different meanings to different people, often depending on their experience with children. It may mean that a child does not babble as much as other 10- to 12-month-olds and likes to grunt in odd ways, or that he or she squeals in situations where other babies would coo or make word-like vocalizations. It may also mean that the child does not engage in reciprocal social games (e.g., peekaboo) with vocalizations, or that he or she is not yet trying to say words or imitate sounds (e.g., animal sounds). If their child does not say any words by 12–18 months, parents frequently consult their pediatrician, and they often become more adamant about seeking help as their child turns 2, particularly if he or she has tantrums or other difficult behaviors. Thus, deficits in communication may often first be present in infancy, be recognized as such in early preschool, and continue throughout adolescence and adulthood (Lord & Risi, 2000). Particularly in firstborn children, deficits in social reciprocity are often not recognized until later and, at least until recently, were most easily diagnosed in older preschool and early school-age children (Lord, 1995; De Giacomo & Fombonne, 1998; Wetherby et al., 2004).

When sufficiently sophisticated spoken language is acquired, children with autism may exhibit stereotyped, repetitive, or idiosyncratic language, as well as speech abnormalities in pitch, intonation, rate, rhythm, or stress (Cohen & Volkmar, 1997). A child with autism might speak in a monotone or with a singsong intonation, so that it is difficult to tell whether he or she is asking a question or making a comment (e.g., saying "This looks like a triangle?" to label something as a triangle). He or she might also repeat phrases that others have said in a stereotyped way, such as "Time to clean up, boys and girls," or recite dialogues from videos and television shows. Children with autism also tend to have difficulty initiating and sustaining conversation with others.

Reduced amounts of spontaneous, developmentally appropriate make-believe or social imitative play are also characteristic of autism. Deficits in play often manifest as the failure to use objects to represent other objects, such as using a stick as a sword or a cup as a miniature swimming pool. However, whether this is due to a true lack of ability, a lack of interest in representational play, or both, is not fully understood (Jarrold, Smith, Boucher, & Harris, 1994). Even when the child is clearly using imagination, a failure to enjoy sharing in pretend play is often present (Leslie, 1992).

Of the impairments included in the communication domain, delays in language comprehension are perhaps most specific to autism. For example, children with autism and fragile X syndrome were best discriminated from children with fragile X syndrome without autism by poorer scores on receptive language measures (Philofsky, Hepburn, Hayes, Hagerman, & Rogers, 2004). This holds true for very young children's deficits in understanding words out of context and for the difficulty that older preschool children with ASD have in understanding sentences (Lord, 1995). Expressive language delays and reduced imaginative play tend to be less helpful in diagnosing young preschoolers than impairments in nonverbal communication. Expressive language delays occur in many other conditions besides autism, and, the frequency and complexity of imaginative play in early preschool varies widely, which makes abnormalities in this area more difficult to detect (Lord, Rutter, & Le Couteur, 1994). By contrast, some of the most consistent impairments exhibited by children with ASD across various situations are impaired use of nonverbal behaviors, such as eye contact, facial expression, and gestures to regulate social interaction (Lord et al., 2000; Lord, Storoschuk, Rutter, & Pickles, 1993).

Children with autism generally show limited interest in other children, such as actively avoiding the approaches of their peers or failing to engage in joint play, but this may be difficult to detect in very young children who do not have contact with many other children. Children with autism also exhibit reduced amounts of showing, giving, and sharing enjoyment, and they initiate joint attention (i.e., directing another's attention to an interesting object that is out of reach just for the purpose of "sharing attention") less frequently than do children with other disorders (Mundy, Sigman, & Kasari, 1990; Mundy, Sigman, Ungerer, & Sherman, 1986).

The third area of functioning affected in children with ASD is restricted and repetitive behaviors and interests, which is the most heterogeneous domain within a diagnosis of ASD. This domain is also strongly affected by development, meaning that different types of behaviors and interests are observed with variable frequency and intensity at different developmental stages. For instance, although restricted and repetitive behaviors may not always be observed in children at age 2 with later diagnoses of ASD (Cox et al., 1999; Moore & Goodson, 2003), they contribute substantially to a diagnosis of autism at age 3 (Lord, 1995). Furthermore, some authors have suggested that one of the major distinctions between a diagnosis of autism and a diagnosis of PDD NOS is repetitive behaviors (Walker et al., 2004).

Children with autism often exhibit repetitive motor mannerisms, such as hand flapping or body rocking, and they may be preoccupied with parts of objects, such as the wheels of toy cars. A child with autism may insist on adhering to specific routines or rituals, such as taking a specific route to school each day, and/or may experience high levels of distress in response to minor changes in his or her environment, such as a parent's new haircut or an open door to a brother's bedroom. Children with autism also often have strong preoccupations, such as a fascination with stop signs or carpet lint, or circumscribed interests, which are typical interests that are abnormal in intensity (e.g., a strong interest in Disney characters).

Particularly when the focus is age-appropriate (i.e., dinosaurs or trains), a circumscribed interest can be difficult to detect in preschoolers with autism, because it is not always clear whether a strong interest is unusual or simply a favorite activity. One way to begin to make this distinction is to assess the degree to which the interest interferes with the child's ability to play with other toys. For example, is it possible to involve the child in activities that do not involve trains, or is he or she only interested in playing games that include that interest? This task may be complicated by the fact that, especially in preschoolers, the amount of time spent on an activity is as much determined by the parent as by the child (e.g., parents may buy toys and organize activities according to their child's interests). Additionally, preschool children with ASD may not yet have enough language to convey the level or nature of their interests, so it may be only after these children begin to talk more fluently that the intensity of their interest(s) becomes apparent (Lord, 1995).

Research suggests that even young preschool children with ASD show at least one restricted or repetitive behavior (Lord et al., 1993; Cox et al., 1999); however, unusual preoccupations and compulsions/rituals are less often reported in 2-year-olds than in older preschool children with ASD (Stone et al., 1999; Moore & Goodson, 2003).

DIFFERENTIAL DIAGNOSIS

One of the primary difficulties in diagnosing ASD in preschoolers is the overlap between features of ASD and features of other childhood psychological disorders, including, but not limited to, expressive and receptive language disorders, mental retardation, reactive attachment disorder, generalized anxiety disorder, and attention-deficit/hyperactivity disorder (ADHD). There is also substantial overlap between the symptoms of ASD and behavioral features of certain genetic conditions, such as fragile X syndrome and Angelman syndrome. Making diagnosis more complicated still is the fact that the disorders that make up the autism spectrum share so many commonalities. Even after a child is determined to be "on the autism spectrum," selecting the most appropriate diagnosis within the spectrum is often difficult.

Asperger Syndrome

According to the DSM-IV, Asperger syndrome is characterized by both qualitative impairments in social interaction and the presence of restricted and repetitive behaviors/interests that are identical to those seen in autism. Unlike autism, however, the definition of Asperger syndrome stipulates that there can be no clinically significant delay in language, cognitive development, or adaptive behavior (except social skills). Also, if an individual meets criteria for autism, CDD, or Rett syndrome, then he or she is to receive that diagnosis instead.

Although the ability of diagnosticians to differentiate between autism and other PDDs has been enhanced by recent advancements in diagnostic technology, there is still disagreement among clinicians and researchers about diagnostic criteria for differentiation within ASDs. Particularly with regard to Asperger syndrome, the field has been burdened by multiple definitions of the disorder and varied diagnostic frameworks, which has made it difficult for professionals to communicate (Ozonoff, South, & Miller, 2000). For example, whereas some research groups adhere to the strict DSM-IV definition when diagnosing Asperger syndrome for research and clinical purposes, other groups do not require that autism first be ruled out before making a diagnosis of Asperger syndrome (Szatmari, Bryson, Boyle, Streiner, & Duku, 2003).

This is an important issue, because the way Asperger syndrome is defined affects the way that autism and PDD NOS are diagnosed; that is, if mild cases of autism are referred to as Asperger syndrome or PDD NOS, then a diagnosis of autism will be more likely related to severe mental retardation (Klin et al., 2005). If Asperger syndrome is defined as any case of mild autism without mental retardation then children with PDD NOS will have lower IQs than if

Asperger syndrome has a narrower definition. If Asperger syndrome is to be useful as a diagnostic category, it is important to agree on one common definition of the disorder to ensure that researchers and clinicians from different centers are speaking a similar language. This is especially important when conducting studies that compare individuals with autism to individuals with Asperger syndrome, because the findings of such investigations are almost impossible to interpret when different diagnostic criteria are used at different sites.

Another disadvantage of having multiple definitions for the same label (or multiple labels for the same definition) is that parents are often left confused about what to make of their child's diagnosis. For example, partially as a result of the popular media, Asperger syndrome has come to be associated with savant skills, high intelligence, strong verbal skills, and other desirable qualities, whereas autism is more commonly associated with mental retardation, aloofness, and a grim prognosis. For parents of a child with ASD, their conceptualization of the disorder, including expectations about the future, is likely to be very different depending on whether the child receives a diagnosis of autism or Asperger syndrome. Parents may elect to have their child classified as having Asperger syndrome, because they hope he or she will eventually acquire strong language skills. Meanwhile, they may not get help to support their child's language development. Because of all of these concerns, current diagnostic guidelines organized by National Institute of Child Health and Human Development (NICHD) and National Institute on Deafness and Other Communication Disorders (NIDCD) multisite studies in the Collaborative Programs for Excellence in Autism (CPEA) recommended that a diagnosis of Asperger syndrome should be made only at or after age 5. Children under age 5 would then receive a diagnosis of autism, PDD NOS, or ASD instead of a diagnosis of Asperger syndrome.

Pervasive Developmental Disorder Not Otherwise Specified

The category of PDD NOS is intended for those children who exhibit severe abnormalities in the development of reciprocal social interaction, as well as either difficulties in communication or the presence of restricted and repetitive behaviors/interests, but do not meet criteria for autism, Asperger syndrome, Rett syndrome, or CDD. Cases in which a child does not meet criteria for autism because of late onset, atypical symptomatology, and/or subthreshold symptomatology are also included in the category of PDD NOS in DSM-IV. Although technically a category that describes atypical autism (ICD-10) or "not quite autism," depending on how specifically autism criteria are interpreted, PDD NOS often ends up functioning like a specific diagnosis (Buitelaar, Van der Gaag, & Klin, 1999). In fact, some studies have indicated that there are substantially more children within this category than in the category of autism (Chakrabarti & Fombonne, 2001).

Some authors have questioned to what degree PDD NOS is on the same continuum as autism (Towbin, 2003). As with Asperger syndrome, this partly depends on how broadly autism is defined, because it will affect whether children with PDD NOS appear to have a mild variant of autism or a qualitatively different disorder (Pomeroy, Friedman, & Stephens, 1991). In a comparison of children with PDD NOS, autism, and Asperger syndrome, children with PDD NOS had levels of functioning between those of children with autism and children with Asperger syndrome, but they exhibited fewer autism symptoms (especially repetitive and stereotyped behaviors) than both the autism and Asperger syndrome groups (Walker et al., 2004).

Most important for preschool children, evidence suggests that diagnoses of PDD NOS in early preschool are less stable than autism diagnoses (e.g., Stone et al., 1999). Not surprisingly, clinicians are able to make more reliable distinctions in 2-year-olds between autism spectrum disorder and nonspectrum diagnoses than between diagnoses of autism and PDD NOS, or PDD NOS and other nonspectrum diagnoses. These results suggest that PDD NOS is indeed on the same continuum as autism; whereas children rarely switch from diagnoses of autism spectrum to nonspectrum, it is not uncommon for children to change diagnoses within the spectrum (e.g., from a diagnosis of PDD NOS to autism; Stone et al., 1999; Lord et al., 2000; Lord, Risi, Shulman, & DiLavore, 2005).

From a clinical standpoint, which specific ASD diagnosis a child under age 3 receives is much less important than the fact that he or she falls somewhere on the autism spectrum. On the other hand, a specific diagnosis of autism sometimes qualifies a child for more services than a diagnosis of PDD NOS. The National Research Council (NRC) Report (2001) strongly recommended that all ASDs be considered within a single educational classification, even though types of interventions may vary greatly depending on the needs and skills of individual children. Clinicians who elect to use a broader term such as ASD or PDD NOS, or a less well-defined term such as Asperger syndrome for preschool children, should be careful not to imply that such a diagnosis means that the child will not someday also meet criteria for autism.

Child Disintegrative Disorder

Child Disintegrative Disorder is characterized by a period of apparently normal development followed by a significant regression around 2 years of age. To receive a diagnosis of CDD, the onset of the disorder must occur between the ages of 2 and 10 years, and the child must exhibit loss of previously acquired skills in two or more of the areas of expressive or receptive language, social skills or adaptive behavior, bowel or bladder control, play, or motor skills. Children with CDD must also exhibit impairments in two out of the three domains in autism (i.e., social interaction, communication, restricted and repetitive behaviors/interests; American Psychiatric Association, 1994).

Despite similarities in behavior, CDD differs from autism both in the timing of onset and the nature of the regression. Whereas children with CDD must have at least 2 years of typical development, abnormalities in children with autism are most often present in the first year of life (Osterling & Dawson, 1994). Furthermore, although about 20% of children with autism experience a regression in language or social behaviors (Lord, Shulman, & DiLavore, 2004), they typically do not lose adaptive or motor skills, as is seen in children with CDD (Volkmar & Rutter, 1995; Luyster et al., 2005). Also, the regression in children with autism is almost always before the age of 24 months (Lord et al., 2004).

Studies comparing children with CDD to children with autism have reported higher rates of epilepsy (Kurita, Osada, & Miyake, 2004; Moursiden, Rich, & Isager, 1999), more restricted and repetitive behaviors (Kurita et al., 2004; Malhotra & Gupta, 2002), and poorer long-term outcomes among children with CDD (Malhotra & Gupta, 2002). However, these findings have been somewhat inconsistent across studies. One question that has been proposed with regard to CDD is whether at least some cases of CDD are simply "late-onset" autism cases. But even in cases of late-onset autism, there is usually some evidence of preonset developmental abnormality, as opposed to apparently normal early development in children with CDD (Volkmar & Cohen, 1989).

Rett Syndrome

Rett syndrome is a neurological disorder that occurs almost exclusively in girls. It is associated with severe to profound mental retardation and physical disabilities (Kerr & Engerstrom, 2001). As is the case with CDD, the early development of children with Rett syndrome is apparently normal. Between the ages of 5 months and 48 months, their progress slows or arrests, and they experience a unique pattern of regression that differs from that experienced in CDD or autism. This regression is characterized by decelerated head growth, loss of previously acquired purposeful hand skills, such as building with blocks or doing simple puzzles, development of stereotyped midline hand movements (e.g., hand wringing or clapping), loss of social engagement, appearance of poorly coordinated gait or trunk movements (children may stop walking), and, if talking, severely impaired language development (American Psychiatric Association, 1994). During toddler and preschool years, children with Rett syndrome may meet behavioral criteria for ASD, though this is less the case in later years, in part because their physical symptoms become more apparent.

According to the current diagnostic classification system of DSM-IV, Rett syndrome falls under the umbrella of ASDs. However, because recent genetic discoveries have linked 80% of cases of Rett syndrome to a mutation in the methyl cytosine–binding protein 2 (MECP2; Amir et al., 1999; Dragich, Houwink-Manville, & Schanen, 2000), there is considerable debate in the field as to whether Rett syndrome still belongs on the autism spectrum. One reason for taking Rett syndrome out of the ASD category is that the term "spectrum" implies that disorders on the spectrum are not necessarily distinct, and may be expressions of the same disorder with varying levels of severity. Since the etiology of Rett syndrome is distinct from that of other ASDs, it is a separate disorder, despite considerable symptom overlap at certain periods of development. On the other hand, some argue that Rett syndrome shares important behavioral similarities with ASDs, and that ASDs actually have a variety of etiologies that may include MECP2, as well as fragile X, tuberous sclerosis, and other as yet not understood genetic patterns. One advantage of classifying Rett syndrome as an ASD is that, in some states in the United States, children with Rett syndrome will have access to more resources, including school services and insurance coverage (because some insurance companies do not cover genetic disorders), if they are diagnosed with an ASD.

A similar dilemma has arisen with genetic disorders such as fragile X syndrome. Approximately 20% of children with fragile X syndrome meet criteria for a diagnosis of ASD (e.g., Hatton & Bailey, 2001). Because the behavioral phenotype of fragile X includes autistic-like behaviors, professionals disagree about whether an additional diagnosis of ASD is appropriate in these children. The question is, when fragile X is characterized by certain "autistic" behaviors (e.g., poor eye contact), are they indicative of a comorbid ASD diagnosis, or simply part of the expression of fragile X syndrome?

These debates raise important questions about the diagnostic conceptualization of ASD. If autism is purely a behavioral disorder that may be a final common pathway from a number of sources, then a diagnosis of ASD should be made, if appropriate, in children whose behaviors result from known etiologies, such as in the case of genetic disorders, as well as unknown etiologies (which is the case for most children with ASD). If, however, autism is considered to be etiologically distinct from other disorders, then it would not be appropriate to diagnose ASD in children with other genetic or medical conditions. In any case, more research is needed to better define the degree to which specific autism symptoms are part of the behavioral phenotype of certain genetic disorders, and whether comorbid ASD diagnoses provide any new information in these populations, such as prognosis or response to different treatments.

EPIDEMIOLOGY

The prevalence of autism has recently become a point of contention, in part due to the rise in the number of autism cases reported during the past decade. For studies published between 1966 and 1991, the median prevalence rate of autism was 4.4 cases per 10,000. The median rate for studies published between 1992 and 2001, by contrast, was 12.7 cases per 10,000 (Fombonne, 2003). A combination of factors, such as increased awareness about the disorder, better diagnostic instruments, and broader diagnostic criteria, has contributed to at least part of the rise in number of autism cases during the past two decades. "Diagnostic substitution," which refers to assigning a label of autism instead of mental retardation for educational purposes, has also been proposed as a contributing factor to higher prevalence estimates, particularly when educational case records are used in epidemiological studies (Croen, Grether, & Hoogstrate, 2002; Wing & Potter, 2002). Some have theorized that environmental agents or components of vaccines are responsible for the increase in prevalence. There is no scientific evidence to support these specific claims, but environmental factors cannot be ruled out completely.

The rate of Asperger syndrome, which has generally been found to be less common than autism, is estimated at 2.5 cases per 10,000, but epidemiological data for Asperger syndrome are quite limited (Fombonne, 2003). One possible explanation for the lack of epidemiological data on Asperger syndrome is that national prevalence estimates are difficult to calculate when studies depend on such different criteria to diagnose the disorder. Similarly, information about PDD NOS is relatively scarce, but cases of PDD NOS are probably more common than autism, in part due to broader, more flexible diagnostic criteria. Fombonne (2003) estimates the current prevalence of PDD NOS at 15 per 10,000. Rates for Rett syndrome and CDD are much lower than other ASDs, with estimated prevalence rates of less than 1 in 10,000 for Rett syndrome (Kozinetz et al., 1993) and 1.1–6.4 per 100,000 for CDD (Fombonne, 2002). In total, the prevalence of ASDs in the general population is estimated to be at least 27.5 per 10,000, though a number of recent studies have reported rates more than twice as high. Bertrand et al. (2001) reported a rate of 6.7 cases of ASD per 1,000 among 3- to 10-year-old children in Brick Township, New Jersey. Similarly, within a population of U.K. preschool children (ages 2 years, 6 months to 6 years, 5 months), Chakrabarti and Fombonne (2001) reported the prevalence at 62.6 per 10,000.

Across 32 epidemiological studies published since 1966, the mean male:female sex ratio among individuals with autism was 4.3:1 (Fombonne, 2003). This finding is consistent with male:female sex ratios found in clinically referred populations (Lord, Schopler, & Revicki, 1982; Volkmar, Szatmari, & Sparrow, 1993). Notably, there is evidence to suggest that gender ratio is strongly associated with mental retardation, with the highest male:female ratios (i.e., at least 5.75:1) reported for individuals in the normal range of intelligence and the lowest male:female ratios (i.e., 1.9:1) reported for individuals with profound mental retardation (Fombonne, 2003; Lord et al., 1982).

Information about the prevalence of autism in different racial and ethnic populations is limited, but epidemiological studies to date have found similar rates across racial groups (e.g., Honda, Shimizu, & Misumi, 1996; Fombonne & Du Mazaubrun, 1992; Mágnússon & Sæmundsen, 2001). Also, despite Kanner's (1943) initial report suggesting a potential link between high parental education and autism, recent epidemiological data have failed to demonstrate a relationship between social class and autism prevalence (Fombonne, 2003).

COMORBID DIAGNOSES AND ASSOCIATED CONDITIONS

Once a diagnosis of ASD is made, it is important to conduct further evaluation to determine whether the child meets criteria for other comorbid psychological disorders or medical conditions. The condition that is most commonly associated with autism is mental retardation, which is defined by a score that is at least 2 standard deviations below the mean on standard measures of intelligence (i.e., Nonverbal IQ < 70). Previous epidemiological studies indicated that approximately three-fourths of children with ASD were mentally retarded (e.g., Fombonne, 2003; Bryson, Clark, & Smith, 1988), but more recent findings suggest that the majority of children on the autism spectrum do not have mental retardation (Bryson & Smith, 1998). In a study of preschool children with ASD (Chakrabarti & Fombonne, 2001), 25.8% had some degree of mental retardation, though a substantially higher proportion of children with autism had mental retardation (69.2%) compared to children with PDD NOS (7.6%) or Asperger syndrome (0%). In a CDC (2001) survey, 50% of 3- to 10-year-old children with autism had IQs less than 70, whereas 40% of children with PDD NOS or Asperger syndrome fell in the mentally retarded range. Thus, it appears that a significantly smaller proportion of children with ASDs are mentally retarded than was previously thought. Among children with ASD, children with diagnoses of autism are more likely to have general cognitive impairments than children with PDD NOS or Asperger syndrome.

Besides assessing developmental level or IQ in young children with ASD, practitioners should rule out other psychological disorders that are sometimes associated with ASD. However, one of the difficulties in doing so is that many of the symptoms of ASD overlap significantly with symptoms of other childhood disorders. For that reason, disorders such as ADHD, anxiety disorders, and communication disorders are not technically diagnosable by DSM-IV criteria if they occur "exclusively during the course of a pervasive developmental disorder" (American Psychiatric Association, 1994). Nevertheless, because not all children with ASD have attention problems, severe anxiety, and/or large discrepancies between their receptive and expressive language and other abilities, assigning comorbid diagnoses can be useful in identifying necessary services for children who do exhibit such difficulties. Therefore, many clinicians give additional diagnoses to child clients with ASD in cases where multiple diagnoses are needed to best describe different aspects of the child's behavior. Secondary diagnoses may also be important for research purposes, especially when comparing possible subgroups within autism. Later in development, in adults with ASD without mental retardation, comorbid diagnoses may significantly affect independence, so it is important to treat secondary symptoms in conjunction with core symptoms of ASD.

Findings from epidemiological studies suggest that 25–30% of individuals with autism have associated medical conditions, including epilepsy, sensory impairment (blindness and/or deafness), and tuberous sclerosis (Bryson

& Smith, 1998). A recent Finnish study found that, out of 187 children (under 16 years) with autism, 12.3% were diagnosed with a medical disorder (Kielinen, Rantala, Tomonen, Linna, & Moilamen, 2004). Studies have also found that gastrointestinal problems occur at a higher rate in children with ASD (Malloy & Manning-Courtney, 2003), particularly in those children who have experienced a regression (Richler et al., in press). Other medical problems commonly associated with ASD include ear infections (Konstantareas & Homatidis, 1987), feeding difficulties (Schreck, Williams, & Smith, 2004), and sleep disturbances (Honomichl, Goodlin-Jones, Burnham, Gaylor, & Anders, 2002), which may be associated with autism severity (Schreck, Mulick, & Smith, 2004).

Several genetic disorders, such as fragile X syndrome, Williams syndrome, Angelman syndrome, Kleinfelter syndrome, Turner syndrome, and Prader–Willi syndrome have been found to occur more commonly in individuals with autism than in the general population. Previous studies proposed that the rates of disorders such as neurofibromatosis, congenital rubella, phenylketonuria (PKU), Down syndrome, and cerebral palsy are higher in individuals with autism (e.g., Nordin & Gillberg, 1996), but these associations have not yet been supported by more recent epidemiological data (Fombonne, 2003). It is not clear whether genetic disorders and medical problems are as prevalent in populations with equal levels of mental retardation as they are in ASD populations. In other words, because these disorders are more common in individuals with lower IQs, there may not be a specific association with ASD that is separate from the association with mental retardation.

The proportion of children with ASD who have associated medical problems varies widely between studies. Depending on the sources of referral and recruitment, and the age at which the children with ASD were identified, studies have yielded different estimates for various medical conditions. A child with ASD who has medical problems is more likely to be followed first by a medical specialist (e.g., a child neurologist) and may obtain services under that classification, and he or she may not be identified as having an ASD until he or she is quite a bit older. By contrast, a child with ASD who does not have any medical problems may be more likely to be referred to a speech and language pathologist or a psychologist, and may receive a communication disorder or ASD diagnosis at a younger age. Because of such referral trends, the percentage of children with ASD who have additional medical diagnoses is much higher in some samples than in others.

ETIOLOGY

Based on sibling studies of children with autism, most researchers agree that autism has a strong genetic component, but there is currently no genetic test for ASD. Brain imaging studies have indicated structural abnormalities in individuals with autism in multiple areas, including the cerebellum, but there is not yet agreement about what is necessary or sufficient to cause ASD (e.g., Akshoomoff et al., 2004). Recent imaging studies have used functional magnetic resonance imaging (fMRI), although this method has not yet been used with young children with ASD. Children with autism also tend to have larger heads and greater brain volumes than matched controls, which suggests that there is something abnormal about head/brain growth in children with ASD.

ASSESSMENT

As is the case with all childhood disorders, accurate diagnosis of ASDs begins with gathering data from multiple sources. Because ASD is often first suspected in very young children and/or in children who have impaired communication abilities (so that they cannot self-report), adult reports of the child's behavior are of particular importance. Obviously parents or guardians are usually in the best position to provide information about their child's behavior, but other adults (e.g., early interventionists, day care or preschool teachers, speech therapists) may also be able to provide useful information about the child's behavior in various settings. For a comprehensive discussion of practice parameters and diagnostic instruments, see Filipek, Accardo, and Ashwal (2000), Klinger and Renner (2000), and Lord and Corsello (2005).

Parent Interviews

Several instruments have been designed to aid professionals in gathering information from adults that is useful in making a diagnosis of ASD (see Table 12.1). These instruments come in different formats and have various advantages and disadvantages. Thus, the decision to use one instrument over another should be based on multiple considerations, including time, money, and accessibility of the informant.

Many clinicians are accustomed to using an open-ended interview format when gathering information about their pediatric clients, but when ASD is suspected, it is often helpful to use a more structured format to ensure that all of the necessary information is obtained. One way to accomplish this is to use a semistructured interview, because it allows for gathering all the necessary information and also enables the clinician to use his or her clinical judgment and ask additional questions when necessary. The semistructured interview preserves the conversational element of the traditional open-ended interview, which facilitates rapport building between clinician and client.

The most widely used and well-established semistructured interview designed to diagnose ASD is the Autism Diagnostic Interview—Revised (ADI-R; Le Couteur, Lord, & Rutter, 2003). One advantage of using the ADI-R is that it helps parents understand the types of impairments associated with ASD. It also provides quantifiable scores related to severity of symptoms in three domains (i.e., communication, reciprocal social interaction, and restricted and

TABLE 12.1. Autism Screening and Diagnostic Instruments

Instrument	Format	Purpose	Best age	Training?	Advantages	Disadvantages
Autism Diagnostic Interview—Revised (ADI-R)	Semistructured parent interview	Research and clinical diagnosis	18 mo+	Yes	Comprehensive picture of child	Time consuming
ADOS	Administered by clinician	Research and clinical diagnosis	18 mo+	Yes	Creates structured, standardized, social content	Based on single observation
Autism Behavior Checklist (ABC)	Parent questionnaire	Screening, measures change		Yes	May be useful as measure of treatment	Does not map onto standard diagnostic criteria
Childhood Autism Rating Scale (CARS)	Administered by clinician	Screening	2–12 yr	Yes	Quick and easy; widely used; well established	Does not map onto standard diagnostic criteria
Children's Communication Checklist (CCC)	Parent/teacher questionnaire	Identify pragmatic language problems		No	Differential diagnosis; assesses broader phenotype	Relatively new measure
CSBS DP Infant Toddler Checklist Caregiver Questionnaire Behavior Sample	Checklist Questionnaire administered by clinician	Screening, assess play and communication difficulties	6–24 mo 6–24 mo 6–24 mo	No No Yes	Covers a range of communication difficulties	Does not address ASD directly
DISCO	Semistructured parent interview	Diagnose ASDs and comorbidities	4 yr+	Yes	Assesses a wide range of conditions	Lengthy; limited psychometrics

(continued)

265

TABLE 12.1. (*continued*)

Instrument	Format	Purpose	Best age	Training?	Advantages	Disadvantages
Gilliam Autism Rating Scale (GARS)	Parent checklist			No	Quick; easy to use	Does not map onto standard diagnostic criteria
M-CHAT	Screener	General population screening	Toddlers	No	Quick; easy to use	Need more data
Psychoeducational Profile—Revised	Administered by clinician	Obtain intervention recommendations	3–5 yr	Yes	Provides clinically useful information	Minimal psychometrics
Social Communication Questionnaire (SCQ)	Parent questionnaire	Screening for research	3 yr+	No	Quick; similar types of questions as ADI-R	Low sensitivity in preschoolers
Social Responsiveness Scale (SRS)	Parent questionnaire	Identify social difficulties		No	Covers a broad range of social behaviors	Lengthy
Screening Test for Autism in Two-Year-Olds (STAT)	Administered by clinician	"Level 2" Screening	24 mo	No	Easy to use and code	Limited to 2-year-olds
3di	Computerized parent interview	Diagnose ASDs and comorbidities	24 mo+	Yes	Assesses non-ASDs; scored by computer	Relatively new; small norming sample

repetitive behaviors), as well as separate algorithms for verbal and nonverbal children. Disadvantages of the ADI include its length (2–3 hours) and training requirement, as well as its tendency to overdiagnose ASD in children with nonverbal mental ages less than 2 years, or with severe to profound mental retardation.

The Diagnostic Interview for Social and Communication Disorders (DISCO; Wing, Leekam, Libby, Gould, & Larcombe, 2002) is another semistructured interview designed to obtain information about a child's developmental history and current patterns of behavior. Like the ADI, the DISCO is intended to aid in the diagnosis of ASD; however, it can also be used to diagnose other developmental disorders, as well as nonspectrum psychiatric disorders.

The Development, Diagnostic and Dimensional Interview (3di; Skuse et al., 2004) is a newly developed standardized interview that is administered with the help of a computer. Based on the responses entered, the computer indicates which set of questions to ask, and the interviewer reads the questions exactly as they are written. The 3di is intended to assess autism severity and symptoms of comorbid conditions (e.g., fragile X syndrome, tuberous sclerosis, ADHD); thus, it is broader in scope than the ADI-R. In spite of high validity and reliability estimates, the original validation sample for the 3di included limited numbers of preschool children, nonverbal children, or children with mental retardation. Therefore, the authors suggest that the 3di be used together with independent child observational assessments, such as the Autism Diagnostic Observation Schedule (ADOS; Skuse et al., 2004).

The Vineland Adaptive Behavior Scales (VABS; Sparrow, Balla, & Cicchetti, 1984) is a parent interview about everyday adaptive behavior that can be used together with one of the aforementioned diagnostic interviews. The VABS is not designed to diagnose ASD per se, but it provides information about a child's adaptive (and maladaptive) behaviors that can be useful in forming diagnostic impressions, as well as recommendations for intervention. Adaptive behavior has been shown to be an area of weakness for children with ASD, because these children almost always have lower VABS scores than would be expected based on their IQs (Carter et al., 1998; Loveland & Kelley, 1991). Furthermore, some researchers suggest that children with ASD follow a particular profile on measures of adaptive behavior, which could be used to identify children with possible ASD (Carter et al., 1998; Loveland & Kelley, 1991; Paul et al., 2004).

Questionnaires and Checklists

When time constraints or lack of accessibility to the informant prevent the use of an interview for gathering information, a questionnaire or checklist can be used instead. Questionnaires and checklists can also be used for preassessment screening. When parental consent is provided, questionnaires can be useful in gathering information from teachers and other helping professionals about the child's behavior outside of his or her home environment.

Several questionnaires and checklists have been developed for the purpose of measuring social and communication impairments in children suspected of having ASDs (see Table 12.1). The Autism Behavior Checklist (ABC; Krug, Arick, & Almond, 1980) and the Gilliam Autism Rating Scales (GARS; Gilliam, 1995) are examples of measures intended to identify children with ASD, though each has significant limitations in terms of the degree to which its scores correspond to standard clinical diagnoses. The Childhood Autism Rating Scale (CARS; Schopler, Reichler, DeVellis, & Daly, 1980), another autism diagnostic measure that was originally scored based on clinician observation, is now commonly used as a parent checklist. When using the CARS with 2- and 3-year-old children, specificity is improved by raising cutoffs (Lord, 1995).

Some more recently designed instruments, such as the Children's Communication Checklist (CCC; Bishop, 1998), attempt to capture individuals with symptoms that overlap with the phenotype of ASD (i.e., individuals who do not meet full criteria for a diagnosis of ASD but exhibit some symptoms of the disorder). Originally designed for teachers but now validated for use with parents (Bishop & Baird, 2001), the CCC is intended to differentiate between children with ASDs and those with pragmatic language disorders (Bishop & Baird, 1998). The Social Responsiveness Scale (SRS; Constantino, 2002), another relatively new questionnaire, is intended to serve as a measure of severity of social deficits among children with ASD.

Regardless of the format used to gather information about a child, it is important to collect data about the child's medical and developmental history, including information about early language acquisition and age of symptom onset. This can then be used in conjunction with data obtained through interviews and/or questionnaires in making differential diagnoses between ASDs and other disorders.

Child Observation Measures

In addition to adult reports about the child's behavior, direct observation of the child is another important component in making a diagnosis of ASD. Although in the past a number of important research studies relied solely on parent report to assign participants to diagnostic categories, diagnosis of ASD for clinical purposes (and ideally for research purposes as well) should never be made without observing the child. Even though parents are often excellent observers and reporters of their child's behavior (and getting better informed all the time), they have seldom seen the range of behavior associated with ASD that is required to make observations for the purpose of diagnosis (though semistructured interviews may help with this to some extent). Some parents may underreport atypical behaviors because of the child's tendency to behave "better" with family members, particularly the primary caregiver. Research also suggests that parents may have a more difficult time identifying abnormalities in their firstborn children than in later-born children (De Giacomo & Fombonne, 1998).

Many clinicians conduct observations in a relatively free-form manner, watching the child play and looking for aberrant behaviors that would be useful in making a diagnosis. The problem with this type of observation is that a relaxed and unstructured setting may or may not elicit the types of behaviors often exhibited by children with ASD. For example, a preschooler with autism may not appear to be particularly unusual when allowed to play by himself with toys he likes, but when the clinician attempts to play with him or introduce new toys, he may resist her attempts at social interaction or respond inappropriately. Similarly, a preschooler who exhibits no repetitive behaviors in the absence of toys may begin spinning wheels on toy cars or lining up figurines once those materials become available. In the same way that mental retardation should not be diagnosed before administering a standardized test and gathering evidence of impairment in everyday adaptive functioning, ASD should not be diagnosed or definitively ruled out before observing a child's behavior within a number of different kinds of social contexts. Because these contexts may not always arise within an office visit, setting up scenarios during an evaluation that are likely to elicit behaviors associated with ASD can provide information not available in other ways (see Table 12.1).

One tool designed to aid clinicians in eliciting behaviors necessary for making a diagnosis of ASD is the Autism Diagnostic Observation Schedule (ADOS; Lord, Rutter, DiLavore, & Risi, 1999). The ADOS comprises a standard series of tasks that assess abilities and impairments in the areas of communication, reciprocal social behavior, and restricted and repetitive behaviors. The ADOS is organized into four different modules that correspond to various levels of language (i.e., Module 1 for nonverbal children, Module 2 for children with phrase speech, Module 3 for children and adolescents with fluent speech, and Module 4 for adults with fluent speech). Most preschoolers who are being assessed for ASD receive a Module 1 or Module 2, but Module 3 is the most appropriate measure for typically developing 4- to 5-year-olds. The ADOS takes approximately 45 minutes to administer, and with training, it can be relatively easily incorporated into a standard clinical assessment battery. The goal of the ADOS is to create a positive social environment within which the clinician deliberately manipulates the level of social scaffolding to see what the child can do. Also, because many of the activities are play-based, children usually enjoy completing the ADOS, thus allowing the clinician (and the parents) the opportunity to see the child when he or she is happy and engaged.

In working with a younger, preschool population, the Screening Tool for Autism in Two-Year-Olds (STAT; Stone, Coonrod, & Ousley, 2000) is another clinician-administered observation measure that assesses a subset of the areas found within the ADOS for a more specific age group. The STAT is composed of a series of items administered by a clinician and scored on a pass–fail basis. An algorithm provides diagnostic classifications for autism.

The Communication and Symbolic Behavior Scales Developmental Profile (CSBS DP; Wetherby & Prizant, 2002) is a three-part assessment that evaluates communication and play skills in young children. It is intended for children with functional communication levels between 6 months and 2 years, but it may be administered to children as old as 6, if their mental age is less than 2 years. The behavior sample is a brief, face-to-face evaluation that is intended to be administered to children who perform below age level on the CSBS DP Infant–Toddler Checklist (see below). Like the ADOS, the CSBS DP behavior sample is a play-based assessment that creates opportunities for the child to interact with the examiner and the caregiver; however, it is scored by watching a videotape of its administration. The behavior sample can be supplemented with the CSBS DP Caregiver Questionnaire, which provides additional information about the child's behavior.

Screening Instruments

Some professionals, such as pediatricians or epidemiological researchers, may use screening instruments with their pediatric populations. These instruments, such as the Checklist for Autism in Toddlers (CHAT; Baird et al., 2000), Modified Checklist for Autism in Toddlers (M-CHAT; Robins, Fein, Barton, & Green, 2001), the Social Communication Questionnaire (SCQ; Rutter, Bailey, Lord, & Berument, 2003), and the CSBS DP Infant–Toddler Checklist (Wetherby & Prizant, 2002), are used with toddlers and young preschoolers, and are intended to identify children at risk for a wide range of social and communication difficulties, including ASD. Screening tools are not designed to serve diagnostic purposes. They should be very sensitive, but may not be very specific, and they are meant to target those children who might require further assessment.

Assessment of Very Young Children

Diagnosis of autism in 2-year-olds can be as reliable as diagnosis of 3-year-olds when carried out with standardized instruments, including a parent interview and a structured observation, and done by an experienced diagnostician. At age 2, diagnostic instruments such as the ADI-R and ADOS, are predictive of later behavior, but not as strongly as at age 3 or 4. Thus, the judgment of a clinician experienced not only with autism but also with 2-year-olds is even more crucial at this point than in the later preschool years. Diagnosis of children with milder difficulties, including PDD NOS and atypical autism, is much less reliable (Lord & Risi, 2004; Stone et al., 1999; Moore & Goodson, 2003). Many children who receive more tentative diagnoses at age 2 will eventually develop more easily identifiable behaviors associated with autism, including repetitive behaviors and more obvious social deficits, by the time they are age 3. However, a very small number of children with early PDD NOS diagnoses show such marked improvements that they "grow out of" the autism spectrum. Usually such changes occur very early, that is, between ages 2 and 3, or at the most, by age 5. Because of this variability, it is important that clinicians who have less experience with very young children with autism seek consultation whenever possible and beware of not appearing more certain about a specific diagnosis than the information justifies.

Relatively little is known about diagnosis of autism in children under age 2. Although there are examples of children who showed very clear profiles associated with autism from very early on (Dawson, Osterling, Meltzoff, & Kuhl, 2000; Klin et al., 2004), retrospective reports and video studies suggest that in a substantial number of cases, autistic symptoms become worse in the second year of life. It is also not clear whether there are children under age 2 who meet some criteria for autism but do not continue to show these symptoms into the second year.

Autism screening instruments intended for children ages 18–24 months old have tended to be most effective when administered to children who have already been referred for special services (Robins et al., 2001). In population studies published to date, screeners for autism have tended to show low sensitivity, with relatively good specificity (Baird et al., 2000). Much work is currently in progress concerning identification of autism in children under age 2, but care must be taken, because techniques that theoretically seemed very plausible, such as those used in the CHAT, have not been successful so far.

COGNITIVE AND LANGUAGE TESTING

In the past, it has been argued that many children with ASD are simply "not testable," but much of the difficulty in testing these children has been due to the inappropriateness of the assessment tools being used and/or the clinician's inexperience with working with children on the autism spectrum. Tests that rely too heavily on the use of language, for example, may not be appropriate for measuring the intelligence of children with severe language delays. Similarly, tests that do not effectively separate the measurement of nonverbal from verbal skills often result in underestimates of nonverbal abilities. It is therefore necessary to select assessment tools that yield Nonverbal IQ scores that are not overly influenced by a child's verbal abilities. This is particularly important when testing children suspected of having ASD, because individuals on the autism spectrum often exhibit significant discrepancies between their Verbal and Nonverbal IQs (Joseph, Tager-Flusberg, & Lord, 2002). Some tests that may yield less verbally mediated estimates of nonverbal reasoning skills include the Mullen Scales of Early Learning (Mullen, 1995) and the Differential Ability Scales (DAS; Elliott, 1990). These instruments are not as dependent on verbal skills for motivation and/or for understanding the tasks.

Gathering data about a child's language level, including information about both expressive and receptive language abilities, is another critical component of assessing children with ASD. Language level has significant implications for both treatment and outcome in children with ASD. Many traditional measures of intelligence, such as the Wechsler Preschool and Primary Scales of Intelligence—Third Edition (WPPSI-III; Wechsler, 2002), do not take into account potential differences between expressive and receptive language abilities, so additional language measurements may be needed to construct an accurate profile of verbal intelligence. When such a profile reveals a significant split between a child's expressive and receptive language abilities, interventions need to be specifically designed to address the child's difficulties in each domain.

Language measures, such as the Reynell Developmental Language Scales (Reynell & Huntley, 1987) and the Preschool Language Scales—4th Edition (PLS-4; Zimmerman, Steiner, & Pond, 2002), typically assess receptive and expressive language abilities separately. The Clinical Evaluation of Language Fundamentals—Preschool Edition (CELF-P; Wiig, Secord, & Semel, 1992) is another measure of preschool language skills, but it has a relatively high basal level that makes it inappropriate for moderately to severely language-delayed preschoolers. The Peabody Picture Vocabulary Test—Third Edition (PPVT-III; Dunn, 1997), a measure of single-word receptive vocabulary, may be used as a screener for more general language difficulties, because it is highly correlated with other receptive and expressive language measures in children with verbal mental ages of 2 or more years (Tager-Flusberg, Paul, & Lord, 2005). The PPVT-III does not measure expressive language or comprehension of more complex language, however.

One of the main difficulties in finding assessment tools that are appropriate for use with preschoolers suspected of having ASD is that the majority of child assessment instruments are normed primarily on typically developing children. Such assessment tools presuppose a repertoire of abilities in their test-taking populations, including comprehension of simple spoken language, which is not always characteristic of children with ASD. Moreover, some of the skills necessary for successful test taking are skills that many preschoolers with ASD have not yet developed. For example, even tests designed for very young children require the child to point to an object or picture to indicate a response choice, yet many preschoolers with ASD do not understand pointing or use it as a mode of communication. Another challenge of testing preschoolers with suspected ASD is that they are often quite difficult to engage; thus, it is not always easy to distinguish the child's lack of ability from the clinician's inability to engage the child in an activity. Nevertheless, experienced clinicians have developed ways to work around these difficulties, which attests to the need to have referral sources available with these skills.

To increase the chances of conducting a valid assessment, clinicians should create a testing environment in which the child is most likely to perform at his or her best. This can be accomplished by allowing sufficient time for the assessment, having a parent available for the child if needed, and not introducing too many new adults during the assessment (e.g., "arena" assessments). Clinicians should try to avoid redundancy during testing so as not to fatigue the child unnecessarily and should have an array of motivators (mostly toys or interesting objects) on hand as reinforcers. It is also useful to organize an assessment such that work is interspersed with play. Creating a "first–then" routine for the child (i.e., first do some work, then play with a favorite toy) and using schedules are methods for balancing work with play, and for helping the assessment to run more smoothly. Finally, because children often behave differently in various settings, it is important to speak with teachers, therapists, and so forth, to obtain their impressions of the child's behavior.

LIFE AFTER DIAGNOSIS

After a child has been diagnosed with ASD and data about his intelligence, language level, and associated psychological and medical conditions have been gathered, recommendations should be made to the child's family about appropriate services, useful strategies, and relevant goals. Part of the reason for collecting so much information about each child is that recommendations about intervention rely more on a child's individual profile of strengths and difficulties than on a diagnosis of ASD itself. In other words, because the symptoms of ASD are so variable, both in terms of presentation and severity, there is no single intervention or combination of interventions that will be best for every child with ASD. Therefore, in presenting parents with information about treatment options, as well as talking about what to expect (both in the short and long term), clinicians should discuss the diagnosis of ASD in the context of each child's individual profile.

Despite limited research comparing the effectiveness of different interventions for children with ASD, there is no shortage of treatments claiming to be effective. Whereas some of these interventions are based on widely accepted theories about the core deficits of ASD, others have little or no scientific basis and are viewed by many professionals to be ineffective and/or potentially harmful (e.g., Dawson & Watling, 2000). The most consistent findings in the treatment literature suggest that children with ASD respond well to behaviorally based treatments, such as applied behavior analysis (ABA). Empirical support has been derived for other interventions, including Treatment and Education of Autistic and Related Communication-Handicapped Children (TEACCH), pivotal response training, and verbal behavior training, but direct comparisons of these interventions have not been undertaken. Speech therapy, occupational therapy, music therapy, social skills training, and Floor Time are also frequently employed to address some of the difficulties experienced by children with ASD (e.g., Wieder & Greenspan, 2003). Current research suggests that children with ASD should be actively engaged in specialized programming for at least 20–25 hours per week (National Research Council, 2001). Rather than selecting a single type of therapy, many parents of children with ASD choose to take a multidisciplinary approach to intervention, enrolling their children in a number of different treatments or educational programs (including regular preschool or play dates) simultaneously. Regardless of what mode(s) of intervention are implemented, therapies should be specially designed to address a child's individual needs.

It should be noted that ASDs are both developmental and pervasive. Children with ASD experience various types of difficulties at different points of development that most often affect them throughout their lives. Importantly, though, whereas individuals with ASD continue to experience difficulties in the same three general domains as they develop, the nature of their problems as preschoolers can be strikingly different from the nature of their problems as adults. For example, whereas a preschooler with autism might have difficulty talking, an adult with autism may exhibit more subtle difficulties with the reciprocal (i.e., turn-taking) aspect of conversation. Similarly, a preschooler who has little or no interest in interacting with peers will likely become more interested in social interaction as he or she develops, but will still have difficulty understanding social norms and maintaining typical social relationships.

It should also be noted that, as the term "spectrum" implies, children with ASD comprise an extremely heterogeneous group. Not only do children on the spectrum differ in terms of autism severity (i.e., the number and extent of deficits within each domain), but their profiles are also widely varied when it comes to verbal and nonverbal intelligence, temperament, and the presence of other psychological or medical conditions. The diverse nature of this group is an extremely important consideration both when deciding how to recruit and organize participants in research studies, and when designing and implementing assessments and interventions in clinical settings. Researchers and clinicians must therefore be careful not to view children with ASD as a homogeneous group. Information should be obtained regarding each child's unique pattern of deficits and strengths within the autism diagnostic criteria, as well as any associated cognitive, psychological, or medical features that inevitably affect the nature and course of ASD.

REFERENCES

Akshoomoff, N., Lord, C., Lincoln, A., Courchesne, R., Carper, R., Townsend, J., et al. (2004). Outcome classification of preschool children with autism spectrum disorders using MRI brain measures, *Journal of the American Academy of Child and Adolescent Psychiatry, 43*(3), 349–357.

American Psychiatric Association. (1994). *Diagnostic and Statistical Manual of Mental Disorders* (4th ed.). Washington, DC: Author.

Amir, R. E., Ignatia, B., Van den Veyver, I. B., Wan, M., Tran, C. Q., Francke, U., et al. (1999). Rett syndrome is caused by mutations in X-linked MECP2 encoding mathyl-CpG-binding protein 2. *Nature Genetics, 23,* 185–188.

Baird, G., Charman, T., Baron-Cohen, S., Cox, A., Swettenham, J., Wheelright, S., et al. (2000). A screening instrument for autism at 18 months of age: A 6–year follow-up study. *Journal of the American Academy of Child and Adolescent Psychiatry, 39*(6), 694–702.

Baranek, G. T. (1999). Autism during infancy: A retrospective video analysis of sensory-motor and social behaviors at 9–12 months of age. *Journal of Autism and Developmental Disorders, 29*(3), 213–224.

Bertrand, J., Mars, A., Boyle, C., Bove, F., Yeargin-Allsopp, M., & Decoufle, P. (2001). Prevalence of autism in a United States population: the Brick Township, New Jersey investigation. *Pediatrics, 108*, 1155–1161.

Bishop, D. V. M. (1998). Development of the Children's Communication Checklist (CCC): A method for assessing qualitative aspects of communicative impairment in children. *Journal of Child Psychology and Psychiatry, 39*, 879–891.

Bishop, D. V. M., & Baird, G. (2001). Parent and teacher report of pragmatic aspects of communication: Use of the Children's Communication Checklist in a clinical setting. *Developmental Medicine and Child Neurology, 43*, 809–818.

Bryson, S. E., Clark, B. S., & Smith, I. M. (1988). First report of a Canadian epidemiological study of autistic syndromes. *Journal of Child Psychology and Psychiatry, 29*(4), 433–445.

Bryson, S. E., & Smith, I. M. (1998). Epidemiology of autism: Prevalence, associated characteristics, and implications for research and service delivery. *Mental Retardation and Developmental Disabilities Research Reviews, 4*(2), 97–103.

Buitelaar, J. K., Van der Gaag, R., & Klin, A. (1999). Exploring the boundaries of pervasive developmental disorder not otherwise specified: Analyses of data from the DSM-IV autistic disorder field trial. *Journal of Autism and Developmental Disorders, 29*(1), 33–43.

Carter, A. S., Volkmar, F. R., Sparrow, S. S., Wang, J., Lord, C., Dawson, G., et al. (1998). The Vineland Adaptive Behavior Scales: Supplementary norms for individuals with autism. *Journal of Autism and Developmental Disorders, 28*(4), 287–302.

Centers for Disease Control and Prevention. (2000). *Prevalence of autism in Brick Township, New Jersey, 1998: Community Report.* Atlanta: U.S. Department of Health and Human Services.

Chakrabarti, S., & Fombonne, E. (2001). Pervasive developmental disorders in preschool children. *Journal of the American Medical Association, 285*(24), 3093–3099.

Cohen, D. J., & Volkmar, F. R. (1997). *Handbook of autism and pervasive developmental disorders* (2nd ed.). New York: Wiley.

Constantino, J. N. (2002). *The Social Responsiveness Scale.* Los Angeles: Western Psychological Services.

Cox, A., Klein, K., Charman, T., Baird, G., Baron-Cohen, S., Swettenham, J., et al. (1999). Autism spectrum disorders at 20 and 42 months of age: Stability of clinical and ADI-R diagnosis. *Journal of Child Psychology and Psychiatry, 40*(5), 719–732.

Croen, L. A., Grether, J. K., & Hoogstrate, J. (2002). The changing prevalence of autism in California. *Journal of Autism and Developmental Disorders, 32*(3), 207–215.

Dawson, G., Osterling, J., Meltzoff, A., & Kuhl, P. (2000). Case study of the development of an infant with autism from birth to two years of age. *Journal of Applied Developmental Psychology, 21*(3), 299–313.

Dawson, G., & Watling, R. (2000). Interventions to facilitate auditory, visual, and motor integration in autism: A review of the evidence. *Journal of Autism and Developmental Disorders, 30*(5), 415–421.

De Giacomo, A., & Fombonne, E. (1998). Parental recognition of developmental abnormalities. *European Child and Adolescent Psychiatry, 7*(3), 131–136.

Dragich, J., Houwink-Manville, I., & Schanen, C. (2000). Rett syndrome: A surprising result of mutation in MECP2. *Human Molecular Genetics, 9*, 2365–2375.

Dunn, L. M. (1997). *Peabody Picture Vocabulary Test* (3rd ed.). Circle Pines, MN: American Guidance Service.

Eisenmajer, R., Prior, M., Leekam, S., Wing, L., Ong, B., Gould, J., et al. (1998). Delayed language onset as a predictor of clinical symptoms in pervasive developmental disorders. *Journal of Autism and Developmental Disorders, 28*(6), 527–533.

Elliott, C. D. (1990). *Differential Abilities Scale (DAS)*. San Antonio, TX: Psychological Corporation.

Filipek, P. A., Accardo, P. J., & Ashwal, S. (2000). Practice parameter: Screening and diagnosis of autism: Report of the Quality Standards Subcommittee of the American Academy of Neurology and the Child Neurology Society. *Neurology, 55*(4), 468–479.

Fombonne, E. (2002). Prevalence of childhood disintegrative disorder. *Autism, 6*(2), 149–157.

Fombonne, E. (2003). Epidemiological surveys of autism and other pervasive developmental disorders: An update. *Journal of Autism and Developmental Disorders, 33*, 365–382.

Fombonne, E., & du Mazaubrun, C. (1992). Prevalence of infantile autism in four French regions. *Social Psychiatry and Psychiatric Epidemiology, 27*(4), 203–210.

Gilliam, J. E. (1995). *Gilliam Autism Rating Scale*. Austin, TX: PRO-ED.

Hatton, D. D., & Bailey, D. B., Jr. (2001). Fragile X syndrome and autism. In E. Schopler & N. Yirmiya (Eds.), *Research basis for autism intervention* (pp. 75–89). New York: Kluwer Academic/Plenum Press.

Honomichl, R. D., Goodlin-Jones, B. L., Burnham, M., Gaylor, E., & Anders, T. (2002). Sleep patterns of children with pervasive developmental disorders. *Journal of Autism and Developmental Disorders, 32*(6), 553–561.

Honda, H., Shimizu, Y., & Misumi, K. (1996). Cumulative incidence and prevalence of childhood autism in children in Japan. *British Journal of Psychiatry, 169*(2), 228–235.

Jarrold, C., Smith, P., Boucher, J., & Harris, P. (1994). Comprehension of pretense in children with autism. *Journal of Autism and Developmental Disorders, 24*(4), 433–455.

Joseph, R. M., Tager-Flusberg, H., & Lord, C. (2002). Cognitive profiles and social-communicative functioning in children with autism spectrum disorder. *Journal of Child Psychology and Psychiatry and Allied Disciplines, 43*, 807–821.

Kanner, L. (1943). Autistic disturbances of affective contact. *Nervous Child, 2*, 217–250.

Kerr, A. M., & Engerstrom, I. W. (2001). The clinical background to Rett disorder. In A. M. Kerr & I. W. Engerstrom (Eds.), *Rett disorder and the developing brain* (pp. 1–26). Oxford, UK: Oxford University Press.

Kielinen, M., Rantala, H., Tomonen, E., Linna, S., & Moilanen, I. (2004). Associated medical disorders and disabilities in children with autistic disorder. *Autism, 8*(1), 49–60.

Klin, A., Chawarska, K., Paul, R., Rubin, E., Morgan, T., Wiesner, L., et al. (2004). Autism in a 15-month-old child. *American Journal of Psychiatry, 161*(11), 1981–1988.

Klin, A., Pauls, D., Schultz, R., & Volkmar, F. (2005). Three diagnostic approaches to Asperger syndrome: Implications for research. *Journal of Autism and Developmental Disorders, 35*, 221–234.

Klinger, L. G., & Renner, P. (2000). Performance-based measures in autism: Implications for diagnosis, early detection, and identification of cognitive profiles. *Journal of Clinical Child Psychology, 29*(4), 479–492.

Kolvin, I., Ounsted, C., Richardson, L. M., & Garside, R. F. (1971). Studies in the childhood psychoses: III. The family and social background in childhood psychoses. *British Journal of Psychiatry, 118*(545), 396–402.

Konstantareas, M. M., & Homatidis, S. (1987). Ear infections in autistic and normal children. *Journal of Autism and Developmental Disorders, 17*(4), 587–594.

Kozinetz, C. A., Skender, M. L., MacNaughton, N., Almes, M. J., Schultz, R. J., Percy, A. K., et al. (1993). Epidemiology of Rett syndrome: A population-based registry. *Pediatrics, 91*(2), 445–450.

Krug, D. A., Arick, J. R., & Almond, P. J. (1980). *Autism Screening Instrument for Educational Planning*. Portland, OR: ASIEP Educational Company.

Kurita, H., Osada, H., & Miyake, Y. (2004). External validity of childhood disintegrative disorder in comparison with autistic disorder. *Journal of Autism and Developmental Disorders, 34*(3), 355–362.

LeCouteur, A., Lord, C., & Rutter, M. (2003). *The Autism Diagnostic Interview—Revised (ADI-R)*. Los Angeles: Western Psychological Services.

Leslie, A. M. (1992). Pretense, autism, and the theory-of-mind module. *Current Directions in Psychological Science, 1*(1), 18–21.

Lord, C. (1995). Follow-up of two-year-olds referred for possible autism. *Journal of Child Psychology and Psychiatry, 36*(8), 1365–1382.

Lord, C., & Corsello, C. (2005). Diagnostic instruments in autistic spectrum disorders. In F. R. Volkmar, A. Klin, & R. Paul (Eds.), *Handbook of autism and pervasive developmental disorders* (3rd ed.). Hoboken, NJ: Wiley.

Lord, C., & Risi, S. (2000). Diagnosis of autism spectrum disorders in young children. In A. M. Wetherby & B. M. Prizant (Eds.), *Communication and language issues in autism and pervasive developmental disorder: A transactional developmental perspective* (pp. 22–30). Baltimore: Brookes.

Lord, C., & Risi, S. (2004). Trajectory of language development in autistic spectrum disorders. In M. Rice (Ed.), *Developmental language disorders: From phenotypes to etiologies* (pp. 8–29). Mahwah, NJ: Erlbaum.

Lord, C., Risi, S., DiLavore, P., Shulman, C., Thurm, A., & Pickles, A. (in press). Autism from two to nine. *Archives of General Psychiatry.*

Lord, C., Risi, S., Lambrecht, L., Cook, E. H., Leventhal, B. L., DiLavore, P. C., et al. (2000). The Autism Diagnostic Observation Schedule—Generic: A standard measure of social and communication deficits associated with the spectrum of autism. *Journal of Autism and Developmental Disorders, 30*(3), 205–223.

Lord, C., Rutter, M., DiLavore, P. C., & Risi, S. (1999). *Autism Diagnostic Observation Schedule*. Los Angeles: Western Psychological Services.

Lord, C., Rutter, M., & Le Couteur, A. (1994). Autism Diagnostic Interview—Revised: A revised version of a diagnostic interview for caregivers of individuals with possible pervasive developmental disorders. *Journal of Autism and Developmental Disorders, 24*(5), 659–685.

Lord, C., Schopler, E., & Revicki, D. (1982). Sex differences in autism. *Journal of Autism and Developmental Disorders, 12*, 317–330.

Lord, C., Shulman, C., & DiLavore, P. (2004). Regression and word loss in autistic spectrum disorders. *Journal of Child Psychology and Psychiatry, 45*(5), 936–955.

Lord, C., Storoschuk, S., Rutter, M., & Pickles, A. (1993). Using the ADI-R to diagnose autism in preschool children. *Infant Mental Health Journal, 14*(3), 234–252.

Loveland, K. A., & Kelley, M. L. (1991). Development of adaptive behavior in preschoolers with autism or Down syndrome. *American Journal on Mental Retardation, 96*(1), 13–20.

Luyster, R., Richler, J., Risi, S., Hsu, W., Dawson, G., Bernier, R., et al. (2005). Early regression in social communication in autistic spectrum disorders. *Developmental Neuropsychology, 27*, 311–336.

Mágnússon, P., & Sæmundsen, E. (2001). Prevalence of autism in Iceland. *Journal of Autism and Developmental Disorders, 31*(2), 153–163.

Malhotra, S., & Gupta, N. (2002). Childhood disintegrative disorder. Re-examination of the current concept. *European Child and Adolescent Psychiatry, 11*, 108–114.

Molloy, C., & Manning-Courtney, P. (2003). Prevalence of chronic gastrointestinal symptoms in children with autism and autistic spectrum disorders. *Autism, 7*, 165–171.

Moore, V., & Goodson, S. (2003). How well does early diagnosis of autism stand the test of time?: Follow-up study of children assessed for autism at age 2 and development of an early diagnostic service. *Autism, 7*(1), 47–63.

Moursiden, S. E., Rich, B., & Isager, T. (1998). The natural history of somatic morbidity in disintegrative psychosis and infantile autism: A validation study. *Brain Development, 21*(7), 447–452.

Mullen, E. (1995). *Mullen Scales of Early Learning*. Circle Pines, MN: American Guidance Service.

Mundy, P., Sigman, M., & Kasari, C. (1990). A longitudinal study of joint attention and language development in autistic children. *Journal of Autism and Developmental Disorders, 20*(1), 115–128.

Mundy, P., Sigman, M. D., Ungerer, J., & Sherman, T. (1986). Defining the social deficits of autism: The contribution of non-verbal communication measures. *Journal of Child Psychology and Psychiatry, 27*(5), 657–669.

National Research Council. (2001). *Educating children with autism. Committee on Educational Interventions for Children with Autism.* Washington DC: National Academy Press.

Nordin, V., & Gillberg, C. (1996). Autism spectrum disorders in children with physical or mental disability or both: I. Clinical and epidemiological aspects. *Developmental Medicine and Child Neurology, 38*(4), 297–313.

Osterling, J., & Dawson, G. (1994). Early recognition of children with autism: A study of first birthday home videotapes. *Journal of Autism and Development Disorders, 24*(3), 247–257

Ozonoff, S., South, M., & Miller, J. N. (2000). DSM-IV-defined Asperger syndrome: Cognitive, behavioral, and early history differentiation from high-functioning autism. *Autism, 4*(1), 29–46.

Paul, R., Miles, S., Cicchetti, D., Sparrow, S., Klin, A., Volkmar, F., et al. (2004). Adaptive behavior in autism and pervasive developmental disorder—Not otherwise specified: Microanalysis of scores on the Vineland Adaptive Behavior Scales. *Journal of Autism and Developmental Disorders, 34*(2), 223–228.

Philofsky, A., Hepburn, S. L., Hayes, A., Hagerman, R., & Rogers, S. J. (2004). Linguistic and cognitive functioning and autism symptoms in young children with fragile X syndrome. *American Journal on Mental Retardation, 109*(3), 208–218.

Pomeroy, J. C., Friedman, C., & Stephens, L. (1991). Autism and Asperger's: Same or different? *Journal of the American Academy of Child and Adolescent Psychiatry, 30*(1), 152–153.

Reynell, J. K., & Huntley, M. (1987). *Reynell Developmental Language Scales manual.* Windsor, UK: NFER-Nelson.

Richler, J., Luyster, R., Risi, S., Hsu, W., Dawson, G., Bernier, R., et al. (in press). Is there a regressive "phenotype" of autism spectrum disorder associated with the measles–mumps–rubella vaccine?: A CPEA study. *Autism and Developmental Disorders.*

Robins, D. L., Fein, D., Barton, M. L., & Green, J. A. (2001). The Modified Checklist for Autism in Toddlers: An initial study investigating the early detection of autism and pervasive developmental disorders. *Journal of Autism and Developmental Disorders, 31*(2), 131–144.

Rutter, M., Bailey, A., Lord, C., & Berument, S. K. (2003). *Social Communication Questionnaire.* Los Angeles, CA: Western Psychological Services.

Schopler, E., Reichler, R. J., DeVellis, R. F., & Daly, K. (1980). Toward objective classification of childhood autism: Childhood Autism Rating Scale (CARS). *Journal of Autism and Developmental Disorders, 10*, 91–103.

Schreck, K. A., Mulick, J. A., & Smith, A. F. (2004). Sleep problems as possible predictors of intensified symptoms of autism. *Research in Developmental Disabilities, 25*(1), 57–66.

Schreck, K. A., Williams, K., & Smith, A. (2004). Comparison of eating behaviors between children with and without autism. *Journal of Autism and Developmental Disorders, 34*(4), 433–438.

Skuse, D., Warrington, R., Bishop, D., Chowdhury, U., Lau, J., Mandy, W., et al. (2004). The development, diagnostic and dimensional interview (3di): A novel computerized assessment for autism spectrum disorders. *Journal of the American Academy of Child and Adolescent Psychiatry, 43*(5), 548–558.

Sparrow, S., Balla, D., & Cicchetti, D. (1984). *Vineland Adaptive Behavior Scales.* Circle Pines, MN: American Guidance Service.

Stone, W., Coonrad, E., & Ousley, O. (2000). Screening Tool for autism in Two-Year-Olds

(STAT): Development and preliminary data. *Journal of Autism and Developmental Disorders, 30*(6), 607–612.

Stone, W. L., Lee, E. B., Ashford, L., Brissie, J., Hepburn, S., Coonrod, E., et al. (1999). Can autism be diagnosed accurately in children under 3 years? *Journal of Child Psychology and Psychiatry, 40*(2), 219–226.

Szatmari, P., Bryson, S. E., Boyle, M. H., Streiner, D. L., & Duku, E. (2003). Predictors of outcome among high functioning children with autism and Asperger syndrome. *Journal of Child Psychology and Psychiatry, 44*(4), 520–528.

Tager-Flusberg, H., Paul, R., & Lord, C. (2005). Language and communication in autism. In F. R. Volkmar, R. Paul, A. Klin, & D. Cohen (Eds.), *Handbook of autism and pervasive developmental disorders, Vol. 1. Diagnosis, development, neurobiology, and behavior* (3rd ed., pp. 335–364). Hoboken, NJ: Wiley.

Towbin, K. E. (2003). Strategies for pharmacologic treatment of high functioning autism and Asperger syndrome. *Child and Adolescent Psychiatric Clinics of North America, 12*(1), 23–45.

Volkmar, F., & Cohen, D. (1989). Disintegrative disorder or "late-onset" autism? *Journal of Child Psychology and Psychiatry, 30,* 717–724.

Volkmar, F. R., & Rutter, M. (1995). Childhood disintegrative disorder: Results of the DSM-IV Autism Field Trial. *Journal of the American Academy of Child and Adolescent Psychiatry, 34*(8), 1092–1095.

Volkmar, F. R., Szatmari, P., & Sparrow, S. S. (1993). Sex differences in pervasive developmental disorders. *Journal of Autism and Developmental Disorders, 23*(4), 579–591.

Walker, D. R., Thompson, A., Zwaigenbaum, L., Goldberg, J., Bryson, S. E., Mahoney, W. J., et al. (2004). Specifying PDD NOS: A comparison of PDD NOS, Asperger syndrome, and autism. *Journal of the American Academy of Child and Adolescent Psychiatry, 43*(2), 172–180.

Wechsler, D. (2002). *Wechsler Preschool and Primary Scales of Intelligence—Third Edition.* San Antonio, TX: Psychological Corporation.

Werner, E., Osterling, J., & Dawson, G. (2000). Brief report: Recognition of autism spectrum disorder before one year of age: A retrospective study based on home videotapes. *Journal of Autism and Developmental Disorders, 30*(2), 157–162.

Wetherby, A. M., & Prizant, B. M. (2002). *Communication and Symbolic Behavior Scales Developmental Profile (CSBS DP) manual.* Baltimore: Brookes.

Wetherby, A., Woods, J., Allen, L., Cleary, J., Dickinson, H., & Lord, C. (2004). Early indicators of autism spectrum disorders in the second year of life. *Journal of Autism and Developmental Disorders, 34,* 473–493.

Wieder, S., & Greenspan, S. I. (2003). Climbing the symbolic ladder in the DIR model through Floor Time/interactive play. *Autism, 7*(4), 425–435.

Wiig, E. H., Secord, W. A., & Semel, E. (1992). *Clinical Evaluation of Language Fundamentals—Preschool.* San Antonio, TX: Psychological Corporation.

Wing, L., & Potter, D. (2002). The epidemiology of autistic spectrum disorders: Is the prevalence rising? *Mental Retardation and Developmental Disabilities Research Reviews, 8,* 151–161.

Wing, L., Leekam, S. R., Libby, S. J., Gould, J., & Larcombe, M. (2002). The Diagnostic Interview for Social and Communication Disorders: Background, inter-rater reliability and clinical use. *Journal of Child Psychology and Psychiatry, 43*(3), 307–325.

World Health Organization. (1992). *International Classification of Diseases* (10th ed.). Geneva: Author.

Zimmerman, I. L., Steiner, V. G., & Pond, R. E. (2002). *The Preschool Language Scales—4th edition.* San Antonio, TX: Psychological Corporation.

Part III

Assessment and Intervention in the Preschool Period

13

Neuropsychological Assessment

CHRISTINE MRAKOTSKY and AMY K. HEFFELFINGER

Neuropsychological assessment of the preschool child has presented a long-standing challenge; fortunately, however, interest, necessity, and the opportunity to evaluate young children have increased dramatically during the last decade. Early identification of neurological, neurodevelopmental, and mental disorders has been on the forefront of medical intervention, federal research agendas, and public policy. Nevertheless, despite the critical importance of assessment in informing diagnosis and treatment, the formulation of age- and developmentally appropriate assessment models has been slow, and adequate instruments are still scarce.

Fortunately, there has been a steep increase in efforts to design developmentally appropriate assessment techniques and approaches in recent years. More measures are now becoming available to improve the diagnostic process. Most importantly, however, models that incorporate the understanding of brain systems, functional and neural development, and the child's biological and environmental context with findings from tests and observations are becoming widely adopted in neuropsychological practice. The goal of the assessment is hereby not only to generate a diagnosis but also to inform intervention planning and risk management. Neuropsychological assessment has thus become a critical component in diagnosis and treatment of preschool conditions, including psychiatric, neurological, and medical disorders, and the impact of underprivileged environments.

This chapter discusses conceptual frameworks and assessment models, as well as addresses current issues and limitations in preschool assessment. An overview of specific neurobehavioral domains and their assessment is provided, with assessment methods reviewed for each domain.

THEORETICAL FRAMEWORK FOR PRESCHOOL
NEUROPSYCHOLOGICAL ASSESSMENT

Conceptual Models of Neuropsychological Assessment

Neuropsychological assessment is not purely the administration of psychological tests. It is a complex "clinical process whose goals are to determine a diagnosis as well as to guide the development and implementation of a management plan" (Bernstein & Waber, 2003, p. 773). There are many factors—both internal and external—to consider when evaluating a young child. A conceptual framework that provides a working hypothesis is thus critical to guide the assessment process (including the selection of instruments). Early conceptual approaches to the assessment of brain–behavior relationships in children were largely derived from adult models; those appropriate for the neuropsychological development in children have lagged behind (Wilson, 1992; Hooper, 2000). Adult-based models, however, have significant limitations when applied in pediatric populations, because they assume brain functions to be static and lack the integration of *development*. This is particularly problematic for the assessment of preschool children, whose specific brain functions are developing rapidly, at different rates, and with different qualities. Development of cognitive and neuropsychological abilities is hardly a continuum throughout childhood, and abilities often change qualitatively, as well as quantitatively, even between preschool and early school age, complicating their assessment. Neurodevelopmental assessment aims to integrate knowledge from all relevant disciplines, including developmental psychology, clinical psychology, neuropsychology, neurology, developmental neurobiology, and cognitive neurosciences. Although few formal assessment approaches are available that are designed for the preschool child specifically (Wilson, 1992; Rey-Casserly, 1999), current child models that address the aforementioned limitations provide valuable foundations for the younger age groups.

The lack of developmental considerations in neuropsychological assessment of children as pointed out by Fletcher and Taylor (1984), has led to the formulation of normative developmental approaches incorporating brain, behavior, and developmental variables (Fletcher & Taylor, 1984; Taylor & Fletcher, 1990; Rourke, Fisk, & Strang, 1986). They described several problematic assumptions in pediatric neuropsychology that limit the validity of assessment results, including the erroneous beliefs that (1) behavioral outcome of brain-related disorders in adults is similar in children, (2) tests designed for adults measure the same skills in children, (3) specific behavioral deficits are directly reflective of brain disease, and (4) behavioral deficits present brain impairment on a continuum. Fletcher and Taylor's *functional organization approach* (1984) highlights the development of a child's cognitive ability structure at the core of the assessment process, with a specific emphasis on processes of change. It also integrates different types of variables underlying development, including brain-related and context (moderator) variables. The importance of distinguishing between behaviors that are the basis of a neurodevelopmental disorder and those that are secondary symptoms related to the disorder is therein underscored. The emphasis also lies on how deficits interfere with normal development rather than on identifying which brain areas are deficient. Normative developmental approaches have been critiqued for their focus on the child's cognitive ability structure in the here and now, as contrasted with a view of the child him- or herself as the core of analysis (Bernstein, 2000). When working with young children in particular, it is essential to consider each child unique, taking past development, neurological and medical history, as well as family factors into account.

A conceptual framework that overcomes some of these limitations and puts the child as a "whole" at the core of analysis incorporating developmental and neuropsychological theory is the *neurodevelopmental systems approach* formulated by Bernstein and colleagues (Bernstein, 2000; Holmes-Bernstein & Waber, 1990). This model is particularly suitable for application in preschool children, because it analyzes behavioral development with regard to brain development and environmental demands in a comprehensive, holistic way. The core strategy of this approach is the integration of information from several sources (history, observation, test performance) with neurodevelopmental theory. The wealth of clinical data generated through this approach is invaluable to the assessment of an age group that is difficult to assess with the few standardized measures available.

A triad of *brain–context–development* interactions build the framework of the systems approach. One of the main principles therein is that the *brain* is "the necessary—albeit not sufficient—substrate of behavior" (Bernstein, 2000, p. 413). The brain is the major substrate for learning and behavior at all levels, not only at the cognitive but also at the regulatory, emotional, and social levels. It is thus critical for the developmental neuropsychologist to understand the role of neural substrates underlying behavior (and "when" and "how" these systems develop). At the "brain" level this encompasses general knowledge of neural systems and brain functions, both in adults and children, including localization of function and behavioral output in the case of insult to a certain brain region.

Furthermore, the developmental systems approach emphasizes the importance of *context*, with the premise that the brain does not operate and develop in isolation but in constant interaction with the environment (Bronfenbrenner, 2005; Bronfenbrenner & Ceci, 1994; Greenough, Black, & Wallace, 1987). Thus, the context within which a child demonstrates a certain behavior (or skill) plays a critical role for interpretation of this behavior; that is, analysis of the demands and conditions under which preschool children are able to manage their behavior and the world around them plays an important role in diagnosis and is critical to risk assessment and management. The success of brain-context transactions determines the child's adaptation to the environment; failure to adapt to this environment (and not the behavior itself) is what constitutes a learning disorder (Holmes-Bernstein & Waber, 1990). Context variables are not limited to the situational context of the assessment (setting, task properties, role of the examiner) but include the child's genetic makeup (including age and gender), previous history, and other environmental factors (socioeconomic, cultural, social). Evaluation of context variables is critical to elucidate the source of observed difficulties to avoid, for example, misdiagnosing lack of exposure to learning materials as a lack of ability or deficit. In contrast, children who have a real deficit may go undiagnosed, because they do not demonstrate the problem behavior (i.e., inattention) in the assessment setting. In this case, careful analysis of factors within the assessment versus "real-world" (preschool, home) setting is needed to elucidate such a finding not only for diagnosis but also for planning effective interventions. The most common observation in preschool assessment is that the structure of the assessment setting (quiet room with few distractions, work with structured materials, one-to-one interaction, individual attention from the examiner, praise vs. the loud and busy classroom setting or the different but often equally challenging experience of a busy home with less routinized transactions from activity to activity) often facilitates a child's ability to focus, maintain engagement with the task and situation, and sustain overall performance. In addition, performance can significantly depend on task properties such as level of task structure and task complexity. So, for example, the shy, inattentive preschooler or the child with language difficulties may be able to answer questions that require a simple "yes–no" or single-word response (i.e., in naming tasks) but may struggle to elaborate his or her responses on questions with an open-ended answer format or those requiring production of more complex language. Similarly, children may comfortably copy block designs when a model is placed in front of them, but they may struggle to organize and integrate information independently on puzzle tasks in which no such model is provided.

In the preschool period, the most important feature that yields a true "picture" of the child is that of *development* (at both the brain and the behavior level). Brain processes and abilities are not static but develop and change over time, and in response to the environment. Particularly during the first 5 years, neural systems and cognitive functions develop rapidly (for details, see Heffelfinger & Mrakotsky, Chapter 3, this volume). Therefore, clinicians working with young children have to gain thorough knowledge of both cognitive and brain development. Early brain development includes both progressive (neuron proliferation and migration, synaptogenesis, myelinization) and regressive processes (programmed cell death, synapse elimination, pruning) (Bourgeois, Goldman-Rakic, & Rakic, 1994, 2000; Rakic, 1995). These processes are genetically predetermined, but they are also crucially dependent on the child's exposure to and experience with the world around him or her (Greenough & Alcantara, 1993). Errors at each level of these processes can cause serious neurodevelopmental deviations. For example, errors in migration of neurons are believed to be associated with a range of developmental and psychiatric disorders (e.g., autism: Bailey et al., 1998; Piven et al., 1990).

More rapid changes occur early in development for certain abilities and brain regions, whereas the onset and development for others can be later and more protracted. For example, synaptogenesis increases dramatically at birth, although critical periods (when neural connections are still undifferentiated, hence highly plastic and also more vulnerable to change) differ for specific brain regions, with basic sensory systems (e.g., the visual cortex) reaching critical periods much sooner than those subserving higher cognitive functions (e.g., parietal and frontal regions) (Huttenlocher & Dabholkar, 1997). Knowledge about the timing of *when* neural processes occur and specific systems develop is paramount to the understanding of developmental deviations both at the brain and behavior level, since the high plasticity of the brain during early development also poses a risk for greater vulnerability to adverse influences and developmental deviation. Younger children are often more vulnerable to insult, adverse effects, or intensive treatments during critical periods of development. For example, young age at diagnosis has been a robust risk factor for late cognitive effects of central nervous system (CNS) treatment in children with leukemia (Cousens, Waters, Said, & Stevens, 1988; Waber et al., 2001). Similarly—and contrary to long held beliefs about early reorganization— early diffuse brain lesions can have more pervasive consequences on neurocognitive development than later diffuse lesions (Ewing-Cobbs, Levin, Eisenberg, & Fletcher, 1987; Ewing-Cobbs et al., 1997). It is thus critical to know whether an injury or deviation occurred prenatally, during the first few months, or at age 4 years, all of which have different implications for neurodevelopmental course and outcome.

Deficits in functions may, however, not always emerge immediately but may become more apparent as the child develops and seeks to respond to increasing demands in the learning environment. Thus, although a child with relatively minor compromise in basic cognitive and behavioral skills may be able to perform comfortably in preschool, he or she may not be able to sustain that level of function in school as demands for attention, inhibitory control, organization, and independent learning increase. This developmental phenomenon can give the appearance of decline, if one attends only to standardized scores, but it in fact represents *adaptive* problems as age-level demands increasingly stress areas of weakness (Mrakotsky & Waber, 2006).

When assessing young children, it is thus essential to understand not only *what* is developing and *when*, but also *how* and in *what context*. Several core questions can guide the clinician: What is developmentally appropriate for a certain age? How does the child at each developmental stage adapt to his or her natural environment? Does the child meet the developmental challenges expected for his or her age and does so consistently across settings, or does the behavior differ between preschool and home settings? The developmental history to date must be integrated in the analysis as much as the child's current presentation, with contextual variables carefully evaluated for both.

Approaches to Assessment Strategies

From a measurement standpoint, early approaches often used a single, global measure to predict outcome. Fixed versus flexible battery approaches have been long debated in the neuropsychological assessment of children. "Fixed battery" approaches are strictly controlled series of well-normed psychological tests, with well-established psychometric properties, but their rigid course does not allow for the descriptive information necessary for intervention planning, which has limited their use for the assessment of children, particularly those with complex medical disorders (Baron, Fennell, & Voeller, 1995). Flexible battery approaches are now the common standard in pediatric assessments, because they allow for a more flexible and eclectic response to the individual child's needs and the referral question; they most often consist of a routine set of screening measures that is supplemented by selected tests in a decision tree fashion to accommodate and integrate clinical questions, observations, and previous findings.

An example for such a model highlighted in the adult literature is the *process approach* (Kaplan, 1988, 1990). An initial set of tests is utilized to sample specific behaviors, and supplemental measures are added, based on these findings. At its core, the process approach is a strategy for assessment (originally that of brain-injured adults) that enriches standardized assessment procedures with detailed analyses of the process by which an individual tackles a task (including behavior and error analysis) in the context of the presenting brain-based disorder. The emphasis thereby lies on qualitative observation of a person's cognitive and problem-solving style. This approach can be very useful for the assessment of children, because it provides a wealth of clinically relevant data; however, it was originally not formulated to incorporate developmental principles.

A flexible battery approach designed for preschool children is Wilson's *branching model* (Wilson, 1992), wherein the clinical evaluation of the young child is guided by a hypothesis-testing strategy based on the child's pattern of performance on an initial set of higher-order cognitive tasks supplemented with additional assessment of specific areas of weakness. Hooper (2000) describes an empirical approach that delineates specific neuropsychological core domains relevant to preschool children (motor, tactile–perceptual, attention, language, visual processing, memory, executive functions). Many flexible and systemic approaches utilize strategies that review such neurobehavioral systems or domains by integration of data from multiple sources (Bernstein, 2000; Rey-Casserly, 1999; Wilson, 1992). Neuropsychological assessment of preschoolers has to be comprehensive (capturing all domains of functioning) and integrated. This requires integration of test, observation, and report, as well as history data (e.g., medical, developmental, educational) into domains of functioning (e.g., attention, language). Assessment should never be limited to test data alone or to one specific domain (i.e., IQ), but requires thorough understanding of brain–behavior relationships that incorporates assessment findings with "real-world" behavior and previous history. The role of parents and teachers as informants to this process is paramount. Such strategy results in a meaningful "picture" of a child's pattern of strengths and weaknesses, their etiological sources, and practical information for interventions that will be most effective in the individual child's context or environment.

NEUROPSYCHOLOGICAL ASSESSMENT OF SPECIFIC ABILITIES

The comprehensive neuropsychological assessment of the preschool child includes evaluation of general cognitive abilities and adaptive skills, as well as assessment of specific neuropsychological abilities, including sensory–motor, attention, executive functions, language, visual–spatial, and memory abilities. In addition, thorough evaluation of the young child's psychological status and socioemotional functioning is critical for better understanding of the child as a "whole." At present, formal assessment of all mentioned areas still presents a challenge due to the limited availability of developmentally appropriate standardized tests for the preschool age. Data from history and behavior observations are thus invaluable components of the assessment (in accord with previously described models; Bernstein, 2000; Rey-Casserly, 1999; Wilson, 1992).

General Cognitive Ability

The construct of *general cognitive or intellectual ability* is one of the most controversial in (neuro)psychological assessment (for detailed reviews see Sattler, 2001; Sternberg, Grigorenko, & Bundy, 2001; Thorndike, 1997). Nevertheless, intelligence tests are ingrained in psychological assessment and often are the only or main cognitive measure used by school systems to assess a child's need for services. This is because they provide a well-researched statistical basis and are known to a wide range of professionals. "Intelligence" has numerous definitions, from those based on factor-analytical theory (Spearman, 1904; Thurstone, 1938; Catell, 1963) to more pragmatic, test-based IQ concepts, including Binet and Simon's mental age score (1905, 1916), Stern's ratio measure (1912), and Wechsler's deviation quotient (1949). In general, it is understood as the ability to comprehend, reason, solve problems, plan, and adapt effectively to the environment. Whether intelligence is defined by a single factor of general cognitive ability (g; Spearman, 1904, 1923; Wechsler, 1939, 1949) or a set of multiple, relatively independent abilities (i.e., Thurstone, 1938; Guilford, 1956), most intelligence tests distinguish between subcomponents of abilities (verbal vs. nonverbal/spatial; fluid vs. crystallized; simultaneous vs. sequential) that ultimately produce one global IQ or ability score. The use of such global score in developmental assessment and diagnosis is problematic, because it combines performance on subtests assessing a variety of functions and does not elucidate the child's pattern of strengths and weaknesses that is much more informative for diagnosis and treatment. In addition, tests of cognitive ability for preschoolers tend to vary in composition of subtests, normative data, and other psychometric properties, and can be insensitive to individual differences. They also highly depend on educational and cultural background (Flanagan & Alfonso, 1995; Greenfield, 1997; Sternberg et al., 2001).

Limitations in Predictive Power of Intelligence Tests for Young Children

One of the main concerns in interpreting global assessments of cognitive abilities in young children is their limited predictive validity and reliability; that is, test findings in very young children are often variable and unstable over time, and are in general not predictive of future intelligence (Neisworth & Bagnato, 1992; Sternberg et al., 2001). Although IQ scores become more stable during the preschool period, their predictive power for later functioning is not fully established until school age (Neyens & Aldenkamp, 1996). This carries the obvious risk of misdiagnosis in either direction (positive and negative). In the latter case, due to the lack of predictive validity, clinicians may be tempted to reason or wish away impaired performance, leading the family to have increased hope; however, more globally impaired performance on cognitive measures during the preschool period *is* typically related to future difficulties. It is our experience that those preschoolers performing below age expectation on a range of measures and domains (i.e., cognitive concepts, language, adaptive functioning) will likely not perform within age expectation when assessed at school age. In summary, global "IQ" scores should always be interpreted as an estimate of current function, not future potential. In fact, parental ability, socioeconomic status (i.e., parental education, occupation, and family income) and early home environments have been found to be better predictors for preschool and later cognitive functioning than IQ measured through tests during early childhood (Aylward, 1988; Espy, Molfese, & DiLalla, 2001; Molfese, Holcomb, & Helwig, 1994; Sameroff, Seifer, Barocas, Zax, & Greenspan, 1987).

Finally, abilities and skills assessed with standardized tests are often not reflective of the child's demands and functions in the "real world"; thus, test findings are only meaningful if integrated with history and observational data from the child's natural environment. Table 13.1 provides an outline of variables in observation and history that should be explored, in addition to standardized tests, when assessing cognitive abilities in preschoolers.

Probably the most commonly used instruments for the preschool age are the Wechsler Intelligence Scale for Children, third revision (WPPSI-III; Wechsler, 2002), the Differential Abilities Scale—Preschool Level (DAS; Elliot, 1990), and under some circumstances the Kaufman Assessment Battery for Children (K-ABC; Kaufman & Kaufman, 1983), although they vary in underlying IQ concept and subtest composition. The Bayley Scales of Infant Development, second edition (BSID-II; Bayley, 1993) and the Mullen Scales of

TABLE 13.1. Common Standardized Tests and Assessment Methods for General Cognitive Ability

Standardized tests		Observations (examiner, parent, teacher)	History (developmental, medical, psychological, educational)
Test	Age range (years: months)		
WPPSI-III	2:6–7:3	• Problem-solving behavior	• Developmental milestones including early cognitive concepts (color, shape, size)
DAS—Preschool	2:6–5:11	• Knowledge and generation of basic cognitive concepts	• Acquisition of preacademic skills (numbers, letters)
K-ABC	2:6–12:5		
McCarthy	2:6–8:6		
SB-5	2:0–85	• Depth of elaboration	
BSID-II	1–42 months	• Exploratory behavior	• Interests (wide or narrow)
Mullen	0–68 months	• Quality of symbolic play	• Previous test results
			• Family history of learning and developmental disorders

Note. WPPSI III, Wechsler Preschool and Primary Scale of Intelligence—Third Edition; DAS–Preschool, Differential Ability Scales—Preschool Level; K-ABC, Kaufman Assessment Battery for Children; McCarthy, McCarthy Scales of Children's Abilities (McCarthy, 1972); SB-5, Stanford–Binet Intelligence Scale, Fifth Edition; BSID-II, Bayley Scales of Infant Development, Second Edition; Mullen, Mullen Scales of Early Learning. Adapted by permission from Rey-Casserly (1999). Copyright 1999 by Allyn & Bacon.

Early Learning (Mullen, 1995) are developmental scales not based on traditional IQ concepts, and are used in younger children. Nevertheless, all of these instruments include reasoning and problem-solving measures of some sort that are reflective of cognitive ability. Typically, these are represented in the nonverbal domain as tasks of visual–spatial/constructional and integration ability (block construction and puzzle-building tasks), as well as tasks of early conceptual thinking and reasoning (picture–concept matching and matrix reasoning tasks). Important in the interpretation is, however, that most of these tasks are dependent on other abilities (language, attention, motor, speed). In the verbal domain, cognitive ability might be most reflected by tasks of verbal concept formation (finding conceptual word categories) and word reasoning/riddle tasks in which the child has to abstract, generate, and integrate underlying concepts through clues. There are also knowledge-based (i.e., vocabulary and fact knowledge) and language-related tasks (i.e., comprehension of directions, object naming) that measure "verbal ability" to varying degrees; however, their interpretation as intellectual measures per se has been less clear. Assessment of general cognitive ability in preschoolers should always also include thorough observation of problem-solving approaches to tasks and in the natural environment (i.e., during play), as well as depth of elaboration of responses (i.e., basic or more sophisticated). Generalization of information or strategies to other tasks and situations is also an important indicator for conceptual thinking. Level of exploration of the environment or specific materials, level of imaginative play, including appropriate use of toys, and information about early cognitive development from the child's history, are all critical components of cognitive assessment.

Motor/Sensory Skills

Motor and sensory skills consist of a range of functions that are essential for performance on most cognitive tests and functioning in the natural environment. Motor skills are divided into gross and fine motor skills, with the former referring to broader functions of motor control (i.e., ambulation, posture, balance, coordination), whereas the latter refer to "small" movement control and level of eye–hand coordination (i.e., pencil control, manipulation of small objects).

Qualitative observation of motor skills in addition to quantitative assessment, is very important in the evaluation of preschoolers (see Table 13.2). Children may perform adequately on measures of fine motor skills (i.e., speed and dexterity), but may be overly clumsy, have difficulty manipulating objects at midline, or may have overt lateralizing motor preferences that may indicate the need for a neurological or occupational therapy evaluation. Hand preference should also be assessed. Although not firmly established until school age, most children show a preference much earlier. Unusually early or late hand preference can, however, suggest neurological dysfunction. Left-handedness particularly in the absence of positive family history, can be suggestive of early insult.

One caveat in assessing motor skills, however, is that preschoolers often have disorganized or seemingly unusual motor movements that would be considered "atypical" in school-age children. Examples of fairly common atypical movements are toe walking, mirror movements (involuntary reciprocal movement on novel tasks, with the contralateral resting limb mirroring that of the active limb), motor overflow, and stereotypies such as finger fluttering. Although all of these can be indications for developmental delay or atypical development, they can also appear in children without known clinical cause. Therefore, a clinical diagnosis should not be made based purely on motor findings.

Attention

Attention is not a single construct, but comprised of several components, including the ability to orient, to focus/select, and to sustain attention (Cohen, 1993; Posner & Peterson, 1990). Attention can and should be evaluated in all preschoolers undergoing evaluation, due to the high prevalence of attentional difficulties in developmental, neurological, and psychiatric disorders. Although standard observation and parent–teacher reports provide ample and very useful information regarding a child's attention (the latter in the context

TABLE 13.2. Common Standardized Tests and Assessment Methods for Motor Skills

Tests, rating scales	Observations	History
Broad Motor Scales • McCarthy Motor Scale • BSID-II Motor Scale • VABS Motor Domain • SIB-R Motor Scales	*Gross motor* • Posture, gait, balance, coordination (gait and bimanual)	• Developmental motor milestones (standing, walking, drawing, etc.) • Establishment of hand preference (timing)
Fine motor tasks • Purdue Pegboard • WRAVMA Pegboard • NEPSY Fingertip Tapping	*Fine motor* • Graphomotor control and quality, pencil grip, speed, and dexterity	• Family history of left-handedness • Evidence of atypical movements
Visual/graphomotor tests • VMI • DAS Copying • NEPSY Visuomotor Precision	*Lateralization* • Hand preference, bimanual coordination, crossing midline	• Findings from physical and occupational therapy evaluations
Praxis tests • NEPSY Imitating Hand Positions • K-ABC Hand Movements	*Praxis* • Demonstration of learned movements (combing hair, waving good-bye)	
Sensory–perceptual tests • Finger Localization Tactile • Form Recognition	*Sensory–perceptual* • Response to textures, tactile experiences	

Note. VABS, Vineland Adaptive Behavior Scales (Sparrow, Balla, & Cicchetti, 1984); SIB-R, Scales of Independent Behavior—Revised (Bruininks, Woodcock, Weatherman, & Hill, 1996); Purdue Pegboard (Tiffin & Asher, 1948; Wilson, Iacovello, Wilson, & Risucci, 1982); WRAVMA, Wide Range Assessment of Visual–Motor Abilities (Adams & Sheslow, 1995); NEPSY, NEPSY: A Developmental Neuropsychological Assessment (Korkman, Kirk, & Kemp, 1997); VMI, Beery–Buktenica Developmental Test of Visual–Motor Integration (Beery, 1997). All other test abbreviations as in Table 13.1. Adapted by permission from Rey-Casserly (1999). Copyright 1999 by Allyn & Bacon.

of the natural environment), few standardized measures are available to substantiate these findings (see Table 13.3).

The basic level of arousal and alertness is the first aspect to observe when assessing a young child. This can be a potential problem for children with significant neurological conditions (i.e., seizures) or those on medication. In addition, observation and parent–teacher report of attentional focus to tasks and over time are critical, because these processes can be highly variable between preschoolers and between settings (i.e., school vs. test setting). Cancellation or scanning tasks (i.e., NEPSY Visual Attention; Korkman, Kirk, & Kemp, 1997) can give insight into the preschooler's level of inattentiveness and impulsivity, providing information about omission (omitting a target) and commission errors (falsely marking a nontarget). The NEPSY Visual Attention task can be a very useful measure of attention; however, the overall scaled score is often less informative, because it includes both "time of completion" and "number of errors." Therefore, a child that performs very

TABLE 13.3. Common Tests and Assessment Methods of Attention

Tests, rating scales	Observations	History
Focused attention—auditory tests • NEPSY Auditory Attention • DAS Recall of Digits *Focused attention—visual tests* • NEPSY Visual Attention • WPPSI-III Symbol Search *Sustained attention* • GDS • K-CPT • TOVA Preschool Version *Parent–teacher rating scales* • Conners Rating Scales-R • BRIEF-P Subscales	• Arousal, alertness, orientation, regulation, inhibitory control, focus to specific materials (i.e., task, toys), sustained attention over time (throughout assessment or circle time)	• Course of attentional development (history of impulsivity, distractibility) • Attention limiting medical factors (i.e., medication) • Emotional problems affecting attention • Sleep patterns • Family history of attention problems

Note. GDS, Gordon Diagnostic System (Gordon, McClure, & Aylward, 1996); K-CPT, Conners' Kiddie Continuous Performance Test (Conners, 2001); TOVA, Test of Variables of Attention (Greenberg, 1996); BRIEF-P, Behavior Rating Inventory for Executive Functions—Preschool Version (Gioia, Espy, & Isquith, 2003). All other test abbreviations as in previous tables. Adapted by permission from Rey-Casserly (1999). Copyright 1999 by Allyn & Bacon.

quickly but makes many errors can score well, because fast completion time will cancel out error scores—a scenario commonly observed with impulsive preschoolers. The supplementary scores, which provide percentile classifications, can give detailed information about time of completion, inattentive, and impulsive errors separately. Auditory attention tasks (i.e., NEPSY Auditory Attention for ages 5 years and up) can be more problematic, because they often pose notable language demands, as well as rule learning, inhibitory, and shifting ability, complicating their interpretation. Based on clinical observation, many children have difficulty understanding the instructions or remembering them throughout such task. Of the very few alternatives, auditory span tasks (i.e., DAS Recall of Digits) can prove useful.

Standardized computerized and structured observation measures of sustained attention (continuing performance tests, go–no-go paradigms) can also be informative. These should, however, never be given as the sole attention measure, because they often yield average performance due to the high variability of normative data in this age group and are thus prone to false negatives. In addition, most computerized continuous performance tests currently available are long and tedious, and many preschoolers struggle to complete them, which limits their usefulness when time and duration of assessment is a factor. One possible approach is to first have parents and teachers complete questionnaires about their child's attention (i.e., Conners Rating Scales—Revised; Conners, 1996), observe the child's attention carefully during testing, and complete shorter measures of attention. If there continue to be questions about a possible deficit, then administration of a continuous performance task may be helpful.

Executive Functions

Executive functions refer to a variety of higher-order regulatory and metacognitive control processes necessary for adaptive and goal-oriented behavior. These functions include the abilities to anticipate, plan, organize, monitor, shift, and control behavioral–emotional responses, and are primarily mediated by prefrontal brain systems (Stuss & Benson, 1986; Welsh, Pennington, & Groisser, 1991). In young children, assessment of these higher-order skills was for a long time neglected, because they were assumed not to develop until later in childhood given the preschooler's "dysexecutive" presentation and high-normal variability of functions. Basic aspects of executive functions (inhibition, flexibility, and working memory), however, develop earlier than more complex metacognitive functions (problem solving, planning) and can thus be assessed in preschoolers (Diamond, 1991; Espy, 1997; Espy, Kaufman, Glisky, & McDiarmid, 2001; Espy, Kaufman, McDiarmid, & Glisky, 1999). Regulatory capacities in particular are critical to the preschooler's adaptation to his or her environment. Impairment of executive control processes is a common symptom in psychiatric and neurodevelopmental disorders (i.e., attention-deficit/hyperactivity disorder [ADHD], autism spectrum disorders), and is often already manifest in rudimentary executive functions during the preschool years, underscoring the need for early assessment.

Assessment of executive functions in preschoolers has been plagued by very limited availability of appropriate measures and the general criticism of limited ecological validity of formal tests. Assessment must therefore always include observation and parent–teacher report of "real-world" behavior. This should encompass observation and history of behavior regulation (i.e., impulsivity), emotional control (i.e., tolerance to frustration), flexibility (i.e., managing transitions), working memory (i.e., being able to remember things for a few minutes), and basic planning, rule-learning, and problem-solving skills. Standardized tests that are appropriate and sensitive to executive function deficits in preschoolers are scarce (see Table 13.4). Tower tasks are sometimes used to assess more complex planning and problem-solving abilities, but their sensitivity and interpretation is often questionable (i.e., NEPSY Tower). Verbal fluency tests are useful to assess speed of output, retrieval, and lexical organization. A range of tasks now in development is derived from developmental and cognitive neuroscience paradigms. Piaget's classic *A-not-B/ delayed response* and *alternation* tasks have been extensively researched in the context of prefrontal cortex functions (Diamond & Goldman-Rakic, 1989; Diamond, 1991; McEvoy, Rogers, & Pennington, 1993) and measure basic working memory, inhibition, and shifting abilities. The *Day–Night Test* (Gerstadt, Hong, & Diamond, 1994), based on the classic Stroop paradigm, was designed to examine inhibition and switching in young children; how-

TABLE 13.4. Common Tests and Assessment Methods for Executive Functions

Tests, rating scales	Observations	History
Inhibition, switching • Shape School • Day–Night Test • Trails-P • Alternation Task	*Behavior regulation* • Inhibitory control, activity level, emotional control, frustration tolerance, adjustment to transitions	• Early regulatory skills (sleep, emotion regulation) • History of behavior/ emotional problems (impulsivity, mood swings)
Working memory • A-not-B Task • Delayed Response Task	*Metacognitive* • Processing speed, divided attention, switching, working memory, initiation, planning, rule learning, goal-directed problem solving	
Fluency • NEPSY Verbal Fluency		
Rule learning, planning • NEPSY Tower • Spatial Reversal • BRIEF-P		

Note. NESPY, Korkman, Kirk, & Kemp (1997); BRIEF-P, Behavior Rating Inventory of Executive Function— Preschool Version (Gioia, Espy, & Isquith, 2003). Adapted by permission from Rey-Casserly (1999). Copyright 1999 by Allyn & Bacon.

ever, it has proven too difficult for children under 5 years old. Espy and colleagues (Espy, 1997, 2004; Espy, Kaufmann, et al., 2001) are currently developing a battery of tasks appropriate for preschoolers. *The Shape School* (Espy, 1997), a colorful storybook assessing inhibition and switching processes, has proven sensitive to maturation. TRAILS-P (Espy & Cwik, 2004), based on the Trail Making Test, examines processing speed, switching, and inhibition. Despite these exciting advances, clinicians still have to rely on observation and parent report, because most of these measures are not yet standardized and commercially available. One parent rating scale that has proven very useful and sensitive because it assesses regulatory and early metacognitive components of executive functions in the natural environment is the Behavior Rating Inventory of Executive Function—Preschool Version (BRIEF-P; Gioia, Espy, & Isquith, 2003) for 2- to 5-year-olds.

Language and Language-Related Processing

Language abilities are broadly divided into receptive and expressive language, with the former encompassing all processes related to comprehension of language and the latter referring to the communication of spoken language. Expressive language and speech are differentiated, in that speech is the mechanical aspect of oral language production, whereas language refers to the communication of meaningful symbols (Benson & Ardila, 1996). The importance of language assessment in the mental health setting becomes apparent when considering the notable comorbidity of psychiatric disorders in children with language impairment. Language impairment can also be an indicator for significant developmental or neurological compromise (i.e., early injury; Bates, 2005).

Language assessment should thus always include a parent interview about acquisition of language milestones (i.e., first words, first two-word phrases), as well as the course of language development and possible etiology of compromise. Children's hearing should be checked through an audiological exam. Observation of language and speech parameters during the assessment is critical to substantiate findings from standardized tests that are often limited to basic language tasks. This includes screening of phonological (sound) processing, comprehension of conversational versus complex language, spontaneous language output and conversational fluency, verbal social pragmatics, as well as a range of speech parameters (see Table 13.5). Comprehension problems are often readily evident if the child requires frequent modification of instructions on standardized tasks. There are many standardized assessment tools marketed for speech and language therapists, as well as psychologists. Assessment should include formal testing of receptive and expressive language, and contain more than just examination of basic receptive and expressive vocabulary. Vocabulary tasks, such as confrontation naming or single-word understanding, can often be inflated by the child's experiences, such as involvement in speech and language therapy or exposure to a highly enriched language environment. It is not uncommon that children's perfor-

TABLE 13.5. Common Tests and other Assessment Methods of Language Abilities

Tests, rating scales	Observations	History
Broad language • PLS-4 • CELF-Preschool 2 • TOLD-2 *Receptive/phonological* • PPVT-III • DAS Verbal Comprehension • NEPSY Language subtests *Expressive* • EOWVT • WPPSI-III, DAS Vocabulary subtests • NEPSY Language subtests • VABS Communication	• Hearing • Comprehension of conversation, directions • Spontaneous language • Quality of conversation • Elaboration of verbal responses; vocabulary usage, syntax, grammar • Speech parameters: articulation, prosody, volume, rate and rhythm, fluency of word usage	• Developmental language milestones • Oral–motor development • Medical history (i.e., ear infections) • Communicative skills (use of language to relate experiences) • Signing, gesturing of needs • Play with language content (word games, stories) • Speech therapy report

Note. PLS-4, Preschool Language Scale, Fourth Edition (Zimmerman, Steiner, & Pond, 2003); CELF–Preschool 2, Clinical Evaluation of Language Fundamentals—Preschool, Second Edition (Semel, Wiig, & Secord, 2004); TOLD-2, Test of Language Development—Second Edition (Newcomber & Hammill, 1988); PPVT-III, Peabody Picture Vocabulary Test, Third Edition (Dunn & Dunn, 1997); EOWVT, Expressive One-Word Picture Vocabulary Test (2000 ed., Gardner, 2000). All other test abbreviations as in previous tables. Adapted by permission from Rey-Casserly (1999). Copyright 1999 by Allyn & Bacon.

mance on these measures is elevated, whereas that on measures of more complex grammatical and syntactical language is compromised. Careful note taking and examination of language samples (i.e., exact communications with
parent or examiner, storytelling) is often the only alternative in the absence of
formal complex language measures for preschoolers. Verbal subtests from intelligence scales not only provide valuable information about the child's fund
of verbal knowledge and verbal reasoning skills, but also provides answers to
open-ended questions that can serve as language samples. Finally, language
assessment must account for dialectical derivations between regions, race,
and ethnicity. Within this context, bilingual assessment presents a particular
challenge.

Nonverbal/Visual–Spatial Processing

Visual–spatial processing refers rather loosely to a range of cognitive and
perceptual processes involved in recognition of objects, localizing and attending to objects in space, and understanding the spatial relationships of
the different parts of an object or pattern (Stiles, 2001). Assessment of this
broad class of abilities includes *perceptual* (recognition), *visual–constructional* (manipulation), and *visual–motor* (drawing) tasks that involve spatial
components (see Table 13.6). The most commonly used tests for preschoolers include form matching, block design, jigsaw puzzles, and shape-copying
tasks. Most of these tasks have been found to be sensitive to neurological
compromise, and have gained a central role in clinical neuropsychology.
Their interpretation is, however, often complicated by the different skills required to complete such multifactorial tasks (i.e., sensory perception, speed,
attention to visual detail, visual–motor coordination, planning, organization). In addition, most measures of so-called "nonverbal" processing are
not purely nonverbal, but contain considerable language content; pictorial
and design material can be labeled, and strategies on visual–construction
tasks can be verbally mediated (i.e., "left–right," "up–down"). Careful task
analysis is thus essential for interpretation of test scores and subdomains assessed.

Before assessing visual–perceptual or visual–spatial skills, it is essential to
ensure that primary visual systems are intact. In addition, visual–perceptual
skills that are not captured by standardized tests, yet are relevant for the diagnostic cluster, can often be easily observed throughout the assessment session.
These can include not only observation of the child's navigation in topo-
graphic space (i.e., finding the way back to the testing room) but also recognition of objects, faces, and familiar persons, as well as nonverbal aspects of
social communication, which can be critical indicators for autism spectrum
disorders. In addition, qualitative observation on constructional and drawing
tasks provides invaluable insight into a child's problem-solving and planning
strategies.

TABLE 13.6. Common Tests and Assessment Methods of Visual–Spatial/
Nonverbal Abilities

Tests, rating scales	Observations	History

Visual–perceptual
• WRAVMA Matching
• Beery Matching
• K-ABC Gestalt Closure
 	
Visual–constructional
• Block Design tasks
  (WPPSI-III, DAS,
  NEPSY, K-ABC)
• Puzzle tasks (WPPSI-III,
  K-ABC)
 	
Reasoning
• DAS Picture Similarities
• WPPSI-III Picture Concepts
• WPPSI-III Matrix
  Reasoning
• RCPMT
 	
Visual–motor integration
• WRAVMA Copying
• VMI
	• Visual acuity, visual
	  field, visual scanning
	• Face/object recognition
	• Navigation in and
	  exploration of space
	• Localization of objects
	• Problem-solving strategy
		• Development of visual–
		  constructional and spatial
		  skills (i.e., puzzles, blocks)
		• Interest in building toys
		• Navigation of home and
		  day care environment
		• Neurological and medical
		  history
		• Occupational therapy
		  report

Note. RCPMT, Raven's Coloured Progressive Matrices Test (Raven, 1965). All other test abbreviations as in
previous tables.) Adapted by permission from Rey-Casserly (1999). Copyright 1999 by Allyn & Bacon.

Because most measures of visual–spatial processing, however, require
eye–hand coordination and copying (from a person, stimulus, or picture) under time pressure, they can have limited validity for children with speed,
praxis, or motor impairments. For example, some young children with developmental delays such as pervasive developmental disorder have inherent difficulty with tasks that require copying the examiner. The assessment thus needs
to also include a parent interview about "real-world" visual–spatial skills
(i.e., play with building toys, navigation of the home or preschool environment), and integrate these with test results. In addition, observation of other
visual–spatial problem-solving tasks, including age-appropriate puzzles, building, and computer games, can be useful.

Memory and Learning

Memory refers to a variety of processes to acquire, retain, and retrieve information. The hallmark memory models (Schacter & Tulving, 1994; Squire,
1982; Tulving, 1972) distinguish broadly between *declarative/explicit* (conscious memory) and *implicit/procedural* (incidental unconscious learning)
memory. Declarative memory is further divided into *semantic* memory (fac-

tual knowledge) and *episodic* memory (events and facts with relevance to personal experience), and has been closely linked to the hippocampal formation. Measures to assess these skills often include paragraph recall, list-learning, and design-learning tasks. There are also temporal aspects of memory that are important to consider for clinical assessment: *Short-term* memory is the ability to hold information online for a very short time period (seconds to minutes) before it is encoded and later retained, whereas *long-term* memory refers to consolidation and storage over time. Retrieval of information can be assessed through free recall and recognition tasks; the latter require more basic processes, and poor performance is thus indicative of greater memory compromise.

Contrary to previous assumption, early memory systems, including habit learning/implicit, preexplicit, and early explicit memory, start to develop during the first year of life, with adult-like functions maturing throughout the preschool years (Luciana & Nelson, 1998; Nelson, 1994, 1997; see Heffelfinger & Mrakotsky, Chapter 3, this volume, for details). Preschoolers are thus quite able to perform basic memory tasks. As Baron (2004) points out, however, typical amnestic disorders are relatively rare in children, and more in-depth assessment can help elucidate the etiology and source of memory complaints often presented by parents. In young children, these often reflect other deficits, such as inattention, language impairment, limited knowledge and use of strategies, or emotional problems that should be of particular concern to preschool mental health clinicians because they can interfere with early learning and knowledge acquisition.

Standardized measures of memory for preschool children are sparse, and availability of age-appropriate tests lags behind those of other specific domains, despite a breadth of knowledge on memory development during the preschool age and its tremendous importance during these early years of rapid knowledge acquisition and learning. Broad memory scales assessing several aspects of memory are only available for older preschoolers (age 5 years and up) (see Table 13.7). Some neuropsychological and cognitive scales include memory subtests applicable to younger age ranges, but these are very scarce. It is also critical to evaluate what type of memory is assessed by a specific task (i.e., recall vs. recognition), whether the learning material is visual or verbal–auditory, and whether it provides context (i.e., story) or is noncontextual (i.e., word list). Memory assessment in children typically includes paragraph recall and list-learning tasks, but these are very limited for preschool-age children. Basic memory assessment in preschoolers can include short-term memory tasks such as digit span or sentence repetition tasks, as well as picture recognition tasks. Knowledge-based tests from cognitive scales and naming tests can also be useful, because they often require long-term storage and retrieval components. In addition, history, observation, and behavior probes (i.e., retelling a story or recent event, remembering names of people) in the assessment and the natural environment are important components in the absence of appropriate standardized measures.

TABLE 13.7. Common Tests and Assessment Methods of Memory

Tests, rating scales	Observations	History
Broad memory scales • CMS (5+ years) • WRAML-2 (5+ years) *Declarative memory* • CVLT-C (5+ years) • DAS Recall of Objects (4+) • DAS Recognition of Pictures • NEPSY Narrative Memory, Memory for Names, Memory for Faces • K-ABC Face Recognition, Spatial Memory, Word Order *Short-term memory span* • DAS Recall of Digits • NEPSY Sentence Repetition • K-ABC Number Recall	• Memory for names, faces, objects, places, and topographical location • Memory for everyday events, special events (birthdays, etc.) • Ability to learn and retain information over time (including parent, teacher report) • Flexible versus rote memorization	• Development of early memory skills (recognition of familiar faces; ability to learn names, places, events, etc.) • Acquisition and retention of basic knowledge, nursery rhymes, stories, movie content, etc.

Note. CMS, Children's Memory Scale (Cohen, 1997); WRAML-2, Wide Range Assessment of Memory and Learning, Second Edition (Sheslow & Adams, 2004); CVLT-C, California Verbal Learning Test—Children's Version (Delis, Kramer, Kaplan, & Ober, 1994). All other test abbreviations as in previous tables. Adapted by permission from Rey-Casserly (1999). Copyright 1999 by Allyn & Bacon.

Preacademic Skills

Preacademic skills are all those early skills necessary for scholastic achievement and school readiness, including early letter and number skills essential for reading, spelling, and math. Most preschoolers are able to recognize letters and symbols, form letters and write their name, count, add, and understand basic quantitative concepts. Assessment of these skills is necessary to identify children at risk for later learning disabilities.

For example, dyslexia—the difficulty learning to read and spell—is typically not diagnosable until the end of first or second grade; however, several precursors for risk for dyslexia exist already during the preschool years or even earlier. These include problems with phoneme awareness, articulation, sequencing of syllables, word finding, and learning color and letter names. Children who are exposed to books through adult reading in home or school environments, should be able to recognize all upper- and lowercase letters by the end of kindergarten (Pennington & Lefly, 2001). If they do not, they are at risk for developing reading difficulties and may require immediate reading intervention. Similarly, children with early difficulties in understanding quantitative and number concepts, basic numerical operations (addition), and simple visual–spatial relations may be at risk for later math difficulties. Assessment should hence always encompass a careful history of precursors for such learning difficulties, as well as observation and behavioral probes beyond what is provided through standardized tests (see Table 13.8). The clinician's

TABLE 13.8. Common Tests and Assessment Methods of Achievement

Tests, rating scales	Observations	History
• WJ-III Achievement • K-ABC Achievement Scale • WPPSI-III Arithmetic • DAS Matching Letter-Like Forms, Early Number Concepts	• Naming colors, letters, and numbers • Phoneme and sound–symbol awareness • Letter formation • Counting, basic addition and quantitative concepts	• Acquisition of early number concepts, alphabet, letter formation, signs • Exposure to and interest in books, letter and number games • Educational history • School reports

Note. WJ-III, Woodcock–Johnson Psychoeducational Battery, Tests of Achievement, Third Edition (Woodcock, McGrew, & Mather, 2001). All other test abbreviations as in previous tables. Adapted by permission from Rey-Casserly (1999). Copyright 1999 by Allyn & Bacon.

knowledge of expected development in these areas, as well as the developmental course of specific learning disabilities, is critical to the assessment and intervention planning process.

Socioemotional/Adaptive Skills

Socioemotional skills and adjustment to the environment build the critical foundation for a child's well-being and learning. In simple terms, children need to feel confident and competent to master the daily developmental challenges they face. A child who is not happy is less likely to get involved with activities and peers, and may thus have limited opportunities for important

TABLE 13.9. Common Standardized Tests and Assessment Methods of Adaptive and Emotional/Personality Functioning

Tests, rating scales	Observations	History
Emotional/personality • Draw-a-person • CAT *Behavior rating scales* • CBCL1.5–5 • BRIEF-P Emotional Control *Adaptive skills (parent rating)* • VABS • SIB-R	*Emotional/social* • Range of affect, mood Social interactions • Interpersonal boundaries • Social pragmatics • Adjustment to new situations and people • Content of symbolic play, narratives, drawings *Adaptive skills* • Self-advocacy, self-help skills (dressing, hygiene, mobility, etc.)	*Emotional/social* • Emotional development (temperament, regulation) • Separation, attachment • Family relationships • Peer interactions • Family history of psychiatric disorders *Adaptive skills* • Development of independence, self-help skills, toilet training, etc.

Note. CAT, Children's Apperception Test (Bellak & Bellak, 1987); CBCL 1.5–5, Child Behavior Checklist 1.5–5 (Achenbach & Rescorla, 2000). All other test abbreviations as in previous tables. Adapted by permission from Rey-Casserly (1999). Copyright 1999 by Allyn & Bacon.

learning experiences. Comprehensive neuropsychological assessment needs to include a brief evaluation of the preschooler's emotional status and development, regulatory skills, and adaptive/independence skills. Most of the emotional assessment techniques for preschoolers use structured behavioral observation and parent interview (for an overview, see Table 13.9); however, observation of play and social interactions, as well as historical data, contribute important diagnostic information (for a detailed review on assessment of socioemotional development see Chapters 1 and 2, this volume).

SOME FURTHER CONSIDERATIONS AND LIMITATIONS IN PRESCHOOL ASSESSMENT

Referrals and Assessment Goals

Clinicians in outpatient settings for preschoolers often encounter developmental and behavioral problems as primary referral reasons for neuropsychological assessment. Referral requests increasingly include evaluation of emotional adjustment to existing cognitive or behavioral problems. There has been increased emphasis on the need for early diagnosis of mental and developmental disorders as a basis for early intervention. The primary goal of the assessment is to inform not only diagnosis but also risk assessment and intervention planning. Assessment must be "resource-oriented," with the goal of describing a child's strengths and competencies, as well as identifying weaknesses, to provide effective recommendations and refocus parents' and teachers' attention on what the child *is* capable of doing, instead of overconcentrating on his or her deficits.

Normal Variability of Development

Rapid yet unsteady development is inherent to the nature of the preschool child. Although normative approaches, with outlines for "what develops when," are very useful to guide the assessment process, consideration needs to be given to the significant variability of skills within this age range and within the child (i.e., from day to day). Skills may develop at different ages, at different rates, and out of sequence. This carries major implications not only for reliability (including stability), validity (including prognostic) (see the section of this chapter on general cognitive abilities), and norms of assessment instruments, but also for our understanding of what is considered normative ("extreme normal behavior"—e.g., hyperactivity) versus atypical behavior (behavior not occurring in "normal development"—e.g., stereotypic behavior).

Assessment Setting and Process

In preschoolers, even more so than in older children, the nature of the child poses considerable challenges for the assessment process. Young children have typically less physical and attentional stamina, and require more emotional nurturing than do older children and those who are used to school routines. They often require frequent breaks and several brief assessment sessions to be able to comply with assessment demands. Multiple sessions also provide an opportunity to see the child on different occasions and thus get a more valid appreciation of his or her abilities, rather than a one-time "snap-shot." Careful consideration of variables in the testing environment (i.e., structure, manipulative materials, "noise-free" room) and assessment process (i.e., individual attention, rewards) that facilitate a child's compliance and, therefore, performance is a key element not only in the assessment itself but also in diagnosis and management planning.

Considerations for the Assessment of "True" Abilities

When assessing the young child, one must consider the commonly encountered challenges that may affect the validity of the assessment. A child needs intact sensory and motor skills (i.e., to be able to see, hear, speak, and move) to be able to perform tasks requiring higher cognitive abilities. Whereas developmentally normative limitations (i.e., limited attention, articulation problems) can notably impact a child's performance, and thus mask his or her true ability in any given area, specific neurological, neurodevelopmental, or psychiatric disorders can cause functional impairment that may make standardized psychometric assessment difficult. "Clinical limit testing" (i.e., removing time limits on timed tasks, providing extra cues) in conjunction with observation and thorough history are then essential to get an estimate of the child's true abilities.

Some of the most commonly encountered limitations in the assessment of preschool developmental and mental health populations include the following: For example, preschoolers with mental illness (i.e., ADHD or mood disorders) often demonstrate fine motor and speed difficulties such as slowing, planning, and sequencing deficits. Naturally, they can struggle on tasks primarily measuring fine motor skills, but they are likely to also have difficulties on all tasks that rely on these basic skills (i.e., visual–motor integration, visual–spatial construction). In interpreting test scores on such higher-order tasks, it is thus critical to consider the source of difficulty, because the actual compromise is in basic motor skills or slowed processing, and not in those skills assumed to be measured by the test. Similarly, oro-motor difficulties often result in poor articulation and speech production, which is not indicative of an expressive language problem itself, although children may have a hard time expressing themselves on standardized language tasks. Difficulties in one skill (i.e., articulation) commonly assigned to a specific domain (i.e., language) may have more far-reaching implications for other domains (i.e., motor and planning skills). Difficulties with language (both receptive and expressive), on the other hand, affect performance on all tasks with language demands, including verbal knowledge, reasoning, and memory—and, as a matter of fact, on all tasks with verbal instructions (including so-called "non-verbal" measures). If a child is not able to process complex language, he or she will have difficulty understanding instructions, verbal questions, and other verbal–auditory material (stories, sentences); if children struggle to correctly produce and sequence complex sentences, they are likely to have difficulty demonstrating their knowledge and repeating verbal information (stories, etc.). In both scenarios, the child's poor performance should not be interpreted as an indicator of primary deficits in verbal knowledge or memory per se.

Most commonly, however, attention can be highly variable in preschoolers, which is often normative depending on the level of difficulty of presented material and time required to maintain attention. Because of this, accurate assessment of preschoolers often requires several short testing sessions rather than one long one. Interpretation of results also requires careful examination of on-task behavior and task-complexity of each test to ensure that poor performance was not primarily caused by difficulty in focusing and sustaining attention.

CONCLUSION

In summary, there are many factors to consider when assessing the skills and abilities of a young child. This chapter has provided an overview of the most salient conceptual models and techniques for assessment of individual neuropsychological domains. Most importantly, the neuropsychological assessment is not defined purely by the administration of tests, but is a complex clinical process that requires skilled integration of test, observational, and historical data, with knowledge from multiple disciplines about brain–behavior relationships and development thereof. This is particularly salient in light of limited standardized measures for preschool children. Promising developments are now, however, in progress to expand the volume of developmentally appropriate instruments.

ACKNOWLEDGMENT

We would like to gratefully acknowledge the editorial assistance of Jane Holmes Bernstein, PhD, Department of Psychiatry, Children's Hospital, Boston.

REFERENCES

Achenbach, T. A., & Rescorla, L. (2000). *Child Behavior Checklist for Ages 1. 5–5.* Burlington: Achenbach System of Empirically-Based Assessment, University of Vermont.

Adams, W., & Sheslow, D. (1995). *Wide Range Assessment of Visual–Motor Abilities—Manual.* Wilmington, DE: Jastak.

Aylward, G. (1988). Infant and early childhood assessment. In M. Tramontana & S. Hooper (Eds.), *Assessment issues in clinical neuropsychology* (pp. 225–248). New York: Plenum Press.

Bailey, A., Luthert, P., Dean, A., Harding, B., Janota, I., Montgomery, M., et al. (1998). A clinicopathological study of autism. *Brain, 121,* 889–905.

Baron, I. S. (2004). *Neuropsychological evaluation of the child.* New York: Oxford University Press.

Baron, I. S., Fennell, E. B., & Voeller, K. K. S. (1995). *Pediatric neuropsychology in the medical setting.* New York: Oxford University Press.

Bates, E. (2005). Plasticity, localization, and language development. In S. T. Parker, J. Langer, & C. Milbrath (Eds.), *Biology and knowledge revisited: From neurogenesis to psychogenesis* (pp. 205–253). Mahwah, NJ: Erlbaum.

Bayley, N. (1993). *Bayley Scales of Infant Development* (2nd ed.). San Antonio, TX: Psychological Corporation.

Beery, K. E. (1997). *The Beery–Buktenica Developmental Test of Visual–Motor Integration: Administration, scoring, and teaching manual* (4th ed.). Parsippany, NJ: Modern Curriculum Press.

Bellak, L., & Bellak, S. S. (1987). *Children's Apperception Test.* Larchmont, NY: CPS.

Benson, D. F., & Ardila, A. (1996). *Aphasia: A clinical perspective.* New York: Oxford University Press.

Bernstein, J. H. (2000). Developmental neuropsychological assessment. In K. O. Yeates, M. D. Ris, & H. G. Taylor (Eds.), *Pediatric neuropsychology: Research, theory, and practice* (pp. 405–438). New York: Guilford Press.

Bernstein, J. H., & Waber, D. P. (2003). Pediatric neuropsychological assessment. In T. E. Feinberg & M. J. Farah (Eds.), *Behavioral neurology and neuropsychology* (2nd ed., pp. 773–781). New York: McGraw-Hill.

Binet, A. (1916). New methods for the diagnosis of the intellectual level of subnormals. In E. S. Kite (Trans.), *The development of intelligence in children.* Vineland, NJ: Publications of the Training School at Vineland. (Originally published in 1905 in *L'Année Psychologique, 12,* 191–244)

Bourgeois, J. P., Goldman-Rakic, P. S., & Rakic, P. (1994). Synaptogenesis in the prefrontal cortex of rhesus monkeys. *Cerebral Cortex, 4*(1), 78–96.

Bourgeois, J. P., Goldman-Rakic, P. S., & Rakic, P. (2000). Formation, elimination and stabilization of synapses in the primate cerebral cortex. In M. Gazzaniga (Ed.), *The new cognitive neurosciences* (pp. 45–53). Cambridge, MA: MIT Press.

Bronfenbrenner, U. (2005). The bioecological theory of human development. In U. Bronfenbrenner (Ed.), *Making human beings human: Bioecological perspectives on human development* (pp. 3–15). Thousand Oaks, CA: Sage.

Bronfenbrenner, U., & Ceci, S. (1994). Nature–nurture reconceptualized in developmental perspective: A bioecological model. *Psychological Review, 101,* 568–586.

Bruininks, R. H., Woodcock, R. W., Weatherman, R. F., & Hill, B. K. (1996). *The Scales of Independent Behavior–Revised.* Itasca, IL: Riverside.

Cattell, R. B. (1963). Theory of fluid and crystallized intelligence. *Journal of Educational Psychology, 54,* 1–22.

Cohen, M. J. (1997). *Children's Memory Scale.* San Antonio, TX: Psychological Corporation.

Cohen, R. A. (1993). *Neuropsychology of attention.* New York: Plenum Press.

Conners, C. K. (1996). *Conners' Rating Scales—Revised.* San Antonio, TX: Psychological Corporation.

Conners, C. K. (2001). *Conners' Kiddie Continuous Performance Test.* North Tonawanda, NY: Multi-Health Systems.

Cousens, P., Waters, B., Said, J., & Stevens, M. (1988). Cognitive effects of cranial irradiation in leukemia: A survey and meta-analysis. *Child Psychology and Psychiatry, 29,* 839–852.

Delis, D., Kramer, J. H., Kaplan, E., & Ober, B. A. (1994). *California Verbal Learning Test—Children's Version.* San Antonio, TX: Psychological Corporation.

Diamond, A. (1991). Guidelines for the study of brain–behavior relationships during development. In H. Levin, H. Eisenberg, & A. Benton (Eds.), *Frontal lobe function and dysfunction* (pp. 339–378). New York: Oxford University Press.

Diamond, A., & Goldman-Rakic, P. S. (1989). Comparison of human infants and rhesus monkeys on Piaget's AB task: Evidence for dependence on dorsolateral prefrontal cortex. *Experimental Brain Research, 74,* 24–40.

Dunn, L. M., & Dunn, L. M. (1997). *Examiner's manual for the Peabody Picture Vocabulary Test* (3rd ed.). Circle Pines, MN: American Guidance Service.

Elliott, C. D. (1990). *Differential Ability Scales.* San Antonio, TX: Psychological Corporation.

Espy, K. A. (1997). The Shape School: Assessing executive function in preschool children. *Developmental Neuropsychology, 13,* 495–499.

Espy, K. A. (2004). Using developmental, cognitive, and neuroscience approaches to understand executive control in young children. *Developmental Neuropsychology, 26*(1), 379–384.

Espy, K. A., & Cwik, M. F. (2004). The development of a Trail Making Test in young children: The TRAILS-P. *Clinical Neuropsychologist, 18*(3), 411–422.

Espy, K. A., Kaufman, P. M., Glisky, M. L., & McDiarmid, M. D. (2001). New procedures to assess executive functions in preschool children. *Clinical Neuropsychologist, 15,* 46–58.

Espy, K. A., Kaufman, P. M., McDiarmid, M. D., & Glisky, M. L. (1999). Executive functioning in preschool children: Performance on A-not-B and other delayed response format tasks. *Brain and Cognition, 41,* 178–199.

Espy, K. A., Molfese, V. J., & DiLalla, L. F. (2001). Effects of environmental measures on intelligence in young children: Growth curve modeling of longitudinal data. *Merrill–Palmer Quarterly, 47*(1), 42–73.

Ewing-Cobbs, L., Fletcher, J. M., Levin, H. S., Francis, D. J., Davidson, K., & Miner, M. E. (1997). Longitudinal neuropsychological outcome in infants and preschoolers with traumatic brain injury. *Journal of the International Neuropsychological Society, 3*(6), 581–591.

Ewing-Cobbs, L., Levin, H. S., Eisenberg, H. M., & Fletcher, J. M. (1987). Language functions following closed-head injury in children and adolescents. *Journal of Clinical and Experimental Neuropsychology, 9*(5), 575–592.

Flanagan, D. P., & Alfonso, V. C. (1995). A critical review of the technical characteristics of new and recently revised intelligence tests for preschool children. *Journal of Psychoeducational Assessment, 13*(1), 66–90.

Fletcher, J., & Taylor, H. (1984). Neuropsychological approaches to children: Toward a developmental neuropsychology. *Journal of Clinical Neuropsychology, 6,* 39–56.

Gardner, M. F. (2000). *Expressive One-Word Picture Vocabulary Test—2000 Edition.* Novato, CA: Academic Therapy.

Gerstadt, C. L., Hong, Y. J., & Diamond, A. (1994). The relationship between cognition and action: Performance of children 3½–7 on a Stroop-like Day–Night Test. *Cognition, 53,* 129–153.

Gioia, G. A., Espy, K. A, & Isquith, P. K. (2003). *Behavior Rating Inventory for Executive Function—Preschool Version.* Lutz, FL: Psychological Assessment Resources.

Gordon, M., McClure, F. D., & Aylward, G. P. (1996). *Gordon Diagnostic System interpretive guide* (3rd ed.). DeWitt, NY: GSI Publications.

Greenberg, L. M. (1996). *Test of Variables of Attention.* St. Paul, MN: Attention Technology.

Greenfield, P. M. (1997). You can't take it with you: Why ability assessments don't cross cultures. *American Psychologist, 52,* 1115–1124.

Greenough, W. E., Black, J. E., & Wallace, C. S. (1987). Experience and brain development. *Child Development, 58,* 539–559.

Greenough, W. T., & Alcantara, A. A. (1993). The roles of experience in different developmental information stage processes. In B. de Boysson-Bardies, S. de Schonen, P. Jusczyk, P. McNeilage, & J. Morton (Eds.), *Developmental neurocognition: Speech and face processing in the first year of life* (pp. 3–16). New York: Kluwer Academic.

Guilford, J. P. (1956). The structure of intellect. *Psychological Bulletin, 53,* 267–293.

Holmes-Bernstein, J., & Waber, D. P. (1990). Developmental neuropsychological assessment: The systemic approach. In A. A. Boulton, G. B. Baker, & M. Hiscock (Eds.), *Neuromethods: Vol. 17. Neuropsychology* (pp. 311–371). Totowa, NJ: Humana Press.

Hooper, S. R. (2000). Neuropsychological assessment of the preschool child. In B. Bracken (Ed.), *The psychoeducational assessment of preschool children* (3rd ed., pp. 383–398). Needham Heights, MA: Allyn & Bacon.

Huttenlocher, P. R., & Dabholkar, A. S. (1997). Regional differences in synaptogenesis in the human cerebral cortex. *Journal of Comparative Neurology, 387,* 167–178.

Kaplan, E. (1988). A process approach to neuropsychological assessment. In T. Boll & B. K. Bryant (Eds.), *Clinical neuropsychology and brain function* (pp. 125–167). Washington, DC: American Psychological Association.

Kaplan, E. (1990). The process approach to neuropsychological assessment of psychiatric patients. *Journal of Neuropsychiatry and Clinical Neurosciences, 2*(1), 72–87.

Kaufman, A. S., & Kaufman, N. L. (1983). *Kaufman Assessment Battery for Children: Interpretive manual.* Circle Pines, MN: American Guidance Services.

Korkman, M., Kirk, U., & Kemp, S. (1997). *NEPSY: A developmental neuropsychological assessment.* San Antonio, TX: Psychological Corporation.

Luciana, M., & Nelson, C. A. (1998). The functional emergence of prefrontally-guided working memory systems in four- to eight-year-old children. *Neuropsychologia, 36*(3), 273–293.

McCarthy, D. (1972). *Manual for the McCarthy Scales of Children's Abilities.* New York: Psychological Corporation.

McEvoy, R. E., Rogers, S. J., & Pennington, B. F. (1993). Executive function and social communication deficits in young autistic children. *Journal of Child Psychology and Psychiatry, 34*(4), 563–578.

Molfese, V., Holcomb, L., & Helwig, S. (1994). Biomedical and social-environmental influences on cognitive and verbal abilities in children 1 to 3 years of age. *International Journal of Behavioral Development, 17,* 271–287.

Mrakotsky, C., & Waber, D. P. (2006). Chemotherapy agents for treatment of acute lymphoblastic leukemia. In D. Bellinger (Ed.), *Human developmental neurotoxicology* (pp. 131–147). New York: Taylor & Francis.

Mullen, E. M. (1995). *Mullen Scales of Early Learning.* Los Angeles: Western Psychological Services.

Neisworth, J. T., & Bagnato, S. J. (1992). The case against intelligence testing in early intervention. *Topics in Early Childhood Special Education, 12*(1), 1–20.

Nelson, C. (1994). Long-term retention of memory for preverbal experience: Evidence and implications. *Memory, 2*(4), 467–475.

Nelson, C. A. (1997). The neurobiological basis of early memory development. In N. Cowan (Ed.), *The development of memory in childhood* (pp. 41–82). Hove, East Sussex, UK: Psychology Press.

Newcomber, P. L., & Hammill, D. D. (1988). *Test of Language Development–2.* Austin, TX: PRO-ED.

Neyens, L. G. J., & Aldenkamp, A. P. (1996). Stability of cognitive measures in children of average ability. *Child Neuropsychology, 2,* 161–170.

Pennington, B. F., & Lefly, D. L. (2001). Early reading development in children at family risk for dyslexia. *Child Development, 72*(3), 816–833.

Piven, J., Berthier, M. L., Starkstein, S. E., Nehme, E., Pearlson, G., & Folstein, S. (1990). Magnetic resonance imaging evidence for a defect of cerebral cortical development in autism. *American Journal of Psychiatry, 147*(6), 734–739.

Posner, M. I., & Peterson, S. E. (1990). The attention system of the human brain. *Annual Review of Neuroscience, 13,* 25–42.

Rakic, P. (1995). Corticogenesis in human and nonhuman primates. In M. S. Gazzaniga (Ed.), *The cognitive neurosciences* (pp. 127–145). Cambridge, MA: MIT Press.

Raven, J. C. (1965). *The Coloured Progressive Matrices.* London: Lewis.

Rey-Casserly, C. (1999). Neuropsychological assessment of preschool children. In E. Vazquez Nuttall, I. Romero, & J. Kalesnik (Eds.), *Assessing and screening preschoolers: Psychological and educational dimensions* (2nd ed., pp. 281–295). Needham Heights, MA: Allyn & Bacon.

Rourke, B. P., Fisk, J. L., & Strang, J. D. (1986). *Neuropsychological assessment of children.* New York: Guilford Press.

Sameroff, A. J., Seifer, R., Barocas, B., Zax, M., & Greenspan, S. I. (1987). IQ scores of 4-year-old children: Social–environmental risk factors. *Pediatrics, 79,* 343–350.

Sattler, J. M. (2001). *Assessment of children: Cognitive applications.* San Diego, CA: Author.

Schacter, D. L., & Tulving, E. (1994). *Memory systems.* Cambridge, MA: The MIT Press.

Semel, E., Wiig, E. H., & Secord, W. A. (2004). *Clinical Evaluation of Language Fundamentals—Preschool* (2nd ed.). San Antonio, TX: Harcourt Assessment.

Sheslow, D., & Adams, W. (2004). *Wide range assessment for memory and learning* (2nd ed.). Austin, TX: PRO-ED.

Sparrow, S. S., Balla, D. A., & Cicchetti, D. V. (1984). *Vineland Adaptive Behavior Scales: Interview edition.* Circle Pines, MN: American Guidance Service.

Spearman, C. (1904). "General intelligence," objectively determined and measured. *American Journal of Psychology, 15,* 201–293.

Spearman, C. (1923). *The nature of intelligence and the principles of cognition.* London: Macmillan.

Squire, L. R. (1982). The neuropsychology of human memory. *Annual Review of Neuroscience, 5,* 241–273.

Stern, W. (1912). *The psychological methods of testing intelligence* (G. Whipple, Trans.). Baltimore: Warwick & York.

Sternberg, R. J., Grigorenko, E. L., & Bundy, D. A. (2001). The predictive value of IQ. *Merrill-Palmer Quarterly, 47*(1), 1–41.

Stiles, J. (2001). Spatial cognitive development. In C. A. Nelson & M. Luciana (Eds.), *Handbook of developmental cognitive neuroscience* (pp. 399–414). Cambridge, MA: MIT Press.

Stuss, D. T., & Benson, D. F. (1986). *The frontal lobes.* New York: Raven Press.

Taylor, H. G., & Fletcher, J. M. (1990). Neuropsychological assessment of children. In G. Goldsteni & M. Hersen (Eds.), *Handbook of psychological assessment* (2nd ed., pp. 228–255). Elmsford, NY: Pergamon Press.

Thorndike, R. (1997). The early history of intelligence testing. In D. P. Flanagan, J. L. Genschaft, & P. L. Harrison (Eds.), *Contemporary intellectual assessment: Theories, tests, and issues* (pp. 3–16). New York: Guilford Press.

Thurstone, L. L. (1938). *Primary mental abilities.* Chicago: University of Chicago Press.

Tiffin, J., & Asher, E. J. (1948). The Purdue Pegboard: Norms and studies or reliability and validity. *Journal of Applied Psychology, 32,* 234–247.

Tulving, E. (1972). Episodic and semantic memory. In E. Tulving & W. Donaldson (Eds.), *Organization of memory* (pp. 381–403). New York: Academic Press.

Waber, D. P., Shapiro, B. L., Carpentieri, S. C., Gelber, R. D., Zou, G., Dufresne, A., et al. (2001). Excellent therapeutic efficacy and minimal late neurotoxicity in children treated with 18 grays of cranial radiation therapy for high-risk acute lymphoblastic leukemia: A 7-year follow-up study of the Dana–Farber Cancer Institute Consortium Protocol 87–01. *Cancer, 92*(1), 15–22.

Wechsler, D. (1939). *The measurement of adult intelligence.* Baltimore: Williams & Wilkins.

Wechsler, D. (1949). *Manual for the Wechsler Intelligence Scale for Children.* New York: Psychological Corporation.

Wechsler, D. (2002). *Wechsler Preschool and Primary Scale of Intelligence—Third Edition.* San Antonio, TX: Psychological Corporation.

Welsh, M. C., Pennington, B. F., & Groisser, D. B. (1991). A normative–developmental study of executive function: A window on prefrontal function on children. *Developmental Neuropsychology, 7,* 131–149.

Wilson, B. C. (1992). The neuropsychological assessment of the preschool child: A branching model. In I. Rapin & S. J. Segalowitz (Eds.), *Handbook of neuropsychology: Vol. 6. Child neuropsychology* (pp. 377–394). New York: Elsevier Science.

Wilson, B. C., Iacovello, J. M., Wilson, J. J., & Risucci, P. (1982). Purdue Pegboard performance of normal preschool children. *Journal of Clinical Neuropsychology, 4,* 19–26.

Woodcock, R. W., McGrew, K. S., & Mather, N. (2001). *Woodcock–Johnson III Tests of Achievement (WJ III).* Itasca, IL: Riverside.

Zimmerman, I. L., Steiner, V. G., & Pond, R. E. (2003). *Preschool Language Scale—Fourth Edition.* San Antonio, TX: Harcourt Assessment.

14

Psychopharmacology

JOAN L. LUBY

The idea of prescribing psychotropic agents to preschool children is one that meets with strong social resistance and even aversion. Since pharmacological treatment of young children with serious medical disorders is a common and well-accepted practice, it would seem that implicit in this more specific bias toward psychiatric medications is the underlying disbelief that young children can suffer from serious and impairing mental disorders requiring aggressive medical treatment. Because only a few very specific areas of treatment for mental disorders among young children are under investigation, a high level of caution is well founded at this juncture in light of the absence of safety and efficacy data on the use of these medications for the overwhelming majority of young child mental disorders in young children. However, support for conducting appropriately designed controlled studies of such interventions, which could be potentially effective, may be thwarted by the resistance in principle about the use of these medications and the lack of education about the existence of serious mental disorders in young children—a problem that this edited volume aims to help rectify.

The urgent need for appropriately controlled studies of psychopharmacological interventions in young children is underscored by recent dramatic increases in the prescription of psychotropic medications to preschool children by physicians (Zito & Safer, 2005; Zito et al., 2000). This finding is alarming in light of the absence of safety and efficacy data for this age group but not surprising given the broad range of newer agents now available on the market in the midst of reductions or, in some cases, rationing of mental health care. Many of these newer medication classes, such as the selective serotonin reuptake inhibitors (SSRI), antidepressants, and the atypical antipsychotics, are relatively less complicated to prescribe and generally better tolerated than older drugs of the same class. These features may influence prescribing for

311

practitioners on the "front lines" who may be earnestly attempting to help families whose young children demonstrate out-of-control behaviors, despite the absence of the necessary research to support such interventions in the majority of cases. In keeping with this conclusion, a brief survey has suggested that this prescribing may be done more frequently by general practitioners and less frequently by child psychiatrists. However, the question of what type of practitioners are doing the most prescribing of psychotropics to young children is a compelling one, still in need of further clarification (Coyle, 2000).

During the time period that these dramatic increases in prescribing have occurred, substantial progress in the early detection and age appropriate classification of a number of mental disorders arising in young children has been made (for review see Task Force on Research and Diagnostic Criteria: Infancy and Preschool, 2003, and data as outlined in Chapters 6, 7, and 9, in this volume). The availability of these age-adjusted diagnostic criteria should serve to facilitate the appropriate identification of mental disorders among young children for needed intervention studies. Such very early intervention protocols should include both psychosocial (e.g., psychotherapeutic and/or developmental) and psychopharmacological modalities, alone and in combination for comparison as indicated and appropriate.

Although still a theory that requires controlled empirical testing, mental heath intervention earlier in life may offer the possibility of capturing a window of opportunity for more effective treatment. Such an enhanced early intervention efficacy model is supported by the known greater neuroplasticity of the brain during the preschool period. Along these lines, preliminary empirical support for such a model is also available in the area of autistic spectrum disorders, in which early and intensive behavioral interventions appear to have unique efficacy when applied before the age of 5 years (see Bishop & Lord, Chapter 12, this volume, for more details).

A number of safe and effective pharmacological treatments for specific psychiatric disorders in older children are now available. In particular, in the areas of anxiety disorders, numerous controlled studies, including double-blind, placebo-controlled studies, are now available. These investigations have established greater efficacy of active medication compared to placebo in childhood anxiety disorders. In particular, efficacy has been established in both tricyclic antidepressants and SSRIs for treatment of obsessive–compulsive disorder (D. Geller et al., 2001; D. Geller et al., 2003; Liebowitz et al., 2002; March & Leonard, 1998; Riddle et al., 2001). Along these lines the efficacy of atypical antipsychotic agents (in particular risperidone) for the treatment of autistic spectrum disorder has also been supported by a large, multicenter, double-blind, placebo-controlled study (McDougle et al., 2005; McCracken et al., 2002).

The pharmacological treatment of childhood depression remains controversial due to the emergence of both negative and positive findings. Furthermore, there has been much recent attention to British data suggesting an increase in suicidality in depressed children and adolescents potentially related to antidepressant use. The U.S. Food and Drug Administration (FDA, 2004) has recently issued a "black-box" warning for SSRI antidepressant use in major depressive disorder. This concern about the treatment of childhood depression with SSRI antidepressants has had a strong impact on practice despite promising data on the use of Prozac in depressed school-age children (Emslie et al., 1997, 1998, 2002; Wagner et al., 2004). New guidelines have been issued that recommend very close follow-up (e.g., weekly) after initiation of antidepressant treatment for any indication in children and adolescents (American Academy of Child and Adolescent Psychiatry, 2004).

In those childhood mental disorders for which the efficacy of pharmacotherapy has been demonstrated for older children, these treatments in many cases serve as important adjuncts to psychosocial interventions in these populations. In fact, such combined therapeutic approaches have become the recommended standard of care for several specific child mental disorders such as attention-deficit/hyperactivity disorder (ADHD; MTA Cooperative Group, 1999) and obsessive–compulsive disorder (March, 2003). With the advent of newer and more tolerable antidepressant and antipsychotic agents, their potential application to younger child populations is more feasible. Importantly for child populations, many of these drugs have greater potential for use due to their less sedating side effects, broader therapeutic windows, and lack of required blood tests to monitor levels during the treatment process. Therefore, the question of whether pharmacological treatments could be safe and effective in specific mental disorders in younger children is a highly compelling one that has been the focus of recent attention (e.g., Greenhill et al., 2003; Vitiello, 2001; Jensen, 1998; Stubbe & Martin, 2000). This is by virtue of both the potential dangers and their potential for unique efficacy, suggesting that this is an area in which very careful study with appropriate, close monitoring and longitudinal follow-up is required.

SPECIAL ISSUES FOR CONSIDERATION IN A YOUNG-CHILD POPULATION

Psychopharmacology and Brain Development in the Preschool Period

A central and unique consideration in the use of psychoactive medications in preschool children is the known greater plasticity of brain during this early period of development. Exciting data from basic neuroscience research have suggested that brain changes overall, as well as "experience-dependent" changes, that is, those arising from external environmental influences, have a more profound impact on brain development prior to the age of 5 years (e.g., Turner & Greenough, 1985; Greenough, McDonald, Parnisari, & Camel, 1986; Greenough, Black, & Wallace, 1987). Findings from animal experiments, data on the rate of recovery from brain injury at different stages of development, as well as functional neuroimaging of human infants in which metabolic processes in the brain are evident, support the validity of this early period of enhanced brain change and activity, or "neuroplasticity" (Chugani,

Phelps, & Mazziotta, 1987; Benes, Taylor, & Cunningham, 2000; Kolb, 1995). Although the details of these processes in human subjects and further, the clinical translation, has not been sufficiently investigated at this point, they raise the possibility of a unique window of opportunity or possible "critical period" for treatment earlier in life. If a "critical period" of greater "experience-dependent" neuroplasticity could be established, it would follow that greater treatment efficacy could potentially apply to both psychosocial and pharmacological modalities among very young children. Alternatively, early plasticity could also lend itself to unique dangers, such as producing undesirable and potentially harder to reverse alterations in brain development.

It has been well established that many of the neurotransmitter systems of the brain targeted by psychoactive medications undergo rapid change in the preschool period (Seeman et al., 1987). Similarly, the related architecture or structure of key brain regions undergoes rapid transformation during this time. For example, the density of neurons reaches its peak by the age of 3, after which the process of selective elimination or "pruning" becomes highly active, until more stable adult synapses and synaptic numbers are reached at age 10 (Huttenlocher, 1990). A similar trajectory of changes in the brain's metabolic activity has been detected by functional imaging studies (Chugani et al., 1997).

Along similar lines, animal studies have detected permanent brain changes in a variety of specific regions in response to early exposure to stress hormones or pharmacological agents during known early "critical periods" of development. For example, depletion of serotonin during the critical period shortly after birth in the rodent results in enduring synaptic deficits and related impairments in learning (Mazer et al., 1997). Similar findings have been detected in dopamine systems in response to Haldol given to rats during the postnatal critical period (Hill & Engblom, 1984). Although these data are highly suggestive and may be pertinent to the study of early human brain change and development, there is insufficient evidence at this point to support the notion that similar robust and discreet "critical periods" exist in regions of the brain known to be associated with emotions and behaviors in humans or other primates. However, these studies underscore the need for caution and careful design as they call to our attention the possibility that neuroplasticity could give rise to increased opportunity for either positive or negative brain changes.

Age-Specific Ethical Concerns

Although it seems clear that studies of psychoactive agents for the treatment of specific, severe, and impairing psychiatric disorders in young children are warranted, unique ethical concerns arise. One major issue that pertains to any intervention research in young children is their inability to consent or, more appropriately, assent to participation due to cognitive immaturity. Whereas this issue arises in any research involving young-child subjects, however, it becomes increasingly important with the increasing potential risks of pharmacological treatment research protocols. However, as in all medical research, concerns about such risks must always be balanced by consideration of potential benefits. Based on the substantial demonstrated benefits of these treatments in older children and adults, as well as the known chronic and relapsing course of these disorders, the risk–benefit ratio would support active treatment research programs for young children in this area with several classes of agents.

THE EMPIRICAL DATA BASE ON PRESCHOOL PSYCHOPHARMACOLOGY

Using available medical publication search programs, I have attempted to collect a comprehensive list of all studies done to date on the use of psychotropic agents specifically in preschool populations (see Tables 14.1–14.3). Based on the dearth of available data in this area, the tables include a broad range of available publications, including single-case studies and small open-label trials in addition to placebo-controlled studies, to help inform the issues. Reflecting the focus of the investigations done to date, these studies are organized into three separate tables. Table 14.1 addresses all studies of psychostimulants and related medications for the treatment of ADHD in preschool populations. Table 14.2 addresses treatment studies of autistic spectrum disorders among preschool populations. Table 14.3 addresses studies of bipolar disorder treatment in larger samples of older children that also include a substantial number of preschool children. These younger children have been the focus of study or have been included in larger studies despite the relative dearth of empirical data on the phenomenology of the disorder at this young age (see Luby & Belden, Chapter 10, this volume). Although still small, there is a relatively larger, available database in these three diagnostic areas.

The early pharmacological treatment of autism has also received relatively more attention that any other early-onset psychiatric disorder. This is related to the fact that validation of this early-onset disorder has been well established for some time. Despite this, the data base is still an insufficient to direct treatment confidently among preschool populations.

PRESCRIBING PSYCHOTROPICS TO PRESCHOOLERS: BALANCING CAUTION WITH REASON

Currently only four psychotropic agents are FDA approved for use in psychiatric disorders in children under the age of 6 (see Table 14.4). With the exception of two stimulants, Dexedrine and Adderall, both approved neuroleptic agents (Thorazine and Mellaril) are no longer commonly utilized by practitioners due to the availability of newer, better-tolerated "atypical antipsychotics" with superior side effect profiles, as previously discussed.

TABLE 14.1. Psychostimulants and Related Medications for ADHD

Authors	Drug	Age (N)	Study design	Time frame	Diagnostic assessment	Primary results	Side effect or safety issues
Conners (1975)	Methylphenidate	6 yr (N = 53)	Double-blind, parallel design; MPH 11.8 mg/day	42 days	Clinician diagnosis and psychological testing	27/29 children improved.	Minimal side effects, with a trend toward elevated blood pressure.
Schleifer et al. (1975)	Methylphenidate	3–5 yr (N = 26)	Double-blind, placebo-controlled crossover; MPH 2.5–30 mg/day	28–42 days	Clinician diagnosis	Improved on mother report.	Increased social withdrawal and dysphoria.
Cohen, Sullivan, Minde, Novak, & Helwig (1981)	Methylphenidate	Mean age 5 yr, 2 mo (N = 24)	Open label; MPH 10–30 mg/day	20 wk	Con. Suite	MPH no better than no treatment.	More solitary play.
Barkley, Karlsson, Strzelecki, & Murphy (1984)	Methylphenidate	4 yr–5 yr, 11 mo (N = 54)	Double-blind, placebo-controlled crossover; MPH 0.3 mg/kg/day; MPH 1 mg/kg/day	21–30 days	Con. Suite and W-W-P ARS	"Normalizing" of hyperactive subjects with more positive mother interactions.	The higher the dose, the more frequent side effects.
Barkley (1988)	Methylphenidate	3–5 yr (N = 27)	Double-blind, placebo-controlled crossover; MPH 0.3 mg/kg/day; MPH 1 mg/kg/day	21–30 days	Con. Suite, W-W-P ARS and the HSQ	45% decrease in off-task behaviors on higher dose only.	Mothers reported more side effects when child was on MPH compared to placebo.
Speltz, Varley, Peterson, & Beilke (1988)	Dextroamphetamine	4 yr (N = 1)	Double-blind case study; DEX 2.5 mg/ twice daily; DEX 5 mg, twice daily	77 days	Clinician diagnosis	Decrease in tantrums and aggressive oppositionality.	Increased whining, listlessness, solitary play, and abdominal pain; decreased appetite.
Alessandri & Schramm (1991)	Dextroamphetamine	4 yr (N = 1)	Open-label case study; DEX 5 mg/day	16 wk	Con. Suite and clinician diagnosis	Improved attention and social functioning.	More solitary and parallel play.

Study	Medication	Age (N)	Design; dose	Duration	Measures	Outcome	Side effects
Mayes, Crites, Bixler, Humphrey, & Mattison (1994)	Methylphenidate	3–5 yr (N = 69)	Single-blind, ABA design; MPH 0.3 mg/kg/day with increases of 2.5–5 mg	24 days	Clinician diagnosis	71% of preschool-age children responded to MPH.	51% had side effects: irritability, decreased appetite, lethargy, and dysphoria.
Hagino et al. (1995)	Lithium	4–6 yr (N = 20)	Open label; Li 300–1,200 mg/day	6–37 days	Clinician diagnosis	60% had central nervous system, gastrointestinal, genitourinary, and ocular side effects; 40% had "nuisance" side effects; 20% had "serious" side effects.	The appearance of side effects was associated with higher lithium levels and larger lithium doses.
Avci, Diler, & Tamam (1998)	Fluoxetine	2 yr, 5 mo (N = 1)	Case study; FL 5 mg/day	3 mo	Clinician diagnosis	Resolution of specific phobia, panic attacks.	No mention of side effects.
Harmon & Riggs (1996)	Clonidine patch	3–6 yr (N = 7)	Open label; 1 clonidine patch every 5 days	24 mo	Clinician diagnosis	Reduced aggression, hyperarousal, and sleep difficulties.	Mild local irritation and erythema under the patch, noncompliance.
Lee (1997)	Guanfacine	2–3 yr (N = 4)	Case study; Guan 0.25–0.5 mg, twice daily	6 mo	CBC, Con. Suite and clinician diagnosis	Improved behavior and decreased hyperactivity, impulsivity, and aggression.	No mention of side effects.
Monteiro-Musten, Firestone, Pisterman, Bennett, & Mercer (1997)	Methylphenidate	4 yr–5 yr, 11 mo (N = 31)	Double-blind, placebo-controlled crossover; MPH 0.3 mg/kg/day; MPH 0.5 mg/kg/day	21–30 days	Dx for C & A-Ps and the S, N, and P Checklist	90% of subjects improved.	Side effects were mild and clinically negligible.
Byrne, Bawden, DeWolfe, & Beattie (1998)	Methylphenidate and dextroamphetamine	Mean age 5 yr, 2 mo (N = 16)	Open label; MPH 15–20 mg/day DEX 7.5–15 mg/day	5 mo	CDI, CPRS, and clinician diagnosis	Improved attention and social relations; decreased problem behaviors.	No mention of side effects.

(continued)

TABLE 14.1. (*continued*)

Authors	Drug	Age (N)	Study design	Time frame	Diagnostic assessment	Primary results	Side effect or safety issues
Firestone, Munsten, Pisterman, Mercer, & Bennett (1998)	Methylphenidate	4–6 yr (N = 54)	Double-blind, placebo-controlled crossover; MPH 0.3 mg/kg twice daily; MPH 0.5 mg/kg, twice daily	21–30 days	Dx for C & A-Ps, S, N, and P Checklist and the Con. Suite	97% experienced some side effects while receiving placebo; severe side effects were reported in less than 10%, with as many reports of severe side effects on placebo as on low and high doses.	The most common side effects were irritability, anxiety, proneness to crying, and insomnia.
Handen, Feldman, Lurier, & Murray (1999)	Methylphenidate	4–5 yr (N = 11)	Double-blind, placebo-controlled, crossover; MPH 0.3–0.6 mg/kg dose from four times to three times daily	21 days	PBQ, Con. suite, and clinician diagnosis	73% of preschool children with developmental disabilities and ADHD improved.	45% experienced social withdrawal and irritability.
Ghuman et al. (2001)	Methylphenidate and dextroamphetamine	3–5 yr (N = 27)	Chart review; MPH 0.55–1.16 mg/kg; DEX 0.43–0.6 mg/kg	24 mo	Clinician diagnosis	74% improved at 3 mo; 70% improved at 12 and 24 mo.	63% had side effects; 11% had to stop medication due to side effects: irritability, dysphoria, headache, and dullness.

Note. Abbreviations for Tables 14.1–14.3: Con. Suite, Conners' Parents Questionnaire, Conners' Abbreviated Teacher Rating Scale, Conners' Parent Rating Scale–Revised, Conners' Parent–Teacher Questionnaire or Hyperactivity Index of Conners' Parent Rating Scale; W-W-P ARS, Werry–Weiss–Peters Activity Rating Scale; HSQ, Home Situations Questionnaire; CBC, Child Behavior Checklist; Dx for C & A-Ps, Diagnostic Interview for Child and Adult-Parents; S, N, and P Checklist, Swanson, Nolan, and Pelham Checklist; CDI, Child Development Inventory; CPRS, Children's Psychiatric Rating Scale; PBQ, Preschool Behavior uestionnaire.

318

TABLE 14.2. Medications for Autism Spectrum Disorders

Author (year)	Drug	Age	Study design	Time frame	Diagnostic assessment	Primary results	Side effect or safety issues
Anderson et al. (1984)	Haloperidol	2.33–6.92 yr (N = 40)	Double-blind, placebo-controlled		GDS, CPRS, Con. Suite, CGIS	Significant decrease in behavioral symptoms and general clinical improvement; improvement in discrimination learning.	No mention of side effects.
Anderson et al. (1989)	Haloperidol	2 yr–7 yr, 6 mo (N = 45)	Double-blind, placebo-controlled, crossover design	14 wk	CPRS, CGIS	No effect on discrimination learning; significant reduction in maladaptive behaviors.	
Findling, Maxwell, & Witznitzer (1997)	Risperidone	5–9 yr (N = 6)	Open label; Rsp 0.75–1.5 mg/day	8 wk	Clinician diagnosis	All subjects had an improvement of autistic behaviors reflected by lower CPRS and CGI severity scores.	Most common side effects were weight gain and sedation.
Schreier (1998)	Risperidone	5–16 yr (N = 11)	Open label; 0.25–3.0 mg/day	24 mo	Clinician diagnosis	73% responded to risperidone.	Most common side effects were weight gain and sedation.
Posey, Walsh, Wilson, & McDougle (1999)	Risperidone	23–29 mo (N = 2)	Case study; 0.25–1.25 mg/day	13 mo	Clinician diagnosis	Risperidone reduced aggression and improved social relatedness in both cases.	One child experienced tachycardia complications, which were resolved by a dose reduction.

(continued)

TABLE 14.2. (*continued*)

Author (year)	Drug	Age	Study design	Time frame	Diagnostic assessment	Primary results	Side effect or safety issues
Masi, Cosenza, Mucci, & Brovedani (2001)	Risperidone	3–6 yr (N = 10)	Open label; 0.25–0.50 mg/day	16 wk	Clinician diagnosis	100% had a reduction in target symptoms; CPRS reduced by a mean of 12%, most improved: quality of the relationship, stability of affects, control of stereotypics and fidgetiness.	Minor side effects reported: increased appetite, tachycardia, fever, fatigue, and apparent sadness.
Masi, Cosenza, Mucci, & DeVito (2001)	Risperidone	3–6 yr (N = 24)	Open label; 0.25–0.75 mg/day	16 wk	CARS and clinician diagnosis	21% showed improvement in CPRS and 14% improved in CARS total scores; behavioral control and affect regulation improved > 25%.	54% were free of any side effects; a few experienced transient increase in heart rate, weight gain, and a brief episode of dystonia.
Snyder et al. (2002)	Risperidone	5–12 yr (N = 110)	1-wk, single-blind, placebo-controlled, followed by 6-wk, double-blind, placebo-controlled; 0.02–0.06 mg/kg per day	7 wk	NCBRF, ABC, BPI, CGIS, MCVLT, and a continuous performance task	Risperidone appears to be well tolerated and effective in children with subaverage IQs and severe disruptive behaviors.	Most common side effects: somnolence, headache, appetite increase, and dyspepsia.

TABLE 14.3. Medications for Bipolar Disorder: Studies That Include Children Younger than 6 Years of Age

Author (year)	Drug	Age	Study design	Time frame	Diagnostic assessment	Primary results	Side effect or safety issues
Youngerman & Canino (1978)	Lithium	3–19 yr (N = 46)	Retrospective chart review		Clinical diagnosis	Of the 46, there were 30 positive responses to lithium.	No mention of side effects.
Biederman et al. (1998)	Mood stabilizers	3.5–17 yr (N = 792) (final sample consisted of 49 children)	Chart review		YMRS, K-SADS Epidemiologial Version	Mood stabilizers were associated with significant improvement of manic-like symptoms, while antidepressants, anti-psychotics, and stimulant medications were not; Lithium was most effective	No mention of side effects.
Mota-Castillo et al. (2001)	Valproate and Divalproex	18 mo–5 yr (N = 9)	Clinical case reports		Clinical diagnosis	Provides rationale for use of mood stabilizers rather than stimulants in this population.	No mention of side effects.
Pavuluri, Janicak, & Carbray (2002)	Risperidone, lithium, and topiramate	4 yr, 5 mo (N = 1)	Clinical case report		PAPA, WASH-U-K-SADS	Child became stable on a combination of topiramate and Risperidone; Risperidone as a monotherapy and in combination with lithium resulted in reduced irritability and rage after 1 wk and worsening of depressive symptoms.	Weight gain; child developed polyuria on lithium; most common side effects: cognitive side effects and parasthesia.
Tuzun, Zoroglu, & Savas (2002)	Carbamazepine	5 yr, 2 mo (N = 1)	Case report; 100–300 mg/day; 6.7 μg/mL on 300 mg/day	2 wk	Clinical diagnosis	Mania can be effectively and safely treated with carbamazepine.	No mention of side effects.

(continued)

321

TABLE 14.3. (*continued*)

Author (year)	Drug	Age	Study design	Time frame	Diagnostic assessment	Primary results	Side effect or safety issues
Tumuluru, Weller, Fristad, & Weller (2003)	Lithium	3–5 yr (N = 36)	Clinical case report; retrospective chart review	4.5 yr	Clinical diagnosis	Five children treated with lithium, all five improved.	No mention of side effects.
Scheffer & Niskala Apps (2004)	Mood stabilizers, primarily valproic acid	2–5 yr (N = 31)	Retrospective chart review		Clinical diagnosis, YMRS, CGIS, CGI-S	Treatment with mood stabilizers was clinically effective, with corresponding significant developmental benefits.	Hair loss in one female; elevated liver enzymes on divalproate in one subject.
Biederman et al. (2005)	Olanzapine and risperidone	4–6 yr (N = 31)	Open label; rsp. .25–2.0 mg/day vs. Olanzapine 1.25–10 mg/day	8 wk	YMRS, CGIS, CGI-S, CGI-I, K-SADS Epidemiological Version, CDRS, BPRS	No difference in rate of response with risperidone and olanzapine; treatment with risperidone associated with statistically significant improvement of depressive symptoms.	Most common side effects were increased appetite, headache, and sedation; risperidone associated with increased prolactin levels; significant increase in weight with both agents.

TABLE 14.4. FDA-Approved Drugs for Children Younger Than 5 Years

Drug	Indication	Restrictions
Dexedrine	Narcolepsy, ADHD	Recommended for children ages 3–16 yr.
Adderall	Narcolepsy, ADHD	Has not been tested in children under 6 years of age.
Thorazine	Severe behavioral problems in children	Recommended for children ages 1–2 yr.
Mellaril	Severe behavioral problems in children	Not intended for children under 2; contraindicated in children under 1 yr.

Therefore, at this time, virtually all prescribing to preschool children must be done "off label." Along these lines, the overwhelming majority of psychotropic prescriptions written for preschool children are "off label." Prescribing "off label" means that clinicians cannot give any assurances to parents/guardians about the effects of treatment on growth, development, and basic safety in that regard. It is important to discuss this candidly with caregivers so that they can make a more informed decision before consenting to treatment for their child. Along these lines, it also wise to state this fact explicitly in the written consent for pharmacological treatment form used for the parents of preschool patients.

Based on the available empirical data base, the judicious prescription of stimulant medication to preschool children who present with severe symptoms of ADHD is now a reasonable treatment option. Similar to treatment recommendations for older children with ADHD that are based on empirical data, the combination of medication and behavioral interventions appears to be most effective based on clinical experience for preschoolers as well. However, there is still a great deal we do not know, such as whom to treat with medications and what doses are most effective. Results of the ongoing Preschool Age Treatment of ADHD study (see Steinhoff et al., Chapter 4, this volume) should help to inform these parameters. Furthermore, in the young child, it is important to investigate the possibility that other underlying etiologies (e.g., anxiety or traumatic precipitants) are responsible for the symptoms rather than a core problem with attention. However, when ADHD presents in a severe form in a preschool patient, it is present in multiple settings, without a clear precipitant, and is significantly impairing; thus, the symptoms and therefore the diagnosis are likely to be relatively clear (see Chapter 4, this volume, for more details).

Whereas the two stimulant medications with FDA approval for use in the age group might be attempted first, if these are not effective or well tolerated for any individual child, making a change to other, pharmacologically similar compounds is a reasonable next step. Regardless of which specific medication is selected, it is wise to begin treatment with a short-acting stimulant (of the same type, if available), so that paradoxical responses such as increases in agitation or anxiety (which appear to be somewhat more frequent in younger children) will be transient if they arise. A generic principle that should apply to all medication monitoring in young children is the need to observe closely the patient and therefore to have frequent and regular appointments (weekly to every 2 weeks), as well as frequent phone contact, if needed, especially at the initiation of treatment. Once they are on stable dosing, monthly monitoring of preschoolers is often sufficient; however, less frequent follow-up for such young children is not optimal.

OTHER PRESCHOOL DISORDERS/PROBLEMS
FOR WHICH PSYCHOPHARMACOLOGICAL AGENTS ARE USED

A relatively common reason for referral of a preschooler to a mental health clinic is for impairing irritability and mood dysregulation, impulsivity and aggression that cannot be explained by the diagnosis ADHD or oppositional defiant disorder. The question of whether preschool-age children can manifest mania and/or bipolar disorders is an area under investigation (see Luby & Belden, Chapter 10, for review). This diagnostic question notwithstanding, agents to control extreme and persistent aggression and/or irritability, as well as mood dysregulation, are often needed for young children with these symptoms. It is imperative that a thorough age-appropriate clinical evaluation be performed to be sure that the behavior is not a result of modifiable delays in developmental or psychosocial problems. Once this has been ruled out or addressed therapeutically in an adequate and appropriate manner without sufficient success, it is reasonable to consider a psychopharmacological agent as a next step. It should be noted, however, that it is not appropriate to turn to medications for the control of aggressive, impulsive, or dysregulated behavior in a preschool child without having a comprehensive mental health and developmental evaluation performed.

Alpha agonists such as clonidine and guanfacine have been used with variable success for the control of impulsive behavior (see Table 14.1). Both medications are well tolerated, although Tenex may be preferable for use in younger children due to less sedating side effects. Both medications are safe but require a baseline electrocardiogram (EKG) to ensure that there are no preexisting cardiac abnormalities, as is the standard of care with use in older children. In many cases in which these well-tolerated and safe medications will not sufficiently control severe aggression and/or irritability, low doses of atypical antipsychotics may be tried and may be more effective. However, the decision to use these medications for this indication should not be taken lightly given the greater risk of long-term side effects and the absence of basic data on the effects on growth and development. When these medications are used, it is wise to start at low doses and slowly titrate in an attempt to maintain the lowest possible dose for the shortest duration. To achieve the latter goal, periodic trials on lower doses and, if possible, trials off the medication should be routinely attempted.

Due to their more complex management and side effect profile, the use of mood-stabilizing agents such as lithium carbonate or valproic acid is problematic in young children and generally should not be tried as first-line agents. This is due to the need for frequent blood draws, which are poorly tolerated by preschool children in general, and in many cases a side effect profile that is difficult for young children to tolerate. For example, lithium may produce enuresis during a period when the child is mastering toilet training. The gastrointestinal side effects of valproate may be difficult for young children to tolerate as well. The absence of data both on the effects of these medications on growth and development and on their use in the modulation of mood in young children is also a factor that signals the need for extreme caution.

USE OF MEDICATIONS FOR SLEEP IN PRESCHOOL CHILDREN

As a general rule, medication for sleep is contraindicated in preschool children, because it is developmentally important for young children to learn appropriate self-soothing methods to fall asleep on their own and/or to conquer separation fears that are often an important factor in sleep disturbances at this early developmental period. Principles of basic sleep hygiene (e.g., decreasing stimulation) should always be adhered to as a primary measure. Methods for behaviorally addressing specific sleep disturbances have been described elsewhere (Ferber, 1986).

OBTAINING CONSENT FOR OFF-LABEL PRESCRIBING: SPECIAL CONSIDERATIONS

Obtaining written consent from legal guardians for the prescription of psychoactive medications to children has become a widely used practice. This is particularly important when preschoolers are prescribed medication, the majority of which are off-label, and all of which have inadequate empirical testing. Written consent is useful for the legal protection of the physician, and it is important to take the time to fully inform parents and obtain their consent given the more experimental conditions of treatment. In addition to reviewing possible side effects, the physician should explicitly state and discuss with the parent/guardian the fact that the medication has not been approved by the FDA for this age group. In addition, the possibility of side effects that are not common or known should also be discussed. The overall objective is to focus on informing the parent/guardian of the additional risks incurred by using a medication that is not adequately tested, and the related issue of risk–benefit ratio can be addressed at this time.

CONCLUSION

Preschool psychopharmacology stands out as both an area with the potential for unique promise and as a unique, potentially dangerous area in need of much further research. The urgency of this need is underscored by the epidemic rates of prescriptions of psychoactive agents written for young children in the absence of data to guide this practice. The research available to date merely skims the surface of what is needed and lags far behind the available data bases for older children and for neurological disorders in preschool children. Social stigma relative to the recognition of mental disorders as valid medical conditions continues to stand as an impediment to progress in this area. Given the great strides that the field of mental health has enjoyed through the appropriate use of pharmacotherapy in older populations, this is an unexplored area of great potential promise.

ACKNOWLEDGMENTS

This research was supported by National Institute of Mental Health Grant No. R01 #MR01 MH 064769 to Joan L. Luby, MD.

REFERENCES

Alessandri, S. M., & Schramm, K. (1991). Effects of dextroamphetamine on the cognitive and social play of a preschooler with ADHD. *Journal of the American Academy of Child and Adolescent Psychiatry, 30*, 768–772.

American Academy of Child and Adolescent Psychiatry. (2004, October). *Supplementary talking points for child and adolescent psychiatrists regarding the FDA black box warning on the use of antidepressants for pediatric patients.* Retrieved October 3, 2005, from www.aacap.org/press_releases/2004/ssriemail10_29_041.pdf.

Anderson, L., Campbell, M., Adams, P., Small, A., Perry, R., & Shell, J. (1989). The effects of haloperidol on discrimination learning and behavioral symptoms in autistic children. *Journal of Autism and Developmental Disorders, 19*, 227–239.

Anderson, L., Campbell, M., Grega, D., Perry, R., Small, A., & Green, W. (1984) Haloperidol in the treatment of infantile autism: Effects on learning and behavioral symptoms. *American Journal of Psychiatry, 141*, 1195–1202.

Avci, A., Diler, R. S., & Tamam, L. (1998). Fluoxetine treatment in a 2.5-year-old girl. *Journal of the American Academy of Child and Adolescent Psychiatry, 37*, 901–902.

Barkley, R. A. (1988). The effects of methylphenidate on the interactions of preschool ADHD children with their mothers. *Journal of the American Academy of Child and Adolescent Psychiatry, 27*, 336–341.

Barkley, R. A., Karlsson, J., Strzelecki, E., & Murphy, J. V. (1984). Effects of age and Ritalin dosage on the mother–child interactions of hyperactive children. *Journal of Consulting and Clinical Psychology, 52*, 750–758.

Benes, F. M., Taylor, J. B., & Cunningham, M. C. (2000). Convergence and plasticity of monoaminergic systems in the medial prefrontal cortex during the postnatal period: Implications for the development of psychopathology. *Cerebral Cortex, 10*, 1014–1027.

Biederman, J., Mick, E., Bostic, J. Q., Prince, J., Daly, J., Wilens, T. E., et al. (1998). The naturalistic course of pharmacological treatment of children with manic-like symptoms: A systematic chart review. *Journal of Clinical Psychiatry, 59*, 628–637.

Biederman, J., Mick, E., Hammerness, P., Harpold, T., Aleardi, M., Dougherty, M., et al. (2005). Open-label, 8-week trial of olanzapine and risperidone for the treatment of bipolar disorder in preschool-age children. *Biological Psychiatry.*

Byrne, J. M., Bawden, H. N., DeWolfe, N. A., & Beattie, T. L. (1998). Clinical assessment of psychopharmacological treatment of preschoolers with ADHD. *Journal of Clinical and Experimental Neuropsychology, 20*, 613–627.

Chugani, D. C., Muzik, O., Rothermel, R., Behen, M., Chakraborty, P., Mangner, T., et al. (1997). Altered serotonin synthesis in the dentatothalamocortical pathway in autistic boys. *Annals of Neurology, 42*, 666–669.

Chugani, H. T., Phelps, M. E., & Mazziotta, J. C. (1987). Positron emission tomography study of human brain functional development. *Annals of Neurology, 22*, 487–497.

Cohen, N., Sullivan, M., Minde, K., Novak, C., & Helwig, H. (1981). Evaluation of the relative effectiveness of methylphenidate and cognitive behavior modification in the treatment of kindergarten-aged hyperactive children. *Journal of Abnormal Child Psychology, 9*, 43–54.

Conners, C. K. (1975). Controlled trial of methylphenidate in preschool children with minimal brain dysfunction. *International Journal of Mental Health, 4*, 61–74.

Coyle, J. (2000). Psychotropic drug use in very young children. *Journal of the American Medical Association, 283*, 1059–1060.

Emslie, G., Heiligenstein, J., Wagner, K., Hoog, S., Ernest, D., & Brown, E. (2002). Fluexotine for acute treatment of depression in children and adolescents: A placebo-controlled, randomized clinical trial. *Journal of the American Academy of Child and Adolescent Psychiatry, 41*(10), 1205–1215.

Emslie, G., Rush, J., Weinberg, W., Kowatch, R., Carmody, T., & Mayes, L. (1998). Fluoxetine in child and adolescent depression: Acute maintenance and treatment. *Depression and Anxiety, 7*, 32–39.

Emslie, G., Rush, J., Weinberg, W., Kowatch, R., Hughes, C., & Carmody, T. (1997). A double-blind, randomized, placebo-controlled trial of fluoxetine in children and adolescents with depression. *Archives of General Psychiatry, 54*, 1031–1037.

Ferber, R. (1986). *Solve your child's sleep problems.* New York: Fireside.

Findling, R. L., Maxwell, K., & Wiznitzer, M. (1997). An open clinical trial of risperidone monotherapy in young children with autistic disorder. *Psychopharmacology Bulletin, 33*, 155–159.

Firestone, P., Musten, L. M., Pisterman, S., Mercer, J., & Bennett, S. (1998). Short-term side effects of stimulant medication are increased in preschool children with attention-deficit/hyperactivity disorder: A double-blind placebo-controlled study. *Journal of Child and Adolescent Psychopharmacology, 8*, 13–25.

Geller, B., Hoog, S., Heiligenstein, J., Ricardi, R., Tamura, R., & Kluszynski, S. (2001). Fluoxetine treatment for obsessive–compulsive disorder in children and adolescents: A placebo-controlled clinical trial. *Journal of the American Academy of Child and Adolescent Psychiatry, 40*, 773–779.

Geller, D., Biederman, J., Stewart, S., Mullin, B., Farrell, C., & Wagner, K. (2003). Impact of comorbidity on treatment response to paroxetine in pediatric obsessive compulsive disorder: Is the use of exclusion criteria empirically supported in randomized clinical trials? *Journal of Child and Adolescent Psychopharmacology, 13*(Suppl.), S19–S29.

Ghuman, J. K., Ginsburg, G. S., Subramaniam, G., Ghuman, H. S., Kau, A. S., & Riddle, M. A. (2001). Psychostimulants in preschool children with attention-deficit/hyperactivity disorder: Clinical evidence from a developmental disorders institution. *Journal of the American Academy of Child and Adolescent Psychiatry, 40*, 516–524.

Greenhill, L. L., Jensen, P. S., Abikoff, H., Blumer, J. L., Deveaugh-Geiss, J., Fisher, C., et al. (2003). Developing strategies for psychopharmacological studies in preschool children. *Journal of the American Academy of Child and Adolescent Psychiatry, 42*(4), 406–414.

Greenough, W. T., Black, J. E., & Wallace, C. S. (1987). Experience and brain development. *Child Development, 58,* 539–559.

Greenough, W. T., McDonald, J., Parnisari, R., & Camel, J. E. (1986). Environmental conditions modulate degeneration and new dendrite growth in cerebellum of senescent rates. *Brain Research, 380,* 136–143.

Hagino, O. R., Weller, E. B., Weller, R. A., Washing, D., Fristad, M. A., & Kontras, S. B. (1995). Untoward effects of lithium treatment in children aged four through six years. *Journal of the American Academy of Child and Adolescent Psychiatry, 34,* 1584–1590.

Handen, B. L., Feldman, H. M., Lurier, A., & Murray, P. J. (1999). Efficacy of methylphenidate among preschool children with developmental disabilities and ADHD. *Journal of the American Academy of Child and Adolescent Psychiatry, 38,* 805–812.

Harmon, R. J., & Riggs, P. D. (1996). Clonidine for posttraumatic stress disorder in preschool children. *Journal of the American Academy of Child and Adolescent Psychiatry, 35,* 1247–1249.

Hill, H., & Engblom, J. (1984). Effects of pre- and postnatal haloperidol administrations to pregnant and nursing rats on brain catecholamine levels in their offspring. *Developmental Pharmacology and Therapeutics, 7,* 188–197.

Huttenlocher, P. R. (1990). Morphometric study of human cerebral cortex development. *Neuropsychologia, 28,* 517–527.

Jensen, P. S. (1998). Ethical and pragmatic issues in the use of psychotropic agents in young children. *Canadian Journal of Psychiatry, 43*(6), 585–588.

Kolb, B. (1995). *Brain plasticity and behavior.* Hillsdale, NJ: Erlbaum.

Lee, B. (1997). Clinical experience with guanfacine in 2–and 3-year-old children with attention deficit hyperactivity disorder. *Infant Mental Health Journal, 18,* 300–305.

Liebowitz, M., Turner, S., Piacentini, J., Beidel, D., Clarvit, S., & Davies, S. (2002). Fluoxetine in children and adolescents with OCD: A placebo-controlled trial. *Journal of the American Academy of Child and Adolescent Psychiatry, 41,* 1431–1438.

March, J. (2003). *Pediatric OCD Treatment Study (POTS).* Paper presented at the 156th annual meeting of the American Academy of Child and Psychiatry, San Francisco, CA.

March, J. S., & Leonard, H. (1998). Obsessive–compulsive disorder in children and adolescents. In R. Swinson & M. Antony (Eds.), *Obsessive–compulsive disorder: Theory, research, and treatment* (pp. 367–394). New York: Guilford Press.

Masi, G., Cosenza, A., Mucci, M., & Brovedani, P. (2001). Open trial of risperidone in 24 young children with pervasive developmental disorders. *Journal of the American Academy of Child and Adolescent Psychiatry, 40,* 1206–1214.

Masi, G., Cosenza, A., Mucci, M., & DeVito, G. (2001). Risperidone monotherapy in preschool children with pervasive developmental disorders. *Journal of Child Neurology, 16,* 395–400.

Mayes, S. D., Crites, D. L., Bixler, E. O., Humphrey, F. J., & Mattison, R. E. (1994). Methylphenidate and ADHD: Influence of age, IQ and neurodevelopmental status. *Developmental Medicine and Child Neurology, 36,* 1099–1107.

Mazer, C., Muneyyirci, J., Taheny, K., Raio, N., Borella, A., & Whitaker-Azmitia, P. (1997). Serotonin depletion during synaptogenesis leads to decreased synaptic density and learning deficits in the adult rat: A possible model of neurodevelopment disorders with cognitive deficits. *Brain Research, 760,* 68–73.

McCracken, J. T., McGough, J., Shah, B., Cronin, P., Hong, D., Aman, M. G., et al. (2002). Risperidone in children with autism and serious behavioral problems. *New England Journal of Medicine, 347*(5), 314–321.

McDougle, C. J., Scahill, L., Aman, M. G., McCracken, J. T., Tierney, E., Davies, M., et al. (2005). Risperidone for the core symptom domains of autism: Results from the study by the Autism Network of the Research Units on Pediatric Psychopharmacology. *American Journal of Psychiatry, 162,* 1142–1148.

Monteiro-Musten, L., Firestone, P., Pisterman, S., Bennett, S., & Mercer, J. (1997). Effects of methylphenidate on preschool children with ADHD: Cognitive and behavioral functions. *Journal of the American Academy of Child and Adolescent Psychiatry, 36*, 1407–1415.

Mota-Castillo, M., Torruella, A., Engels, B., Perez, J., Dedrick, C., & Gluckman, M. (2001). Valproate in very young children: An open case series with a brief follow-up. *Journal of Affective Disorders, 67*, 193–197.

MTA Cooperative Group. (1999). A 14-month randomized clinical trial of treatment strategies for attention-deficit/hyperactivity disorder: The MTA Cooperative Group. Multimodal Treatment Study of Children with ADHD. *Archives of General Psychiatry, 56*, 1073–1086.

Pavuluri, M. N., Janicak, P. G., & Carbray, J. (2002). Topiramate plus risperidone for controlling weight gain and symptoms in preschool mania. *Journal of Child and Adolescent Psychopharmacology, 12*, 271–273.

Posey, D. J., Walsh, K. H., Wilson, G. A., & McDougle, C. J. (1999). Risperidone in the treatment of two very young children with autism. *Journal of Child and Adolescent Psychopharmacology, 9*, 273–276.

Riddle, M., Reeve, E., Yaryura-Tobias, J., Yang, H., Claghorn, J., & Gaffney, G. (2001). Fluvoxamine for children and adolescents with obsessive–compulsive disorder: A randomized, controlled, multicenter trial. *Journal of the American Academy of Child and Adolescent Psychiatry, 40*, 222–229.

Scheffer, R. E., & Niskala Apps, J. A. (2004). The diagnosis of preschool bipolar disorder presenting with mania: Open pharmacological treatment. *Journal of Affective Disorders, 82*(Suppl.), S25–S34.

Schleifer, M., Weiss, G., Cohen, N., Elman, M., Cvejic, H., & Kruger, E. (1975). Hyperactivity in preschoolers and the effect of methylphenidate. *American Journal of Orthopsychiatry, 45*, 38–50.

Schreier, H. A. (1998). Risperidone for young children with mood disorders and aggressive behavior. *Journal of Child and Adolescent Psychopharmacology, 8*, 49–59.

Seeman, P., Bzowej, N. H., Guan, H. C., Bergeron, C., Becker, L. E., Reynolds, G. P., et al. (1987). Human brain dopamine receptors in children and aging adults. *Synapse, 1*, 399–404.

Snyder, R., Turgay, A., Aman, M., Binder, C., Fisman, S., & Carroll, A. (2002). Effects of risperidone on conduct and disruptive behavior disorders in children with sub average IQs. *Journal of the American Academy of Child and Adolescent Psychiatry, 41*, 1026–1036.

Speltz, M. L., Varley, C. K., Peterson, K., & Beilke, R. L. (1988). Effects of dextroamphetamine and contingency management on a preschooler with ADHD and oppositional defiant disorder. *Journal of the American Academy of Child and Adolescent Psychiatry, 27*, 175–178.

Stubbe, D. E., & Martin A. (2000). The use of psychotropic medications in young children: The facts, the controversy, and the practice. *Connecticut Medicine, 64*(4), 329–333.

Task Force on Research Diagnostic Criteria: Infancy and Preschool. (2003). Research diagnostic criteria for infants and preschool children: The process and empirical support. *Journal of the American Academy of Child and Adolescent Psychiatry, 42*(12), 1504–1512.

Tumuluru, R. V., Weller, E. B., Fristad, M. A., & Weller, R. A. (2003). Mania in six preschool children. *Journal of Child and Adolescent Psychopharmacology, 13*, 489–494.

Turner, A.M., & Greenough, W. T. (1985). Differential rearing effects on rat visual cortex synapses: I. Synaptic and neuronal density and synapses per neuron. *Brain Research, 329*, 195–203.

Tuzun, U., Zoroglu, S. S., & Savas, H. A. (2002). A 5-year-old boy with recurrent mania successfully treated with carbamazepine. *Psychiatry and Clinical Neurosciences, 56*, 589–591.

U.S. Food and Drug Administration. (2004, October). *FDA launches a multi-pronged strat-*

egy to strengthen safeguards for children treated with antidepressant medications. Retrieved September 27, 2005, from www.fda.gov/bbs/news/2004/new01124.html.

Vitiello, B. (2001). Psychopharmacology for young children: Clinical needs and research opportunities. *Pediatrics, 108*(4), 983–989.

Wagner, K., Robb, A., Findling, R., Jin, J., Gutierrez, M., & Heydorn, W. (2004). A randomized, placebo-controlled trial of citalopram for the treatment of major depression in children and adolescents. *American Journal of Psychiatry, 161,* 1079–1083.

Youngerman, J., & Canino, I. A. (1978). Lithium carbonate use in children and adolescents: A survey of the literature. *Archives of General Psychiatry, 35,* 216–224.

Zito, J., & Safer, D. (2005). Recent child pharmacoepidemiological findings. *Journal of Child and Adolescent Psychopharmacology, 15,* 5–9.

Zito, J., Safer, D., dosReis, S., Gardner, J., Boles, M., & Lynch, F. (2000). Trends in the prescribing of psychotropic medications to preschoolers. *Journal of the American Medical Association, 283,* 1025–1030.

15

Play Therapy
Integrating Clinical and Developmental Perspectives

ANNE LELAND BENHAM and CAROL FISHER SLOTNICK

What could be more delightful than a 4-year-old dressed in a costume of incongruous bits—fairy wings, long beads, a superhero cape, and a sword— confidently swooping around and vanquishing the bad guys, saving the baby, flying to the castle in the clouds, and then cooking lunch?

The emergence of fantasy play in 3- to 5-year-olds is a key developmental acquisition that differentiates preschool children from infants and toddlers, and reflects major developmental change across all domains. Preschool children are unique in that they demonstrate increased cognitive, social, emotional, regulatory, language, and motor capacities, yet they are limited by the preoperational structure of their thought and are characterized by continuing reliance on their parents. Developmental transitions for preschool children are especially vulnerable and progress can be supported or stymied by the larger social context (family, peers, school, or physical environment). Behavioral and emotional symptoms become more differentiated and may be identified as clinical disturbances, indicating a need for early intervention, yet guidelines for therapeutic intervention with this age group are sparse.

We present a psychotherapeutic approach for preschool children, informed by this developmental perspective. Our approach attends to the internal mental representations and the behaviors of both child and parent, the role of the environment, and the developmental status of the child. It is based on the transactional model of development (Sameroff, 2004), which views the child and parent as affecting each other through their reciprocal interaction. It is also based on the concept of multiple ports of entry into the child–parent

331

system through which we may effect therapeutic change (Stern, 1995). These may include modifying child or parent behavior, or changing representations by enhancing the parents' and the child's sense of self, other, and relationships. Our approach is an expansion of the infant mental health approach, because the preschool child's emerging capacity for pretend play provides an enhanced port of entry into the child's internal mental representations.

We describe play therapy as a direct intervention for preschool children. Play functions as a window into the child's inner world, is the child's preferred activity, and is considered the best vehicle to facilitate growth. It is a means for self-expression, communication, relationship development, practice, and development of new capacities, both for the typical and for the developmentally delayed child. Play therapy may address (1) feelings (anxiety, sadness, rage), (2) behaviors (inhibited and disruptive), (3) capacity to play (typical, delayed, rigid, disrupted/disorganized, or inhibited), and (4) specific fears and phobias. It is indicated for children with internalizing disorders, for those with externalizing symptoms that coexist with symptoms of anxiety, depression, stress, trauma, or poor self-esteem, and for developmentally delayed children who need help expanding play capacities.

Play therapy can be very useful when the therapist adjusts conceptually and behaviorally to the developmental needs and characteristics of the preschool child and incorporates work with the parents in a central, collaborative role. We borrow up from the infant mental health field's focus on infant–parent psychotherapies and borrow down from the rich field of child play therapy, including the child-centered therapies, psychodynamic psychotherapies, and cognitive-behavioral therapies. We describe many diverse strategies that can be useful therapeutically with preschool children. The resulting eclectic model integrates different approaches tailored to the individual needs of the child and family rather than adhering to one treatment method. A similar model has been described as prescriptive play therapy (Schaefer, 2003).

We describe both the *expressive* and *formative* aspects of play therapy. The expressive aspect refers to the exploration of the child's emotions, beliefs, wishes, and experiences. The formative aspect refers to building a child's capacities, such as coping strategies, self-regulation, and cognitive, language, and play skills. We discuss both indications for these aspects of therapy and specific techniques.

We believe that work with a young child *must* involve work with the parent(s) or primary caregivers as important agents of change. We discuss, and illustrate, the range of possible interventions, which includes treating the parent–child dyad as a unit, treating the child with the parent in the room as observer/participant, and treating the child individually, while meeting with the parents separately in collateral meetings. We use each of these approaches when warranted, borrowing from many established therapy models, some empirically supported and others based on a long and broad history of accepted clinical experience and practice.

THE PRESCHOOLER

Change in the Preschool Years

In the preschool period, from 3–5 years of age, development proceeds rapidly in all domains, including the cognitive, social, emotional, language, and motor domains (refer to Chapters 1–3, this volume). Piaget (1962) describes the emergence of the preoperational stage (ages 2–6), characterized by the underlying development of representational capacities manifested in the emergence of language, imagery, and symbolic reasoning. The preschool period is also characterized by development in emotional competence, including the regulation, expression, and understanding of emotional states (Denham, 1998). These transitions also pertain to the child's relationship to the social environment (Emde, Everhart, & Wise, 2004). Increased developmental competencies raise parental expectations that the preschool child will communicate more clearly, understand adult communication and expectations, engage socially with more competence, comply with directives, and contribute more to the control of his or her own behavior.

Key Characteristics of the Preschool Child

The preschool child has the following unique characteristics that should be taken into account when evaluating adaptive functioning and considering therapeutic intervention:

1. Reasoning has been described as concrete and egocentric (Piaget, 1962). The preschool child's reasoning is associative and one-dimensional (e.g., the child has trouble considering two emotions simultaneously). Recent research indicates that older preschoolers develop the ability to expand their perspective; however, more egocentric thinking may still occur during times of stress. Preschoolers should be considered limited in their ability to think logically and to engage in accurate reality testing (Davies, 2004).

2. Play has a central role in preschool development (Davies, 2004). Play encompasses both functional play with objects and representational play, which includes symbolization, enactment, and storytelling. Increased symbolic capacity provides the opportunity to access readily the child's thoughts and feelings through pretend play and thus through the process of play therapy.

3. Preschoolers acquire the capacity for narrative (Emde, Wolf, & Oppenheim, 2003) through which they can share experiences with another and "co-construct" new, shared meanings about their experiences.

4. Physical and psychological functioning shifts from external toward internal (self) regulation during this time period. This shift allows for increasing self-management of attention, aggression, and emotions (Bronson, 2000). This provides an important opportunity for the child to benefit from direct

psychotherapeutic intervention focused on the development of internal regulatory capacities.

5. Parents are still central in the preschooler's emotional, social, and adaptive functioning, and therefore need to be an integral part of any intervention plan.

INTERVENTION IN THE PRESCHOOL YEARS

Reasons for Intervention

Various circumstances can generate a need for intervention. First, early-onset disorders of infancy, such as disorders of attachment, affect, autism, sleep, feeding, communication, regulation, and posttraumatic stress (Zeanah, 2000; Zero to Three, 1994) often indicate a need for direct intervention. These and additional disorders are diagnosed in the preschool period.

Second, children in the developmental transitions just described are considered vulnerable (Emde et al., 2004). A preschooler's developmental pathway can be either supported or deflected by the social, emotional, or physical environment. Early deviations affect later development in ways that become more difficult to ameliorate, and can lead to psychopathology. These times of transition provide an opportunity for early intervention to prevent more serious deviations at a later age that become more difficult to correct (Emde et al., 2004). Brazelton (1992) describes the normative regression that precedes developmental bursts as "touchpoints" for developmental guidance.

Third, differences in children's temperament (Clark, Tluczek, & Gallagher, 2004; Stifter & Wiggins, 2004; Thomas, Chess, & Birch, 1968) and in parenting styles (Campbell, 2002) can impact parent–child interactions by supporting or hindering a preschooler's functioning. Linder (1993) notes that a "difficult" child may be more challenging to comfort, more demanding of attention, and potentially mismatched with the parent's personality, which may not only increase the risk for psychopathology but also generate a need for therapeutic intervention.

Finally, intervention also may be warranted for preschoolers exhibiting extreme reactions to life transitions (e.g., birth of a sibling, illness, or loss of a family member), parent psychopathology, or significant traumas. This chapter does not cover in detail the important issue of assessment, recently reviewed by DelCarmen-Wiggens and Carter (2004). Psychiatric diagnosis, developmental status, behavioral and emotional disturbance, and family functioning and relationships should all be considered and explored in some manner (Benham, 2000). The resulting comprehensive assessment informs decisions about whether clinical attention is warranted, what the most appropriate treatment modality might be, and how to intervene. Differentiating between age-typical and symptomatic behavior is often a matter of degree and clinical judgment. The distinctions between transient, age-appropriate, or expectable disturbances in emotions and behavior, and clinically significant ones, are necessarily vague in preschool children. Typically, young children are particularly sensitive to family disruptions that threaten their sense of security. Those who have intrinsic developmental disturbances (e.g., delays, pervasive disorders, sensory regulatory difficulties) may be especially vulnerable to disruptions in their environment.

The clinician must attend to the frequency, intensity, chronicity, and social context of the child's emotions or behaviors to determine whether a reported problem represents a clinical disturbance (Campbell, 2002) and warrants intervention. Parental report is critical, but often insufficient, in addressing this issue with reference to a particular behavior or cluster of behaviors. Important assessments are also provided by teacher report and clinician observation of the child at school or in the office. Judgments and diagnoses that do not consider a range of informants and contexts, and a developmental perspective, lead to simplistic treatment decisions that may prove ineffective or possibly even contraindicated (Holmbeck, Greenley, & Franks, 2003).

The family plays a very important role in supporting or undermining a child's healthy adjustment (Cummings, Davies, & Campbell, 2000). The transactional model/multiple ports of entry approach supports the use of parent consultation and guidance to address problems that lack a "caseness" level of disturbance within the child. Parents should still be the first line of defense in helping young children with their response to traumatic events and life changes. However, whether the problem crosses the threshold into "caseness" may be a function of the caregiver's inability to handle transitions, behaviors, or the child's emotional expression appropriately, rather than the degree of child distress or disruption. Furthermore, even "good-enough" parenting may not be sufficient to solve the child's distress, and clinician-guided techniques or interventions may be needed to help the child resolve fears, distress, or symptoms.

Treatment decisions rest on the clinician's conception of the locus of the problem. That locus can be seen as being within the child (DSM-IV approach), within the parent–child relationship, within the family, or within the wider system (e.g., the school or day care setting). We believe, as do Lieberman (2004), Campbell (2002), and Sameroff (2004), that presenting concerns reach a clinical level of significance when there are disruptions in several parameters of the child's functioning.

Emotional and behavioral symptoms in young children are sometimes grouped as externalizing and internalizing problems (Achenbach & Rescorla, 2000). Externalizing behaviors reflect the immaturity of regulatory functions in the process of development, such as impulse control and frustration tolerance. Externalizing disorders involve disruptive behaviors such as fighting, aggressiveness, disobedience, tantrums, overactivity, poor attention, and poor impulse control. Before deciding that a young child with such symptoms qualifies for a diagnosable disorder, a change in environment (e.g., a preschool that does not enforce a 30-minute seated circle time) is often the appropriate first intervention. Symptoms of poor or immature functioning of these self-regulatory functions are a central part of attention-deficit/hyperactivity disorder (ADHD). However, Campbell (2002) warns of the dangers of overdiagnosis and misdiagnosis of ADHD and oppositional defiant disorder in preschoolers with age-appropriate disruptive behaviors.

Internalizing disorders include symptoms such as social withdrawal (when not part of the pervasive developmental disorder spectrum), fearfulness, phobias, anxiety, and sadness. Children with externalizing symptoms are referred for assessment more frequently than are children with internalizing symptoms, due to the disruptive nature of the more easily recognized externalizing symptoms. Disruptive behaviors can also be one manifestation of internalizing disorders such as anxiety and dysthymia in young children, or a reaction to trauma or family disruption. Young children typically exhibit a mixture of internalizing and externalizing symptoms as a response to trauma (Perry, Pollard, Blakley, Baker, & Vigilante, 1995). Research results from two clinics (Thomas & Guskin, 2001; Leventhal-Belfer, Slotnick, Nichols, Blasey, & Huffman, 2000) have shown that the majority of young children presenting with disruptive behavior were diagnosed with sensory regulatory disorders or with internalizing disorders, including traumatic stress disorder and disorders of affect, using Diagnostic Classification 0–3 (DC:0–3) criteria. Co-occurrence of clinically significant levels of both externalizing and internalizing symptoms on the Child Behavior Checklist (Achenbach, 1992) was seen in 45% of these young children (Thomas & Guskin, 2001). These data suggest that when disruptive behaviors are the presenting concern, internalizing symptoms are often present but not easily recognized.

The following brief case study demonstrates three important issues: (1) internal anxiety can underlie externalized aggressive behavior; (2) developmental delay can compound a child's symptomatic behavior; and (3) a change in the school setting can impact a child's behavioral functioning.

Joey, age 3½ years, was referred because of constant fighting with his mother, aggressive outbursts toward peers in preschool, noncompliance, and tantrums. He was distractible and restless in his play and was on the verge of being expelled by his preschool. The clinical interview revealed two sources of stress: (1) marital stress and arguing, but no violence, and (2) his father's motorcycle accident, when Joey was 2, resulting in bruising and a groin injury. His father spent several weeks at home on intravenous therapy, often with Joey in his room. When the therapist asked Joey in a play session if he remembered Daddy's accident, he said that Daddy died and his penis was cut off. The doctor put it back on and made him alive. His mother, in the session, was able to help correct this frightening misperception. The clinician helped Joey to express how frightened he had been at seeing Daddy's bruises, and Joey's mother was available to comfort and empathize with him. As a consequence of this session, Joey's aggressive behavior toward his mother ceased. Identification of a previously unidentified language delay explained, in part, Joey's frustration and his lashing out in school; he could not keep up with peers or express himself clearly in a fast-paced setting. Placement in a special education classroom for communicatively handicapped children greatly improved his school behavior. Marital therapy was recommended to address his parents' problems. This case demonstrates the value of a comprehensive approach. Intervention targeting only the disruptive behavior per se could have missed Joey's posttraumatic and developmental issues.

Theoretical Models That Inform Our Therapeutic Approach

Two parent–child models inform our work. The transactional model of development (Sameroff & Chandler, 1975) describes the ongoing reciprocal effects between parent and child over time and emphasizes the importance of this dynamic in the child's development. Both child and parents are moving on their own developmental trajectories, with each affected by, and potentially changed by, interaction with the other. Therefore, the outcome for the child is a product of both nature (intrinsic factors, e.g., genetics, temperament, neurobiological status, including damage, difference or disease) and nurture (caregiving and other environmental factors). The child is embedded in a larger social context, referred to as the ecological model by Campbell (2002).

A second, related conceptual model of infant–parent relationships underlies therapeutic approaches (Stern, 1995) with implications for preschool children. Stern-Bruschweiler and Stern (1989) proposed a dynamic equilibrium between each member's internal mental representation (R^M = mother, R^I = infant) of their relationship and his or her behavior (B^M = mother, B^I = infant), affecting the enacted interactional relationship between mother and infant ($R^M \leftrightarrow B^M \leftrightarrow B^I \leftrightarrow R^I$). The mother's and the baby's actions constitute overt interpersonal behavior, and their representations of self, other, and relationships are intrapsychic material. Representations influence behavior; reciprocally, behavior influences representations. Therefore, treatments can be directed at all four entities, the parent, the child, their behaviors and their representations, and the associated ports of entry: R^M, B^M, B^I, and R^I.

Direct Therapy with Preschoolers

Although preschool children demonstrate a surge of progress in their expressive language capacity, many are still unable or unwilling to communicate verbally about their inner life in ways most adults can readily understand. Much of their communication occurs via behavior such as withdrawal or tantrums, the etiology and meaning of which can be difficult to decipher. Angry outbursts may reflect aggression, frustration, or anxiety. Behavioral and parent-training approaches that attempt only to change or control the behavior of young children fail to analyze the underlying etiology and meaning of such behavior and may consequently fail to address important underlying issues. A direct approach for understanding the meaning of this behavior is needed.

The preschooler's emerging symbolic capacities enable him or her to engage in representational play, providing a medium for direct treatment not available to infants and toddlers. This constitutes an enhanced port of entry, addressing the child's representations through his or her imaginative play. Play therapy supports the expansion of the child's capacity to communicate in words and play instead of engaging in unmodulated emotional and behavioral discharge. It has the added advantage of putting the child at ease, so that dialogue about a variety of issues can also occur in the safety of the symbolic domain.

In both individual and dyadic (child–parent) treatment models, this enhanced access to the child's representations provides the opportunity to increase the therapist's and parents' understanding of the child. This understanding is the outcome of experiences in individual or dyadic sessions and discussion in parent collateral sessions (see section on models used in working with parents). Expanded parental understanding of the child's representations may have an impact on the family relationships, because representations and behavior influence each other.

PLAY

The Development and Function of Play in Normative Preschool Development

The emergence of fantasy play differentiates preschoolers from infants and toddlers. The preschooler's cognitive development permits emerging flexible use of materials, so that an object can be used to represent another object (e.g., stick for horse), and flexible use of the child's own actions, so that an action can represent a different action (e.g., pretending to eat rather than eating). This flexibility enables the child to develop imagination (Vygotsky, 1978).

For a preschooler, play is naturalistic, spontaneous, pleasurable, and focused on means, not on ends. Play is often described as rule-free, although Vygotsky (1978) points out that even free play is bound by the rules of social roles. Piaget (1962) defined "play" as the predominance of the function of assimilation (adjusting the objects to the child's schema) over accommodation (adjusting the child's schemas to the object) in the interaction between child and environment. The structure of play emerges in a universal developmental sequence (Lidz, 2003; Piaget, 1962; Westby, 2000).

Play provides a range of functions in early development. It is considered a window into all areas of development, as well as a means of expression of a child's individuality (Vondra & Belsky, 1991; Westby, 2000). Play is central in the development of cognition (Lidz, 2003), creative thinking, problem solving, integration of actions, mastery (Linder, 1993a; Russ, 2004; Vondra & Belsky, 1991; Westby, 2000), language development (Lidz, 2003; Linder, 1993a), motor development (Linder, 1993a; Lidz, 2003), symbolic functioning (Vygotsky, 1967) and social–emotional development (Lidz, 2003). Play is egocentric thought that allows the child to relive past experiences and express subjective feelings (Piaget, 1962). Play is a special activity that provides a medium for engagement with others.

Play also provides the context for learning from social interactions. Vygotsky (1967) described an area beyond the child's independent functioning made possible by adult guidance or social interaction with a skillful peer. He called it the "zone of proximal development" and proposed that it leads development with functions that are in partial formation. Learning, then, occurs in social interaction with adults or peers and later becomes internalized. Play is central, in that it creates this zone of proximal development. Adult-mediated play provides the context for the development of an alliance between parent and child that contributes to the development of competence (Cooke & Sinker, 1993) and the facilitation of cognitive development (Bruner, 1982; Vygotsky, 1967), as well as social development (Greenspan, 1995, 1998).

Functions of Play in Psychotherapy

Play can be used in therapy for expression, communication, development of relationships, creation of a miniaturized version of the world, and the development of new capacities. Early psychoanalytic theorists discussed the role of play in the development of social–emotional capacities. Anna Freud (1966) established a correlation between adult free association and a child's free play, in that they both yielded access to instinctual drives. She stated that one of the functions of play was the denial of reality. Furthermore, she analyzed play interruptions as a disruption in free association, indicating the functioning of ego defense mechanisms (coping strategies to manage both instinctual drives and conflict about their expression). She pioneered the analysis of these defense mechanisms to understand the formation of children's symptoms.

Ego psychologist Erik Erikson stated that "play is a function of the ego, an attempt to synchronize the bodily and social processes within the self" (1963, p. 211). He discussed play satiation (as opposed to play disruption) as providing a resolution of conflicts in spontaneous play and deemed it "self-curative." He noted that this ego function of play formed the basis for play therapy. The toddler game of peekaboo is an example of mastery of separation through play.

Many theorists agree that play therapy is the most comfortable avenue for the child's *expression* of feelings, wishes, fears, and experiences (Chethik, 2000; Guerney, 2003) when successful therapeutic rapport is established. This has been referred to as the "expressive" component of psychotherapy (Kernberg, personal communication, July, 2004). Ginsberg (1993) concluded that emotional expression is an essential, if not *the* most essential, component of play therapy. Mechanisms of change include catharsis, the discharge of energy and emotion (Ginsberg, 1993), and abreaction, the reliving of experiences with an appropriate discharge of affect (Levy, 1939; Ormland, 1993;

Terr, 2003). The expression of feeling as a component of therapy is also a central focus of dyadic therapy (Greenspan, 1995), client-centered therapy (Axline, 1947), and trauma therapy (Levy, 1939; Gaensbauer & Siegal, 1995). These basic principles of psychotherapy apply to preschoolers and are discussed in a later section on the expressive component of play therapy.

Play therapy provides a means of *communication*. Play is the child's language, yet it is not limited by the constraints of language (Landreth, 1993). A child has the freedom to communicate less self-consciously about a wide variety of experiences in play. Play therapy allows the clinician not only to ask questions within the play, which the child experiences as less threatening, but also to communicate ideas and suggestions. Most importantly, it allows the therapist an opportunity to decode the meaning of the child's behaviors. For example, in a dyadic session with 4-year-old Chris and his mother, Chris asked the therapist to be a monster, while he and his mother hid under a blanket. After a period of enjoying this play, Chris suddenly looked fearful, became aggressive, and attacked the therapist. This demonstrated that his aggression in the session was defensive, stemming initially from fear rather than anger. The therapist linked his fearful reaction to early traumatic experiences in an orphanage. Decoding this play incident shifted the mother's understanding of Chris's aggression and the focus of therapy to exploration of his fear. Play therapy also provides a medium for the therapist to communicate his or her understanding, clarifications, and interpretation in a way that is more easily understood by the child. The therapist can respond in the context of play symbolism, which provides some distancing, so that the child can tolerate the emotionally evocative content.

Play therapy is also a vehicle for the *development of relationships*. It provides a basis for developing a therapeutic relationship with the therapist (Axline, 1947), who joins the play and thus communicates to the child that he or she can become a participant, that "I can speak his/her special language" (Chethik, 2000, p. 222). In many treatment models, a play therapy approach is used to improve the parent–child relationship (Greenspan, 1995; Guerney, 1993, 2003; Lieberman, 2004; McDonough, 2004; Muns, 2003). Russ (2004) describes a central mechanism of change in therapy as improving object relationships and internal representations.

In play therapy, the child is able to make a *miniaturized version of the world and then manipulate reality*. Erikson notes that "child's play is the infantile form of the human ability to deal with experience by creating model situations and to master reality by experiment and planning" (1963, p. 222). Play therapy is an arena in which to try out alternatives and change endings. Landreth (1993) argues that the major function of play therapy is the transformation of "unmanageable" reality into "manageable" fantasy. Terr (1990) indicates that a child can master the experience of trauma displaced onto play characters, without having to recognize the problem as his or her own. Change is effected through practicing and problem solving until internalization takes place.

Play provides the therapist an opportunity to scaffold the child's functional capacities and *facilitate the development of new capacities*. Developing the child's capacity to play is the focus of the formative function of therapy for children in whom this capacity is blocked by trauma and inhibition; delayed by developmental lags in language, sensory, or social skills; or limited by poor emotional self-regulation or attention. The parent's role in the development of play is considered critical. Greenspan (1995, 1998) has emphasized the critical role of the parent to follow play in a manner that encourages two-way interaction, leading to the parent's introduction of new ideas, words, and affects. This has been formalized as a technique in "Floor Time" to help a child "master the emotional milestones, one by one, in sequential order, starting with the earliest one he hasn't mastered" (Greenspan, 1998, p. 125).

THERAPEUTIC APPROACHES WITH THE PRESCHOOL CHILD: THE LITERATURE

Although this volume explores the current state of knowledge about diagnosis and disorders in preschoolers, most psychotherapeutic literature does not specify a particular intervention for a given disorder or age group. This is a source of much valid criticism in our field. The child psychotherapy literature can be divided into three main groups of treatments, distinguished by the conceptualized role of the therapist, the role of the parents, and the focus of treatment. The first group, individual therapies, focuses on the child–therapist relationship as the agent of change and/or a venue for understanding the child's behavioral or emotional problems. Most include some collateral sessions with parents. This large group includes the "client-centered" therapies (Axline, 1947; Gil, 1991, 2003; Guerney, 1993), psychoanalysis, psychodynamic psychotherapies (Chethik, 2000; Erikson, 1963), and cognitive-behavioral therapy, amended for preschoolers by Knell (1993) and by Cohen and Mannarino (1996b).

A second group of therapies views the parents as the change agent. Here the therapist's role is to train parents (1) to facilitate emotional development and to alter parent–child relationships, as in Floor Time (Greenspan, 1995, 1998), filial therapy (Guerney, 1993, 2003), and theraplay (Jernberg, 1979), and/or (2) to change the child's behavior by effective limit setting (Eyberg, Boggs, & Algina, 1995; Campbell, 2002).

The third group of therapeutic approaches comes from the field of infant mental health and conceptualizes the parent–child (infant) relationship as the therapeutic focus. These therapies range conceptually from focusing on the parent's internal mental representation of the child, and a need to free the dyad from "ghosts in the nursery" (Fraiberg, 1987), to more phenomenologically based approaches for improving a parent's ability to observe, understand, and interact with the child, as in interaction guidance (McDonough, 2004) and Wait, Watch and Wonder (Cohen et al., 1999). Enhanced attachment, interaction, play, and pleasure in the relationship are also the focus of parent–child therapies such as family play therapy (Gil, 1991; 2003) and theraplay (Jernberg, 1979). Van Horn and Lieberman's child–parent psychotherapy (see Chapter 16, this volume) seeks to enhance the parent–child partnership, intimacy, and trust to help the child cope with traumatic experiences and life stressors.

Empirical Research about Play Psychotherapy

Evidence-based research support for psychotherapeutic interventions is uneven, complicated, and controversial. Meta-analyses of diverse psychotherapy research with children of all ages (Casey & Berman, 1985; Weiss & Weisz, 1990; Weisz, Weiss, Han, Granger, & Morton, 1995), involving hundreds of studies, suggest that substantial effects of psychotherapy are detectable, that treatment is better than no treatment (79% of children were better off treated than not treated), but that the estimated amount of benefit explains less than 20% of the outcome variance (Werry & Andrews, 2002; Weiss & Weisz, 1990).

The best-researched interventions are more likely to be laboratory-based, with recruited populations and manualized techniques (Weiss & Weisz, 1990; Russ, 2004). These behavioral approaches tend to show efficacy most clearly and have narrower measurable targets and outcomes, and manualized, and thus reproducible, interventions. Some authors note that clinical cases are often much more complex and multifactorial (McClellan & Werry, 2003; Werry & Andrews, 2002), which can limit the utility of manualized interventions for clinical work.

Very few studies have looked at the preschool population in particular, partly because few treatments have been developed specifically for this age group. Psychotherapy studies of the first two groups described earlier (individual psychotherapy and parent as therapist/change agent) tend to lump broad age ranges together (e.g., ages 2–18 years). The infant–parent relationship focused therapies and Floor Time focus primarily on infants and toddlers.

One evidence-based preschool intervention is derived from the parent training therapy models (Barkley, 1997) targeting overt child behaviors involving aggression and noncompliance. In successful programs for oppositional, defiant preschoolers (Eyberg et al., 1995; Reid, Webster-Stratton, & Baydar, 2004; Webster-Stratton, 1985), parents are taught both limit-setting *and* positive approaches that enhance the parent–child relationship, such as contingent praise, following the child's play, decreasing criticism and vague commands, and ignoring merely annoying behaviors (Campbell, 2002). Participation by fathers improves maintenance of gains from Parent–Child Interaction Therapy (PCIT) at 1 year (Bagner & Eyberg, 2003). Continued parenting self-efficacy and further improvement in child behavior over the next 3½ years has been hypothesized to result from a "reinforcing spiral" of positive parent and child behaviors (Hood & Eyberg, 2003).

Relationship enhancement, part of the PCIT combined parent training approach, is the central focus for infant–parent therapy models that target both parent interactive behavior (Cohen et al., 1999; McDonough, 2004) and parent internal representations of the child (Cramer et al., 1995; Lieberman, Silverman, & Pawl, 2000). Some children show improved attachment as a positive outcome to such therapeutic approaches (Lieberman et al., 2000; Ciccetti, Toth, & Rogosh, 1999). An empirical study applying this concept to older children, ages 6–10 years, was reported by Muratori, Picci, Bruni, Patarnello, and Romagnoli (2003) who targeted the link between parents' representations and distortions about the child and the child's symptoms in an 11-week intervention with parent and child components. They found greater improvement, progression to nonclinical diagnostic status, and a significant 2-year sleeper effect of further improvement in the intervention group compared to matched, nonrandom controls. This model might hold promise for preschoolers given its success with younger and older populations.

Cohen and Mannarino have combined structured parent counseling and child psychotherapy to treat preschool children who have been sexually abused. Children received cognitive-behavioral therapy, including structured play, reframing, safety education, directive problem-solving, and cognitive restructuring techniques; the parents received parent training in parallel (Cohen & Mannarino, 1993). Results indicate that cognitive-behavioral therapy was more effective than nondirective supportive therapy for both short- and long-term outcomes (Cohen & Mannarino, 1996b, 1997). Furthermore, parent emotional distress and parent support were a strong predictor of outcome, indicating the importance of including parents in the intervention plan (Cohen & Mannario, 1996, 1998).

Play therapy per se is the most difficult therapy to research, because interventions are difficult to manualize. Many reviewers believe that play therapy has not yet been adequately evaluated in well-controlled studies (Campbell, 2002; Russ, 2004). Another confounding factor is that the "no-treatment" controls are often treatment refusers who receive an assessment (Russ, 2004) that may actually serve as an initial intervention. Russ noted that in the meta-analyses, many psychotherapy studies that did show treatment effectiveness had play embedded within the interventions but did not specifically isolate its effect. She reviewed "play intervention" studies, which are focused, well-controlled play interventions for a focal problem. She concluded that play itself appears to reduce fears and anxiety, including preschool separation anxiety (Barnett, 1984), even after controlling for the presence of an attentive adult (Russ, 2004). Notably, the Target and Fonagy (1994a, 1994b; Fonagy & Target, 1994) retrospective chart review studies of intensive psychotherapy (one to four times per week) with hundreds of child cases showed the best outcome with younger children (under age 6). Therapy was especially helpful for children with simple phobias, less severe psychopathology, and preschoolers with stress-related diagnoses (posttraumatic stress disorder, and sleep disorder or adjustment disorder). Kot and Tyndall-Lind (2005) conducted a study of children ages 4–10 who witnessed domestic violence; children received individual or joint-sibling play therapy following Axline's nondirective approach. These children had significantly higher post-test self-concept scores and fewer externalizing and total behavior problems on the Child Behavior Checklist compared to a control group.

Holmbeck et al. (2003) argued that developmentally based intervention strategies increase the effect size of treatments. They also suggested that the cognitive-developmental level is an important moderator of treatment effectiveness, and that normative developmental skills such as self-control and emotion regulation may be important targets for intervention. Therapists must think multisystemically and help parents to become developmentally sensitive.

Clinical studies that did not study preschool-age children separately support the short-term client-centered play therapy approach in targeting school performance (Johnson, McLeoud, & Fall, 1997) or recovery from trauma (Webb, 2001). Gil (1991) noted that these nondirective therapies are most beneficial at the beginning of treatment with abused children, who may be hypervigilant and/or very compliant. Victims of abuse may need long-term therapy. Filial therapy, in which the parents are taught to implement client-centered play therapy techniques in regular home sessions, has demonstrated success in studies that assessed broad outcomes with ethnically diverse populations (Sweeney & Landreth, 2003). A meta-analysis of 94 studies showed a larger effect size for filial therapy than for regular client-centered play therapy (Ray, Bratton, Rhine, & Jones, 2001), suggesting the key importance of parent involvement.

PLAY THERAPY TECHNIQUES

Our own recommended therapeutic approach with preschool children utilizes many of the treatment methods reviewed earlier. It supports an eclectic, flexible approach in which we select from and integrate different approaches based on the developmental and emotional needs and capacities of the child and family, and relies on evidence-based research, if available, to select specific treatments. Furthermore, the techniques need to be adapted to the cognitive-developmental level of the preschool child. Schaefer (2003) describes an eclectic, integrative approach as "prescriptive play therapy."

Role of the Therapist

The style of the therapist's engagement with the child may vary, ranging from nondirective to more active or directive. A nondirective approach allows the child to direct the play activity. Here the therapist watches, listens, and reflects the child's play without leading or interpreting. The therapist can join the play as a participant and remain nondirective if he or she either plays in parallel or takes direction from the child. The therapist can also become facilitative and move toward a more active role that involves probing with open-ended questions, making suggestions, proposing or modeling alternatives, or presenting new information. Guided play is also an option; the therapist seeks to elicit salient clinical issues by selecting specific materials or toys, setting up story stems, expanding the play theme, adding play content, or incorporating cognitive-behavioral therapy techniques.

We believe that play therapy is best begun with the therapist in a more quiet, observing role. The child then discovers that play therapy provides freedom, respect, and permission for all thoughts, feelings, and content (but not all behaviors). The therapist follows the child's lead, takes roles in the play, or remains an observer as directed by the child. Early on, and continuing throughout therapy, the clinician attends particularly to play content, recurring themes, and the child's enacted representations of self, family, and relationships. The therapist helps the child to explore his or her feelings, beliefs, reactions, and defenses. These themes are discussed with the child in age-appropriate terms. When directed by the child to be a character, the therapist seeks the child's direction about what that character would feel, want, and say. The therapist must be prepared to jump in, to be lively, and to have fun in a natural and spontaneous manner. The therapist's dual role as observer and player, in which he or she participates in the play but may also step back and comment at times, has been termed "participant–observer" (Harter, 1985).

The therapist aims to create an atmosphere of acceptance and safety that permits the child to be comfortable and revealing. Winnicott (1965) considered the immersion into play as providing a "holding environment," which recreates important aspects of mothering, in which the child experiences acceptance while having his or her needs met. He discussed the creation of a transitional play space (Winnicott, 1968) and said that "psychotherapy takes place in the overlap of two areas of playing, that of the patient and that of the therapist" (Winnicott, 1986, p. 38). The therapist must become a player, must regress and form a link with the child, to develop a therapeutic alliance (Chethik, 2000). The therapeutic alliance with the child is achieved by having the child experience both a positive, real relationship and a nonjudgmental, understanding response to his or her behavior, ideas and feelings. Even with a young child, the therapist can join with the child explicitly to "talk and play, so we can figure out what makes you fight so much" or "understand what is so scary at night" or "have a chance for you and Daddy to play together here."

The therapist includes the parents in this exploration, either within dyadic sessions or in regular collateral sessions. We believe that the therapist's attitude should be that of a collaborator, respecting the parents' knowledge about and understanding of their child even as the therapist may seek to change these ideas. The therapist must also create an emotionally safe place for the caregivers. Parents need to feel safe in expressing privately their ambivalent feelings toward the child, in describing their interactions with the child and others accurately, and in sharing important issues and events in their lives that may impact the child. Parents may see the therapist as helper, parent, guide, critic, rival or in other complex transference reactions. They may experience feelings of gratitude, empowerment, dependence, strong disagreement, or competition with regard to the therapist. The therapist must avoid the risk of appearing to "parent better than the parents," by including and collaborating with them during or soon after sessions. We believe that the attitude and process of collaboration lessens the danger of negative reactions that can derail or terminate therapy. Our ultimate goal is to augment the parents' independent capacity to support their child's healthy functioning.

Table 15.1 lists possible goals for the child and his or her parents in play therapy.

Expressive and Formative Aspects of Play Therapy

Play therapy has two, related aspects. The *expressive* component of play therapy focuses on eliciting and processing therapeutic content (Kernberg, personal communication, July, 2004). Russ (2004) describes this aspect of therapy as a vehicle for change. Mechanisms of change include processes referred to earlier, such as abreaction, the reliving of experiences with an appropriate discharge of affect.

The other component of therapy refers to building the developmental capacities of the child, including ego mechanisms or coping strategies, and

---

TABLE 15.1. Play Therapy Goals for Child and Parents

Goals for child

- Improve emotional and behavioral self-regulation to diminish symptoms.
- Develop a positive sense of self; improve self-esteem.
- Increase coping skills.
- Increase developmental capacities, including the capacity to develop structural and representational aspects of play for self-expression.
- Improve capacity to engage in relationships and strengthen bonds, especially within the family.
- Master the effects of external stressors and trauma.
- Develop flexible, age-appropriate defenses.
- Improve impulse control.
- Enhance communication, including language development and affective expression.
- Decrease behavioral and affective inhibition.
- Increase freedom of play and fantasy.

Goals for the parents

- Understand and accurately see their unique child as an individual.
- Develop empathy.
- Develop and refine parenting skills to help foster the child's growth and development.
- Improve feeling of efficacy in their parenting role.
- Improve the parent–child bond.

related skills (language, cognition, and symbolic play). Kernberg (personal communication) has referred to this as the "supportive" component of play therapy. Russ (2004) describes using play to strengthen play processes. We propose the term *formative* to capture the developmental aspect of therapeutic intervention.

We describe the expressive and formative aspects separately to discuss their indications and specific strategies. However, in reality, most therapies utilize both expressive and formative techniques.

Expressive Components of Play Therapy

The expressive modality in play therapy refers to the exploration of the child's feelings, fears, wishes, traumatic experiences, and conflicts, as expressed in behavior, play, and verbalization. The focus is on the content and meaning of play. The therapist's observation, participation, and interpretation provide the opportunity for a child to express affect, communicate his or her concerns, develop coping strategies, and resolve conflicts. Therapeutic issues may unfold in the child's spontaneous play. In addition, guided play can be utilized to elicit either neutral or clinical thematic content. Content can be expanded for both the developmentally delayed and the neurotypical child. The therapist can add specific toys that are meaningful to the child's experience and/or probe the meaning of the play. Storytelling, used to explore the child's inner world in research studies (Emde et al., 2003), can be used clinically to facilitate communication. The therapist may use story stems (e.g., about school, being in the hospital, getting scared at night, seeing a big dog, hearing adults yell) that are related to the child's particular issues. With either spontaneous or guided play, the therapist carefully observes the child's response, noting play disruptions that indicate too much anxiety. For example, a 4-year-old girl began hitting a baby doll, then suddenly moved to her mother's lap for a hug, suggesting she was overwhelmed by her own aggressive feelings toward her younger sibling.

INDICATIONS FOR THE EXPRESSIVE COMPONENT

Many children experience behavioral and emotional distress and dysregulation. The distress may be externally triggered by events in the family or environment, or it may be the child's reaction to conditions within him- or herself, such as illness or injury, physical differences, developmental limitations, temperamental variables, or psychiatric conditions. Children with internalizing disorders characterized by inhibition, sadness, or anxiety are good candidates for expressive play therapies. Expressive therapies may be very useful in processing trauma and loss. Those with specific fears and phobias or symptoms of hyperarousal in PTSD may benefit from a combination of cognitive-behavioral techniques (Cohen & Mannarino, 1993; Knell, 1993, 2000, 2003) and exploratory play therapy.

The use of the expressive component to facilitate change is recommended for children with a good capacity for fantasy play (Russ, 2004). It is appropriate for preschool children who are developing the capacity to communicate through symbolic means such as play and/or language, and not just through behavioral discharge. To some degree, the use of expressive modalities presumes the existence of capacities that formative elements seek to strengthen.

STRATEGIES AND THERAPEUTIC PROCESS

Classical psychodynamic psychotherapies focus these expressive elements on exploration and interpretation of unconscious conflicts and their expression in transference reactions. We use the expressive modalities of therapy to explore the child's perspective of his or her world and experience. We believe that with young children the therapist plays an active role in facilitating the child's exploration of his or her inner world through play and perhaps also language. When using more typical psychodynamic play techniques, our emphasis is on the child's and therapist's joint exploration of this inner world, with the parent's involvement in the process, rather than on interpretation of the transference. The therapist may interpret or synthesize play, organize narrative, decode meaning for the child, and help the child to make connections between play and his or her own experiences.

Exploration of Inner World. In fantasy play, preschool children represent their real experiences, their feelings about those experiences, and their wishes or fantasy solutions to internal and external problems and conflicts. Typical wishes include "real" ones, such as wishing to be loved more and to be bigger. This may be seen in exaggerations, such as fantasies of being a baby, a princess, or a superman. Here the child is exploring, in fantasy, ways to solve a problem that he or she cannot articulate. "I would be loved if I were like my sister (a baby); if I were beautiful (a princess); if I were really great (a sports star)." "I would not be scared if I had extra powers (a superhero); if I had a protective companion (an imaginary dog); if I were mean and scary (a witch or monster)."

Play therapy involves such enactments of fantasy (acting out a role or character), especially with younger preschoolers. The therapist may gently explore the meaning of these enactments with the child: "Who would superman need to save?," or "How would a princess's family treat her?" The therapist may keep discussions with the child entirely within a play mode or may step outside of the play to talk about feelings and events. The child may ask the therapist to take a role. Often, the therapist will do that via a toy, such as a puppet, doll, or animal, for whom the therapist will talk. The therapist may also help the child try on different roles and identities: "What if superman gets tired of being strong and saving everyone, and just wants to go home to be taken care of by his mom?"

Young children are especially prone to dramatic shifts and alterations in their stories, with bad guys becoming good guys and back again. This may reflect the associative quality of reasoning at the preschool age, the child's experience of adults as confusing and unpredictable, or a defensive attempt to control fears by denial or reversal. The therapist may explore a child's negative self-image by enacting, for example, "the angry boy," and observing the child's response to that character.

Fostering Acceptance. As the therapist treats all of the child's communications with respect—in play, talk, and behavior—the child develops a feeling of safety in communicating about him- or herself. The therapist seeks to help both child and parents understand and accept the child's perceptions and beliefs as valid and real to the child, regardless of content that may be disturbing. This is a precondition for potential therapeutic efforts to address fears, clarify faulty perceptions, or change self-concept. The therapist's acceptance facilitates the parents' acceptance.

Clarifying Distortions. The young child may use play to express beliefs or memories that are distorted because of his or her level of cognitive development. Typical examples include ascribing cause and effect to events occurring in proximity, or the egocentric and magical belief that one's thoughts cause things to happen. Erroneous beliefs may cause great and unnecessary anxiety or distress for the child (e.g., Joey's misunderstanding of his father's accident in an earlier section of this chapter).

Clarifying Behavior. The young child usually cannot say why he or she is behaving in a certain way, which may mystify, worry, or anger the parent. Play therapy may give clues to unlock this meaning, as in the example of Chris's unpredictable aggression (described earlier), that became understood as fear originating in feeling unprotected during early, traumatic experiences in his orphanage.

Verbalization of Affect. An important role of the therapist is to provide or model the verbal expression of feelings displayed in the child's behavior and play. Young children need vocabulary to express a broader and more complex range of emotions, to move beyond "mad" and "happy," which is often their sole repertoire, to include feelings such as sad (avoided in some families), scared, shy, proud, frustrated, silly, embarrassed, and so on. There are wonderful posters of multiple, labeled facial expressions, children's picture books about feelings, and picture cards and games that the play therapist can use to help children recognize and gain confidence in using the language of emotions. Even children who never really adopt it for themselves will attend to the therapist's use of affect language in play, commentary, or interpretations. Young children often participate with therapists in creating their own books about feelings. One precocious 4-year-old used pages from a children's workbook about loss to draw faces of sad or mad feelings, then taped other, happy faces over them. By using this device to express how she hid her reactions to her dad leaving the family and remarrying, she could then discuss her feelings.

Processing Trauma. Expressive elements of play therapy are particularly useful for the treatment of trauma (Terr, 1990), which DSM-IV defines as life-threatening events accompanied by the experience of helplessness (Scheeringa, Chapter 8, this volume). In addition to obvious traumas, many events that are very frightening or traumatic to young children would not qualify as "trauma" according to the DSM-IV definition. Because of their immature language and cognitive understanding, and also their egocentric and faulty sense of cause and effect, young children may retain large and small traumatic experiences in fragmentary, confused images and memories.

Play therapy can be used to elicit and clarify children's perceptions of traumatic events and to help in the resolution of their misperceptions and their emotions. For example, 3-year-old Sara was treated before and after the extreme trauma of her mother's death from a complication of medical treatment. She entered her mother's room to find her unconscious and covered with blood. Sara initially painted pictures all in red and described "Mommy bleeding all over." In her attempt to find solutions to this trauma, Sara developed extensive play about orphaned animals searching for mothers, and many stories in which she was a doctor fixing hurt animals. However, whereas increasing cognitive capacities in an older preschooler may lead to clearer understanding by the child, richer fantasy production can also lead to new distortions. At age 5, Sara announced, "I shot mommy. The bullet went through her and blood came out." She condensed earlier visual memories with television images and her emerging concept of causality that shootings cause death. Here a simple explanation about how she might have come to this false conclusion was sufficient to relieve Sara's distress.

Children use play in therapy to achieve a sense of mastery over frightening experiences of helplessness. They reverse passive roles into active ones in fantasy by subjecting others to their experiences. This is a frequent theme in medical trauma, such as the child's experience of being held down for stitches in the emergency room. Particularly distressing to children are repetitive treatments for prolonged conditions, such as chemotherapy and lumbar punctures for cancer or debridement during burn care. In therapy, these children gleefully or grimly dispense shots and treatment to parents, therapists, or dolls. One little boy with hemophilia, who experienced regular bleeds into his joints, became the sheriff who tied up the doctor–therapist (as the "bad guy") week after week and threatened him with death.

A therapeutic goal is to help these children move from repetitive posttraumatic play to more flexible play in which they can find solutions that reflect a sense of mastery. Through play and talk, the therapist may help the child put traumatic experiences in context and find personal mechanisms of repair or correction of the experience (Terr, 2003). A child may be able to achieve "play satiation" (Erikson, 1963) about trauma allowing the child to move on to focus on other issues.

Co-Construction of Narrative. Play psychotherapy can be useful for the co-creation of a narrative about traumatic events from fragments and disjointed memories, even those from preverbal periods (Warren, 2003). Sasha, who had been adopted from an Eastern European orphanage at age 1½ years, was seen at age 2½ because of multiple fears, tantrums, and a severe sleep disturbance. Sasha named a dark-haired, female dollhouse figure as "Scary" and wanted to avoid her. Initial exploration of what made the figure scary was unrevealing. Sasha was told she could have the scary doll go away, and she proceeded to open the door, throw the doll out, then retrieve the doll to throw it down the hall. Over time, exploration and play with turning out the lights in the office suggested that "Scary" had yelled "No crying" at her at night. Her parents remembered that most of the caregivers in the orphanage were dark-haired Russian women, in contrast to the blond children. Furthermore, they learned that children were punished for crying at night by being put alone in the dark hallway. Together, parents, child, and therapist reconstructed what had been frightening that Sasha could not articulate, and they engaged in play about night and separation. Her symptoms abated. By co-constructing a narrative through play, Sasha, her parents, and the therapist were able to understand and articulate early experiences contributing to her current fears and symptomatic behaviors, resulting in an abatement of these symptoms.

One can see a play progression in therapy from enactment to miniaturization to narrative. The young child moves from enactment to miniaturization when he or she changes from pretending to be the scary aggressive animal (perhaps even having aggression spill out of the play when he or she scratches the play partner while pretending to be a cat) to using a puppet or toy animal that he or she animates. Miniaturization, or play with toy figures, represents a further step in the development of symbolization, which allows the child to achieve some distance from the pressing memory or feeling. This distancing allows more manipulation of the story, such as the introduction of alternative endings by the child or the therapist, to help the child try out solutions in play. Narrative involves a verbal description of events and the accompanying feelings that help the child process stressful experiences. The therapist may need to model this to help facilitate the child's verbalizations. An example of play progression would be Sara's play progression in her processing of her mother's burial. Initially, she painted colorful blotches of paint with black spatters on top. Then she repetitively reenacted the burial using a circle of chairs, placing herself or the therapist lying down in the center. This was miniaturized later when she repeated the same scene with dolls. The paintings could now be understood as depicting the flowers and dirt thrown into the grave. Finally, Sara verbalized a fantasy of getting into the grave with her mother. In developing a narrative, we could discuss her anxiety and horror during the burial, the extent of which had not been at all evident in her calm, serious behavior at the time. Terr believes that for full-blown PTSD, children must eventually vocalize words for the toys' or their own intense emotions to avert the continued tendency to act out their feelings outside the therapy in dangerous or inappropriate ways (Terr, 2003).

Provision of Specific Play Materials to Elicit Content. Therapists can elicit clinical content by arranging specific toys in the room ahead of time or by introducing the toys during the flow of play. This method provides concrete, visual cues helpful to preschoolers who are in earlier stages of symbolic development and may be less threatening than direct, verbal suggestions. These techniques are often needed with preschool children who do not easily express their ideas verbally or are emotionally restricted in reaction to stress or trauma. This approach is applicable both to typically developing children and to children with developmental delays, as long as the developmental level of the child is taken into consideration.

Specific play materials are also useful in time-limited, problem-focused therapy in which specific problems and goals have been formulated with the parents. Some children are affected by stressors such as a move, the birth of a sibling, entrance into a new school, or parental separation/divorce, resulting in a clinical level of symptoms. In these cases, treatment may be problem-focused and short term. A therapist may want to structure the selection of toys to elicit content pertaining to the specific stressor, with specific toys as the stimulus, so that clinical content may emerge more quickly. The therapist needs to monitor the child's reaction carefully to ascertain whether the play is moving too quickly and causing anxiety, which is often expressed by the child's play disruption.

1. *Divorce, moving.* The use of two dollhouses can facilitate the emotional expression of children experiencing stressors such as parental separation, divorce, or moves (Trebing, 2000). This technique was used with Tom, age 3 years, 9 months, whose lesbian parents (whom he called Mama and Mommy) were separating. They were concerned about his aggression (hitting) and anxious symptoms (chewing clothing). Both he and his younger sibling had witnessed arguing between their parents. Tom was seen with his younger sibling, and the two mothers alternated attending the sessions. The therapist also held parent collateral sessions, that were primarily focused on limit setting. Two houses were provided for both the initial assessment sessions and during the 2 months of treatment sessions.

Providing these toy prompts facilitated the elicitation of Tom's story. The therapist asked Tom to identify the two houses. He identified one as Mama's (the new home just established) and one as Mommy's (the family's original home). He described Mama as invisible, explained that they got a divorce, and expressed the wish that she would return to Mommy's house. He then became very aggressive with the toys. Mommy listened to his story but did not set clear safety limits, which were then modeled by the clinician. Tom, who was handed a small boy doll with an angry face to help him enact his anger symbolically, described the boy as bad. This provided an opportunity for the therapist to correct Tom's misperception by wondering aloud whether the boy doll worried that he caused the divorce.

In subsequent sessions, the mad boy doll continued to act aggressively toward both homes. Tom then placed family dolls in a spaceship but did not let the mad boy doll come, acting out a punishment theme. He included both mothers, representing his wish that the family be back together. Finally the mad boy doll was allowed to enter the shuttle, and was reidentified by Tom as a "sad" boy, reflecting the feelings underneath Tom's aggressive behavior. In a later session, Tom was able to use the mad boy doll to explain that he was mad because he wanted to live with Mommy, and mad because he wanted to live with Mama. Use of the two houses and the angry doll allowed the issues to surface quickly, and to be explored and interpreted. Both mothers learned to understand Tom's feelings and to set safety limits to contain his aggression. Tom's aggressive and anxious behavior abated, and therapy was terminated after about 2 months.

2. *Birth of a sibling.* The use of baby toys and accessories can help to facilitate the expression of reactions to the birth of a sibling. Five-year-old Mary presented with regressed, anxious, and aggressive behavior after the birth of a sibling and a change in babysitters. In an initial session, she complained about her busy mother and how long the new baby nursed. Mary then announced that she did not play with baby things. She said, "Part of me wants to be big, part little, because the baby gets all the attention." Baby dolls and baby materials were then offered. Mary began to play the role of a baby and asked the therapist to act as the mother or babysitter. She also took on the role of the "bad" baby, filling a real baby bottle and drinking from it, throwing it, and then dripping water on the therapist. Over the course of several months, Mary slowly progressed through the infant and toddler stages in her play. She spontaneously enacted lying on the floor curled up in a blanket, pretending to be fed and diapered by the therapist, sitting on the therapist's lap and pretending to nurse, sitting as if in a car seat, playing with toddler toys, and looking at baby books, until she finally emerged as a child her own age. One day she announced, "I'm not going to play babies. I want to be a big girl." She used her transference relationship to the therapist-as-mother figure to express and enact both her need to be nurtured like her new sibling and her need to express her anger, stage by stage. The therapist reflected Mary's feelings and gave her many outlets to express anger and jealousy, until they were resolved and her symptoms were reduced. The availability of multiple infant and toddler toys enabled Mary to enact the baby role and to work through these issues. Her mother was seen in collateral sessions. An alternative would have been to include the mother in dyadic therapy sessions (see the section on models used in working with parents).

3. *Separation anxiety and school disruptions.* We provide a toy school-

house, with dolls, for children with separation anxiety, school refusal, or disruptive behavior at school. Peter, a 5-year-old boy with disruptive behaviors, set up story time at school, with the teacher reading a book to the children. Suddenly, the dinosaurs in the storybook came to life and attacked the teacher. Several dolls came to the teacher's rescue, with one of the dolls having been identified previously by Peter as himself. This doll rode on the back of the dinosaur until the dinosaur was conquered, and the teacher and school were saved. This play demonstrated both Peter's negative feelings toward the teacher and his emerging defensive attempt to contain his aggressive impulses in play.

4. *Medical trauma.* Real and toy medical equipment are helpful for children exposed to medical trauma or parental illness. Carly, age 5, was very worried about her mother's chronic medical illness. When a medical kit was provided in a dyadic session, she played doctor, with her mother as patient. This opened up an opportunity for Carly to ask her mother questions about her medical condition and for the mother to respond.

5. *Encopresis.* Play-Doh and tubing, as well as dolls, are helpful materials for preschool children who are encopretic. Encopresis occurs frequently with preschoolers in response to toilet training, experiences of constipation, or as a regressive symptom in response to stress. Manipulating clay provides an outlet for aggressive impulses that may contribute to stool withholding. Pushing clay through tubing can provide practice and mechanical experience for a child who is fearful of elimination. In another approach, the therapist uses a doll to enact elimination using Play-Doh with a toy such as a potty. The therapist may speak for the doll, making sounds or voicing feelings that depict being scared. Next, the child takes control of the Play-Doh, forming and dropping "poops." When the child is ready, they all go to a real bathroom to repeat this play. The child is encouraged to flush the toilet, since this noise is often frightening. Successful toileting at home may resume rapidly. It can be further reinforced by use of a sticker chart, if needed, or more doll play at home. Relaxation techniques such as deep breathing, blowing bubbles, or listening to stories may facilitate letting go on the toilet. These approaches integrate aspects of cognitive-behavioral play therapy and expressive techniques.

6. *Adoption.* Dolls or animals that may represent the family constellation can be particularly helpful for preschool children who have been adopted. They provide the child with an opportunity to communicate feelings about family dynamics. Sam, an adopted child being treated for separation anxiety, who had not been told of the adoption by his parents, revealed to the therapist that he was adopted like a toy calico kitten that did not match the others in the cat family. He explained that he had multiple mothers, an inaccurate portrayal of his adoption story that reflects the preschooler's tendency toward illogical (egocentric) reasoning. This provided an opportunity for the therapist to help the parents present Sam's adoption story and clarify his misconceptions. He made significant progress in being able to separate and attend school once his adoption story was integrated into his self-concept through therapeutic play.

Molly, age 5, had been told her adoption story, but had strong unresolved feelings that she acted out by trying to reject her adoptive parents. Her play with dolls involved a nuclear family taking in so many lost children that they ran out of beds. She also acted out birth parents tossing away their children. This play allowed the therapist to comment on the dolls' feelings, which led Molly to say that she felt thrown away by her birth parents. She made these comments while being held by her empathetic adoptive mother, who provided the security that enabled Molly to express her deeply hurt feelings.

Therapist Inquiry in Play: Story Stem Technique. The story-stem technique was initially developed for assessment of attachment in 3-year-olds (Bretherton, Ridgeway, & Cassidy, 1990). It is now used as a research tool to elicit narratives for the study of young children's inner worlds, including emotions and representations (Emde et al., 2003). The story stem technique has been adapted for use in the evaluation of anxiety (Warren, Emde, & Sroufe, 2000) and in the treatment of trauma (Gaensbauer & Siegel, 1995). The therapist can utilize this technique to conduct more direct probing in the context of play, informed by data from the assessment and/or from play content provided by the child. Toys are set up, the therapist initiates a story, and the child is asked to "Show me or tell me what happens next." This technique represents a more structured extension of the co-construction narrative techniques previously discussed.

We have used the story stem technique in the treatment of diverse presenting problems, such as school refusal. Jessie, a 3-year-old girl, was referred because of her tendency to withdraw socially in the preschool setting. During a treatment session, the therapist set up a story stem using a play school with dolls set in a circle around the teacher for story time and a dollhouse. The therapist depicted a girl running out of the school, then paused. Jessie took this girl doll and acted out her running home to avoid the noise inside the school and then returning to the playground to play with peers. This response enabled the therapist to identify Jessie's withdrawal as a defense against the sensory overload she was experiencing at school, rather than as a primary social problem. Intervention focused on helping her identify these reactions and on helping her parents decide to move Jessie to a smaller, quieter school setting, where her participation and cooperation improved significantly.

Formative Components of Play Therapy

THE THERAPIST AS PLAYER

Scarlett (1994) and Slade (1994) discuss the process of playing as a key component of therapy when so many capacities for symbolization and meaning are only in formation. "For children whose representational abilities are immature or compromised by developmental delays, it often seems to be that the process of playing itself is consolidating and integrative" (Slade, 1994, pp. 81–82). The therapist must focus on playing with the child, rather than on interpretation to help children create structure, develop narrative, learn how to name feelings, and create meaning. Slade argues that some children get therapeutic benefit from the development of more coherent play, without using language or even allowing the therapist to comment about the play. These skills can be carried beyond the therapy, much to the child's developmental advantage.

Many preschoolers, and particularly those challenged developmentally, do not have readily available skills to use play to express and work through problematic issues. They also benefit from the formative aspect of play therapy, in which the therapist and/or parents facilitate the enhancement or development of new capacities. Russ (2004) reviews several studies demonstrating that play skills can be taught to younger preschoolers or lower functioning children. This formative component focuses on building up ego capacities. These include impulse control, tolerance for frustration, management of affect, the capacity to anticipate and reflect, the capacity for sublimation, and communication through play or language (Kernberg, personal communication, July, 2004). Russ (2004) describes building up the ego capacity to create narrative. Greenspan (1997) explains principles of developmental psychotherapy to enhance ego function. Play therapy can also aid in the development of self-regulatory functions, so that the child can learn to control aggression and impulsivity. Parents' involvement in this process is essential. The therapist needs to model techniques and educate the parents about how to enhance these areas of functioning.

INDICATIONS FOR THE FORMATIVE COMPONENT

Indications for the formative component of therapy include both emotional and developmental issues. Some children are emotionally restricted or regressed in response to attachment disorders or to trauma, anxiety, or depression. They utilize less developed ego capacities. For children with externalizing disorders of defiance, aggression, and/or oppositionality, evidence-based research supports an emphasis on parent training both in limit setting and in facilitating play (Campbell, 2002; Eyberg et al., 1995). Whereas parent training techniques offer an external method to help a child develop control, play therapy and parent-facilitated play both can help a child build internal self-regulation. Younger preschoolers are often just developing these capacities and need extra support to consolidate skills. Developmentally delayed and atypical children also have more limited play tools for the expression of emotion and communication. Thus, developmentally delayed children may need supplemental help in the development of self-regulation, as well as play and language. Enhancing these capacities may be a slow process.

STRATEGIES AND THERAPEUTIC PROCESS

Developmental support of play is an inherent part of the therapeutic process with this age group. Awareness of the child's level of language, cognition, coping strategies, symbolic play, and impulse control is central to devising interventions. The therapist can use this awareness to support children's higher-functioning capacities in a variety of ways. Note that this intervention is considered effective only when a child is introduced to behaviors or ideas that stretch *existing* capacities (Vygotsky, 1967). The therapist facilitates acquisition of skills and simultaneously attends to the content and meaning of the child's play.

Enhancement of ego capacities through the child's more flexible use of age-appropriate defenses is a central goal of the formative component of play therapy. Davies (2004) describes defenses as "the normal means for regulating affect and impulse" and notes that "they only become problematic when they become overgeneralized to situations where they are not appropriate or when they supplant other coping mechanisms such as cognitive and interpersonal skills" (pp. 257–258). He describes the preschooler's use of typical defense mechanisms of projection, denial, displacement, and regression to manage stress and anxiety.

In therapy, we want to facilitate flexible coping strategies and appropriate problem solving. This can be addressed through several different strategies: asking questions such as "What would happen if . . . ?", suggesting alternatives, role playing or rehearsing new approaches, and proposing new solutions. Feelings of powerlessness are a daily experience for the young child experiencing events that he or she can neither understand nor control. The sense of helplessness can be profoundly disorganizing. Play therapy can be helpful in supporting a defense or coping strategy of fantasy solutions that restore the children's sense of the possibility of powerfulness, as they work toward other, realistic coping strategies. For example, two brothers were seen when their father was being treated in a distant city for cancer. Martin, the 2½-year-old, had become very clingy toward his mom and would not leave home, whereas his asymptomatic 5-year-old brother expressed his fears verbally and appropriately. The younger child "drew" the melanoma as black blobs on paper, and wished it would go away from Daddy. The therapist talked about chemotherapy and proposed that Martin pretend to tell the melanoma to "go away" by tearing the paper into bits that they (child, therapist, and Mom) then flushed down the toilet together. Martin beamed and wanted to repeat this play. The fantasy solution gave him a sense of control at the representational level. He became more energized at home and eventually returned to school.

We also use components of cognitive-behavioral play therapy (CBPT) to develop coping skills. CBPT is very goal-oriented, targeting the young child's coping skills for problems such as fears or phobias. The therapist uses toys and play for communication about strategies with the child. Knell (1993) developed CBPT for young children ages 2–6 years to integrate cognitive interventions, play therapy, and behavioral therapy. A puppet can be used to verbalize problem-solving skills or act out ways to solve problems. Children are given positive coping statements such as "I can do this" or "There are no ghosts." Bibliotherapy uses books to model problems and solutions. Systematic desensitization is used to reduce anxiety, but calming play scenes or visualizations may need to replace muscle relaxation techniques. Humor, such as dressing the monster in flame-red underwear, can be employed. The therapist involves the child through child-directed joint play, balancing this with the structured goal-directed activities. The parents are encouraged to participate in behavioral interventions, such as contingency management, to remove attention from negative behaviors and reinforce alternative behaviors, and to practice the therapist's cognitive and behavioral methods at home.

Increasing impulse control may be an important formative function of therapy for preschool children because of their tendency to have impulsive reactions. A therapist may need to set safety limits when behavior is out of control (hitting the parent, sibling, peers, or therapist) and to provide the child with alternatives, such as expressing anger in words, pointing to an emotions thermometer which has gradients from calm to very upset, or discharging affect in a safe play activity (throwing a foam ball at a target). Turn taking can be structured in either spontaneous play (e.g., ball play) or more structured preschool board games. Turn taking can also be practiced between siblings in play with regard to sharing toys or deciding the theme in play (e.g., where the family is flying on vacation in the toy airplane). Constructive strategies can be modeled for both child and parent. These include offering alternative toys to trade for the desired one or taking turns using a timer. Environmental manipulations such as reducing or limiting the number of toys taken out are helpful parenting strategies for the child who has trouble staying focused and needs to learn to control distractibility.

Expansion of symbolic capacities in language and play is central to helping the preschooler utilize play therapy. *Expansion of expressive language* is helpful both for the child that functions at age level and for the language-delayed child. Strategies include labeling affect, which often includes pictures or drawings of children with different affective expressions. Language structure and vocabulary can also be expanded using the IN-ter-Reactive Learning (INREAL) approach (Linder, 1993b), which expands capacities through natural conversation. Techniques of SOUL (silence, observation, understanding, listening), mirroring, self-talk, parallel talk, vocal monitoring and reflecting, expansion, and modeling can be incorporated into play therapy. Language pragmatics can also be expanded when children are given words for their actions; for example, when a child grabs a toy truck, the therapist can comment, "You want the truck."

Symbolic play is also important to expand in high-functioning preschool children on the autistic spectrum, because this is the vehicle for both self-expression and peer play. Empirical studies have indicated that creating goals for the expansion of play based on the child's developmental level has enhanced play development in children with autistic spectrum disorders (Rogers, 2005). An initial goal is to *expand the flexible use of specific toys*, because some children present with limited, repetitive schemas. For example, Aaron entered the office one day with a string and only wanted to play cat's cradle.

After 10 minutes of this play, the therapist suggested an alternative use of the string, as a circle inside which dolls could play. Later, the idea of using the string to make letters (an area of knowledge for this child) was introduced. The entire session was devoted to devising multiple ways to use the child's string to broaden his exploration.

Expansion can also be used by the therapist to *introduce a higher level of symbolic* play using the child's toys or by adding new toys. Knowledge of the developmental sequence of play (Westby, 2000) is important, so that the therapist knows what to introduce as the next step. Scaffolding may involve moving the child's play from the sensorimotor stage (i.e., functional play) to an early representational level, or from simple, linked imaginary schemes (stirring a pot, eating food) to more complex, planned imaginary play (planning a tea party). For example, Jack, a child with autism spectrum disorders, was playing with stacking cups and ordering them by size. After several minutes of Jack's repeatedly stacking them, the therapist turned over the cups, showed Jack that the cup's bottoms had different animals on them, and initiated having the animals talk to each other. This child had language and symbolic capacities but was using a less advanced sensorimotor schema to play with the cups. Once the therapist had expanded the use of the cups and introduced a symbolic level of play, Jack engaged with the therapist at this higher level, creating simple conversations between the animals. These conversations provided the therapist an opportunity to learn about issues important to Jack, such as his difficulty making friends, which informed subsequent therapeutic interventions.

In another example, functional play was expanded to symbolic play that included the parent as a play partner. Chin was a boy who connected trains and enjoyed pushing them around the floor. His therapist built a bridge out of Duplos and invited Chin to push the train through the bridge. She then invited Chin's mother to stand with stretched legs to create a different bridge. This not only introduced alternative methods to create bridges but also included Chin's mother in the play and encouraged social interaction. Later the therapist invited the mother to build a train station, so that Chin's train had a destination and could load and unload passengers.

Models in Working with Parents

We recommend a variety of models of therapist–parent interactions in the treatment of preschool children. For us, the decision about which model to use is based on the focus of treatment. The age of the child or strong preferences of the parent are also factors we consider. For many therapists, this decision is based on prior training and theoretical orientation.

Dyadic Sessions

Parent, child, and therapist participate in joint psychotherapy sessions that utilize play but may include some parent–therapist discussion, in the moment, related to the interaction. This model is particularly useful in therapies targeting attachment problems, conflicted child–parent relationships, poor parent attunement, or a difficult-to-engage child. Dyadic and family-focused therapies are indicated when the preschooler's symptoms are more evident at home than at school. They are also recommended in the treatment of trauma (see Van Horn & Lieberman, Chapter 16, this volume; Lieberman & van Horn, 2004), and in preventive interventions at times of stress and change, such as divorce, family illness, and loss.

The therapist and parent level of activity varies, because one or both may be either actively engaged with the child or watching. The therapist may model play with the child and invite the parent to join in, initiating activities that foster parent–child engagement and support each partner's participation. The identification of emotions expressed by the child and his or her play is often a powerful dynamic within the dyadic session. The therapist may not only address conflict when it arises but also may model negotiation strategies for both child and parent *in vivo*. Therapeutic observations that are better discussed privately with the parent may be postponed for at a later time.

The contribution of the psychodynamic infant–parent therapy model, combined with the transactional theory of development, is to focus us on the continued effect of primary relationships on preschoolers even as they move into a wider social world. Parents of referred preschoolers sometimes see their child's difficult behaviors as manipulative ("Out to get me."), or abusive, ("Just like his father."). Such parents are also focused on relationship aspects of the problem, but in a blaming fashion. The assessment and therapy then must distinguish between the "ghosts" aspect (from the couple relationship or from a parent's own childhood relationships with siblings or parents) that led the parent to misperceive the child's intentions and behavior, and other sources of misunderstanding about the child. Assessment may reveal unrealistic developmental expectations (the child is too young to be able to sit quietly through a 2-hour meal in a fancy restaurant), normal variations (the child is a high-energy, active child), temperamental mismatch with a parent, real disorder in the child, a response to trauma, insufficient parental limit setting, or other parenting issues. Often dyadic sessions clarify these misunderstandings more clearly than does parent history alone. In an integrated therapy for a preschooler, "ghost in the nursery" issues for parents, if identified, are addressed in separate parent sessions, or the parent may be referred for individual psychotherapy. These issues can be brought to the parent's awareness and "uncoupled" from the parent's perception of and behavior toward the child.

One author (Benham, 1995) developed a semistructured family play session for use during diagnostic evaluations to explore enacted family relationships and to assess the appropriateness of dyadic therapy. In this play session, the family has 10 minutes of free play and is then instructed: "Build your house, using anything in the playroom. Then choose a figure or an animal to be yourself and put it somewhere in the house, doing something that you usually do. The only rule is everyone must participate." The therapist stays behind a one-way mirror during the free play and house building, then joins the family. Together, family and therapist discuss how the activity felt, what parents observed about the family interaction, and why each member chose the given figure to represent him- or herself. Children are asked what they think of their parents' choices and what figure or animal they themselves would have chosen to be the mommy or the daddy. This technique is used regularly with families of preschoolers; older siblings eagerly participate, and toddlers often play independently or interfere. Many families comment that they have never played together, and that it is fun. This becomes an important motivator for change in the family process. When parents do not protect their preschooler's creations from a younger, destructive toddler (a frequent dynamic), the angry, reactive preschooler is often seen as the "bad child." The therapist can identify such patterns, helping the "bad" child express frustration verbally rather than physically. The therapist can show the parents how to break down the tasks and play appropriately into steps that facilitate their child's participation.

Parent in Session as Observer

This role with parents is particularly useful in early sessions exploring a child's fears or trauma. The therapist may follow the child's spontaneous play or play stimulated by particular materials (e.g., medical equipment). The parent's presence as an observer may fulfill many goals, not only facilitating the parent's understanding of the child's experience and beliefs about distressing events but also enhancing the parent's empathy for the child. Even though the parent may have been physically or emotionally unavailable during the traumatic event, this same parent can now have the experience of providing support and comfort for the child reliving a traumatic experience (Gaensbauer, 2004). The parent may become an active co-creator of a narrative about past events that the child remembers only in fragments. Sometimes parent and therapist seek to make sense of a child's play, behavior, and verbalizations that hint at events occurring prior to adoption of the child, while the child was in an orphanage, a birth home or foster care (see Sasha, p. 351 of this chapter). The therapy often becomes more classically dyadic after this initial exploration of trauma, with active parent participation in the play as a next stage of therapy.

Individual Therapy with Collateral Parent Sessions

A more classic, individual model of play therapy with collateral parent sessions is most applicable to older preschool–kindergarten-age children (5 years and older) but may be useful with some younger preschoolers. Older children have progressed to more independent functioning, and may benefit from a separate relationship with the therapist that allows exploration of their issues. Furthermore, older children may be both more forthcoming when alone with the therapist and more inhibited when parents are present.

In some highly conflicted child–parent relationships, the parent is either overly intrusive or the child cannot move beyond provoking or engaging the parent in repetitive, unproductive interactions. Either scenario may interfere with the child's capacity to play and to make use of therapy. Whereas these issues may indeed be a focus for the therapy, a period of separate sessions may need to precede dyadic work on the relationship. For children who have experienced abuse or trauma at the hands of the parent, or sexual abuse by a trusted adult, the privacy and safety provided by individual sessions may be essential (Gil, 1991).

Work with a Child Alone

We do not see a role for individual therapy with a young child without significant interactions with primary caregivers. Parents unfamiliar with the treatment process may assume or desire that children be treated alone. Reasons for this may need to be explored in parent sessions. The therapist needs to educate parents about the importance of their involvement. The development of a close relationship between child and therapist can be counterproductive to supporting improved family relationships, if the parents are not an integral part of the therapy. The therapist's role is to help the parent meet the child's needs, not to usurp the parents' role.

When a child has no available or functioning primary caregiver to participate, is therapy feasible? Therapy in such a case may be more of a challenge and be limited by incomplete information and adult participation, yet may still contribute to the child's well-being. Sara, a 3-year-old described on page 350, had been in dyadic therapy with her mother because of the mother's cancer and its impact on their relationship. After her mother's sudden, traumatic death, Sara and her dad began dyadic sessions. Soon Dad could not cope with the sessions, nor could he manage Sara because of her needy, aggressive behavior with him, and because of his own grief and anger. However, he was relieved to have her seen individually in intensive therapy for a period of time. Collateral contacts were made with her nanny and with relatives, while the therapist struggled to keep her father in a therapeutic alliance supporting Sara's therapy. After a few months, Sara's dad was willing to return to regular collateral therapy sessions to collaborate in the support and recovery of his daughter.

What about young children in foster care, who have been traumatized by removal and/or by the events leading to separation from their families of origin? Many such children are bounced from emergency foster care homes to supposed long-term placements to therapeutic foster care homes when their behavioral or emotional symptoms become severe. If they are lucky, one social worker or advocate consistently stays involved with them. For these children, sustained individual therapy, with one therapist, can be emotionally life saving. Again, extensive outreach to the primary caregivers, even if they change, is an essential responsibility for the clinician.

Parent Participation in Part of Session

With some older preschoolers, we use a model similar to CBPT. The parent participates in the first 10–20 minutes of the session, during which a specific problem is addressed in a structured way. The cognitive-behavioral portion of the session focuses on behavioral interventions for a discrete problem. The parent reports on progress in the previous week and observes the next steps in intervention, and child and parent agree on goals for the coming week. The parent then exits, and the rest of the hour is an individual play session that may have both unstructured time and therapist-guided elements to address the child's target problem or other issues. These elements also may be integrated in dyadic sessions.

Collateral Sessions with Parents

Full-length, regular, separate sessions with parents or caregivers should be scheduled at least monthly, independent of child sessions for both individual and dyadic therapies. Preschool children are old enough to resent being talked about but are too young to sit alone in the waiting room for an extended time. Children are very sensitive to discussions of their "bad" behavior or private worries. Even though the child should be told that his or her parents have enlisted the clinician on his or her behalf, overhearing adult discussions can impair the child's comfort with the therapist.

Furthermore, separate adult sessions are important because the therapist needs regular information about events in the family and in the child's life, behavioral and emotional ups and downs, school reports, and important adult issues such as impending moves, changes, separations, or other stressors. Therapists also need the parents' permission and participation in collaborating with teachers and other professionals involved in the child's care. The therapist and parents may address issues pertaining to siblings, or to financial or marital difficulties, especially if they impinge on the child. The child and/or the child's therapy may bring into focus old issues for parents about their own childhood and parenting. Parents need an opportunity to discuss feelings and issues about the child that may lead to a change in their internal representation of the child. "Ghosts" (Fraiberg, 1987) that distort their perceptions of the child may become clear to the therapist, who may elect to address them in these collateral sessions.

Integration of Approaches

Sometimes, several approaches are integrated when specific behaviors are targeted for change, and when exploration of the meaning underlying these behaviors is a focus of treatment. The following case example integrates cognitive-behavioral therapy, play therapy, and parent counseling.

Chloe, age 4, an only child, had been evaluated not only for extreme avoidance of certain smells, foods, and physical activities, but also for accompanying controlling behavior, such as tantrums, to force her parents to leave a restaurant when she smelled cheese. After the therapist ruled out obsessive–compulsive disorder and pervasive developmental disorder, Chloe was referred for occupational therapy to treat her sensory reactions and avoidance of gross motor activities. After several months of occupational therapy, with scant progress, the occupational therapist requested a second mental health consultation.

Parent counseling involved exploring the origins of parental overprotectiveness and failure to support or demand more independence from a child who insisted that her mom accompany her at all times. Initially, Mom was asked to read a magazine for 30 minutes at home while Chloe played alone nearby. Mom also needed support to risk this change. Further history taking had revealed Chloe's mild trauma 1 year earlier during a medical examination. In play evaluation and subsequent treatment, Chloe returned to this trauma frequently with medical play and more overt questions and statements, until it seemed resolved in her mind.

The first 10 minutes of each play session involved cognitive-behavioral techniques. Even though Chloe would not do relaxation exercises, the therapist utilized the technique of graduated exposure. The child, the mom, and the therapist made a hierarchy about cheese: talking about it, viewing photos of cheese, using play cheese, touching wrapped slices, and touching and smelling real cheese. Chloe was given bravery points that continued in occupational therapy. After the initial dyadic cognitive-behavioral therapy portion, the rest of each session utilized individual psychodynamic play therapy techniques, directed by Chloe, in which she addressed both the medical issues and her ambivalence about greater independence from her mom. The therapist noted Chloe's increasing freedom in many areas, as reported by both the child and her mom, including overcoming her fear of dogs, learning to ride a bike, playing alone, using outdoor play equipment, and going to restaurants. In later sessions, Chloe celebrated and consolidated a new sense of herself as independent and competent, a self-concept supported by reports from her preschool.

SUMMARY

The convergence of developmental progress, differentiation of problems, and the impact of early developmental deviations provides the rationale for utilizing play therapy for direct intervention with preschool children. The preschool years are marked by significant, qualitative developmental changes in social, cognitive, motor, emotional, and language capacities. As a result, the child's increased capacity for self-regulation increases adults' expectations for emotional and behavioral control. Developmental differences, emotional reactions, and diagnosable conditions present more clearly in preschoolers than in infants and toddlers. Early deviations in developmental pathways affect later development in ways that become more difficult to ameliorate. Emotional and behavioral problems should be identified early and treated psychotherapeutically with direct intervention.

Assessment is essential in determining the need for intervention. The nature, locus, and severity of the problem, and neurodevelopmental, family, and environmental factors all contribute to a treatment plan. Familiarity with a range of psychotherapeutic approaches and with the current, albeit limited, evidence-based research literature about preschoolers is important to treatment planning.

Our treatment approach is informed by a developmental perspective based on the transactional model of development and the concept of multiple ports of entry. This integrated, interactional approach attends to the child and parent, to the behaviors and internal representations of each player, to the role of the external influences in the family and environment, and to the developmental status of the child. We support a prescriptive (Schaefer, 2003) approach in which we select from and integrate different approaches based on the individual needs of the child and his or her family. We recommend a range of interactive styles, ranging from supportive to guiding, depending on the therapeutic needs of the child and family.

Parents are central in the preschooler's functioning and are considered primary agents of change. The role of parents is critical in therapy and needs to be an integral component of any treatment method. The parents can be incorporated flexibly through dyadic, observer, or collateral roles, depending on the needs of the individual family and the nature of the problems addressed. Parents' understanding of the child on both developmental and emotional levels guides them in facilitating their child's progress and decreasing symptoms. Improvement in the child–parent relationship can increase family engagement and capacity for mutual enjoyment. Enhanced behavioral management methods can increase parents' feelings of efficacy.

Evidence-based research supports an emphasis on parent training in play and limit setting for the treatment of externalizing behavior problems. There are additional conditions in which work with parents alone may be insufficient. This can occur because of the child's developmental differences, the parents' lack of understanding, and/or the need to effect change by addressing the child's feelings and experience directly. Sometimes externalizing symptoms coexist with internalizing disorders that may be more difficult to discern. Research supports the use of play to solve problems and reduce anxiety (Russ, 2004). Play therapy is indicated for children with internalizing disorders, for children whose externalizing symptoms may be masking coexisting and less evident internal anxiety, depression, stress or trauma, for children with developmental delay who need help to develop play capacities for coping purposes, and for children with externalizing disorders who need to develop internal self-regulation that can complement parents' external strategies.

Play therapy is especially useful in treating preschool children. It is utilized for direct treatment because play is a primary representational capacity, and it is central in the preschool child's world. Play is an avenue for communication, exploration, creativity, and affective expression. It supports the development of language, cognition, and ego functions. Play is the preferred activity of the child and provides a window into the child's inner emotional life. It demonstrates the child's most advanced capabilities and is considered the best vehicle to facilitate growth and psychotherapeutic change. Play provides a method of engagement, direct access to what the child is thinking and feeling, and a vehicle for change due to the mutual influences between behaviors and representations. It is particularly suited for preschoolers who do not use language as their primary means of self-expression.

Our therapeutic approaches have been described using the dichotomy of the *expressive* and *formative* aspects of therapy, which are often used in combination. In all cases, establishment of a holding environment and a therapeutic alliance with both parents and child is essential in the beginning phase of treatment. The *expressive* component of play therapy is used to effect change for children who have experienced distress in response to either external events or internal conditions and are demonstrating emotional and behavioral dysregulation. It is useful for children who are able to engage in play and to communicate through play and language. Expressive components may emerge spontaneously or be facilitated by a range of guided techniques for both typical and atypical children, as long as their developmental level is considered. These techniques include exploration of a child's inner world, fostering acceptance, clarifying distortions and behavior, verbalizing affect, and processing trauma. Content can be elicited by providing specific play materials and by probing, such as with story stems.

Play therapy can be utilized to strengthen play processes and capacities, an intervention referred to in this chapter as the *formative* component of play therapy. This is useful for the child who utilizes less developed ego capacities due to young age, regression, emotional restriction, and/or developmental delay. Guided play can enhance ego capacities, such as fantasy solutions, increase impulse control, and expand symbolic capacities in both language and play.

Our 4-year-old fairy/superhero is ready to set aside the work of saving the world. She wants to eat her favorite lunch, to cuddle up for a story, to share the triumphs and woes of her day at preschool, and to take a nap. Play therapy can support her capacity to enjoy all of these normal activities within the warmth and security of her relationship with her parents.

REFERENCES

Achenbach, T. M. (1992). *Manual for the Child Behavior Checklist 2–3*. Burlington: University of Vermont.

Achenbach, T. M., & Rescorla, L. A. (2000). *Manual for the ASEBA preschool forms and pro-*

files: An integrated system of multi-informant assessment. Burlington: University of Vermont Department of Psychiatry.

Axline, V. (1947). *Play therapy.* New York: Ballantine.

Bagner, D. M., & Eyberg, S. M. (2003). Father involvement in parent training: When does it matter? *Journal of Clinical Child and Adolescent Psychology, 32*(4), 599–605.

Barkley, R. A. (1997). *Defiant children: A clinician's manual for assessment and parent training* (2nd ed.). New York: Guilford Press.

Barnett, L. A. (1984). Research note: Young children's resolution of distress through play. *Journal of Child Psychology and Psychiatry, 25,* 477–448.

Benham, A. (2000a). The observation and assessment of young children including use of the Infant–Toddler Mental Status Exam. In C. H. Zeanah, Jr. (Ed.), *Handbook of infant mental health* (2nd ed., pp. 249–265). New York: Guilford Press.

Benham, A. (1995b). *Family "Build your house" task.* Unpublished manuscript.

Brazelton, T. B. (1992). *Touchpoints: Your child's emotional and behavioral development.* Reading, MA: Addison-Wesley.

Bretherton, I., Ridgeway, D., & Cassidy, J. (1990). Assessing internal working models of the attachment relationship: An attachment story completion task for 3–year-olds. In M. T. Greenberg, D. Cicchetti, & E. M. Cummings (Eds.) *Attachment in the preschool years: Theory, research, and intervention* (pp. 273–308). Chicago: University of Chicago Press.

Bronson, M. B. (2000). *Self-regulation in early childhood: Nature and nurture.* New York: Guilford Press.

Bruner, J. S. (1982). The organization of action and the nature of the adult–infant transaction. In E. Z. Tronick (Ed.), *Social interchange in infancy: Affect, cognition, and communication* (pp. 23–25). Baltimore: University Park Press.

Campbell, S. B. (2002). *Behavior problems in preschool children, second edition.* New York: Guilford Press.

Casey, R. J., & Berman, J. S., (1995). The outcome of psychotherapy with children. *Psychology Bulletin, 98,* 388–400.

Chethik, M. (2000). *Techniques of child therapy: Psychodynamic strategies* (2nd ed.). New York: Guilford Press.

Ciccetti, D., Toth, S., & Rogosh, F. A. (1999). The efficacy of toddler–parent psychotherapy in increase attachment security in offspring of depressed mothers. *Attachment and Human Development, 1,* 34–66.

Clark, R., Tluczek, A., & Gallagher, K. C. (2004). Assessment of parent–child early relational disturbances. In R. DelCarmen-Wiggins & A. Carter (Eds.), *Handbook of infant, toddler, and preschool mental health assessment* (pp. 25–60). Oxford, UK: Oxford University Press.

Cohen, J., & Mannarino, A. P. (1993). A treatment model for sexually abused preschoolers. *Journal of Interpersonal Violence, 8*(1), 115–131.

Cohen, J., & Mannarino, A. P. (1996a). Factors that mediate treatment outcome of sexually abused preschool children. *Journal of the American Academy of Child and Adolescent Psychiatry, 34*(10), 1402–1410.

Cohen, J., & Mannarino, A. P. (1996b). A treatment outcome study for sexually abused preschool children: Initial findings. *Journal of the American Academy of Child and Adolescent Psychiatry, 35*(1), 42–50.

Cohen, J., & Mannarino, A. P. (1997). A treatment outcome study for sexually abused preschool children: Outcome during a one-year follow-up. *Journal of the American Academy of Child and Adolescent Psychiatry, 36*(9), 1228–1235.

Cohen, J., & Mannarino, A. P. (1998). Factors that mediate treatment outcome of sexually abused preschool children: Six- and 12-month follow-up. *Journal of the American Academy of Child and Adolescent Psychiatry, 37*(1), 44–51.

Cohen, N. J., Muir, E., Parker, C. J., Brown, M., Lojkasek, M., Muir, R., et al. (1999). Watch, Wait and Wonder: Testing the effectiveness of a new approach to mother–infant psychotherapy. *Infant Mental Health Journal, 20*(4), 429–451.

Cooke, J. L., & Sinker, M. (1993). Play and the growth of competence. In C. E. Schaefer (Ed.), *The therapeutic powers of play* (pp. 65–80). Northvale, NJ: Jason Aronson.

Cramer, B. (1995). Short-term dynamic psychotherapy for infants and their parents. *Child and Adolescent Psychiatric Clinics of North America,4*(3), 649–660.

Cummings, E. M., Davies, P. T., & Campbell, S. B. (2000). *Developmental psychopathology and family process: Theory, research and process.* New York: Guilford Press.

Davies, D. (2004). *Child development: A practitioner's guide, second edition.* New York: Guilford Press.

DelCarmen-Wiggens, R., & Carter, A. (Eds.). (2004). *Handbook of infant, toddler, and preschool mental health assessment.* Oxford, UK: Oxford University Press.

Denham, S. (1998). *Emotional development in young children.* New York: Guilford Press.

Emde, R. N., Everhart, K. D., & Wise, B. K. (2004). Therapeutic relationships in infant mental health and the concept of leverage. In A. Sameroff, S. McDonough, & K. L. Rosenblum (Eds.), *Treating parent–infant relationship problems: Strategies for intervention* (pp. 267–292). New York: Guilford Press.

Emde, R., Wolf, D., & Oppenheim, D. (2003). *Revealing the inner worlds of young children.* New York/Oxford, UK: Oxford University Press.

Erikson, E. (1963). *Childhood and society.* New York: Norton.

Eyberg, S. M., Boggs, S., & Algina, J. (1995). Parent–child interaction therapy: A psychosocial model for the treatment of young children with conduct problem behavior and their families. *Paychopharmacology Bulletin, 31,* 83–91.

Fonagy, P., & Target, M. (1994). The efficacy of pscyhoanalysis for children with disruptive disorders. *Journal of the American Academy of Child and Adolescent Psychiatry, 33*(1), 45–55.

Fraiberg, S. (1987). Ghosts in the nursery. In L. Fraiberg (Ed.), *Selected writings of Selma Fraiberg* (pp. 100–136). Columbus: Ohio State University Press.

Freud, A. (1966). *The ego and the mechanisms of defense.* New York: International Universities Press.

Gaensbauer, T. J. (2004). Traumatized young children: Assessment and treatment process. In J. D. Osofsky (Ed.), *Young children and trauma: Intervention and treatment* (pp. 194–216). New York/London: Guilford Press.

Gaensbauer, T. J., & Siegel, C. H. (1995). Therapeutic approaches to post-traumatic stress disorder in infants and toddlers. *Infant Mental Health Journal, 16,* 292–305.

Gil, E. (1991). *The healing power of play.* New York: Guilford Press.

Gil, E. (2003). Family play therapy: The bear with short nails. In C. Schaefer (Ed.), *Foundations of play therapy* (pp. 192–218). Northvale, NJ: Wiley.

Ginsberg, B. C. (1993). Catharsis. In C. E. Schaefer (Ed.), *The therapeutic powers of play* (pp. 107–141). Northvale, NJ: Jason Aronson.

Greenspan, S. I. (1995). *The challenging child.* Reading, MA: Addison-Wesley.

Greenspan, S. I. (1997). *Developmentally based psychotherapy.* Madison, CT: International Universities Press.

Greenspan, S. I. (1998). *The child with special needs.* Reading, MA: Addison-Wesley.

Guerney, L. (1993). Relationship enhancement. In C. E. Schaefer (Ed.), *The therapeutic powers of play* (pp. 267–290). Northvale, NJ: Jason Aronson.

Guerney, L. (2003). Filial play therapy. In C. E. Schaefer (Ed.), *Foundations of play therapy* (pp. 99–142). Hoboken, NJ: Wiley.

Harter, S. (1985). Cognitive-developmental considerations in the conduct of play therapy. In C. E. Shaeffer & K. J. O'Connor (Eds.), *Handbook of play therapy* (pp. 95–127). New York: Wiley.

Holmbeck, G. N., Greenley, R. N., & Franks, E. A. (2003). Developmental issues and considerations in research and practice. In A. E. Kazdin & J. R. Weisz (Eds.), *Evidence-based psychotherapies for children and adolescents* (pp. 21–41). New York: Guilford Press.

Hood, K. H., & Eyberg, S. M. (2003). Outcomes of parent–child interaction therapy:

Mother's reports of maintenance three to six years after treatment. *Journal of the American Academy of Child and Adolescent Psychiatry, 32*(3), 419–429.

Jernberg, A. (1979). *Theraplay: A new treatment using structured play for problem children and their families.* San Francisco: Jossey-Bass.

Johnson, L., McLeod, E., & Fall, M. (1997). Play therapy with labeled children in the schools. *Professional School Counseling, 1*(1), 31–34.

Knell, S. M. (1993). *Cognitive behavioral play therapy.* Northvale, NJ: Jason Aronson.

Knell, S. M. (2000). CBPT for childhood fears and phobias. In H. G. Kaduson & C. E. Shaefer (Eds.), *Short-term play therapy for children* (pp. 3–27). NY: Guilford Press.

Knell, S. M. (2003). Cognitive behavioral play therapy (CBPT). In C. Schaefer (Ed.), *Foundations of play therapy* (pp. 175–191). Hoboken, NJ: Wiley.

Kot, S., & Tyndall-Lind, A. (2005). *Intensive play therapy with child witnesses of domestic violence.* In L. Reddy, T. Files-Hall, & C. Schaefer (Eds.), *Empirically based play interventions for children* (pp. 31–49). Washington, DC: American Psychological Association.

Landreth, G. L. (1993). Self-expressive communication. In C. E. Schaefer (Ed.), *The therapeutic powers of play* (pp. 41–63). New Jersey/London: Jason Aronson.

Leventhal-Belfer, L., Slotnick, C., Nichols, M., Blasey, C., & Huffman, L. (2000). *Understanding disruptive behavior in preschool children: Using the Zero to Three Diagnostic Classification.* Unpublished manuscript, The Children's Health Council, Palo Alto, CA.

Levy, D. (1939). Release therapy. *American Journal of Orthopsychiatry, 9,* 713–736.

Lidz, C. S. (2003). *Early childhood assessment.* Hoboken, NJ: Wiley.

Lieberman, A. F. (2004). Child–parent psychotherapy: A relationship-based approach to the treatment of mental health disorders in infancy and early childhood. In A. Sameroff, S. McDonough, & K. L. Rosenblum (Eds.), *Treating parent–infant relationship problems: Strategies for intervention* (pp. 97–122). New York: Guilford Press.

Lieberman, A. F., Silverman, R., & Pawl, J. H. (2000). Infant–parent psychotherapy: Core concepts and recent developments. In C. H. Zeanah (Ed.), *Handbook of infant mental health* (2nd ed., pp. 472–484). New York: Guilford Press.

Lieberman, A. F., & Van Horn, P. (2004). Assessment and treatment of young children exposed to traumatic events. In J. D. Osofsky (Ed.), *Young children and trauma: Intervention and treatment* (pp. 111–138). New York/London: Guilford Press.

Linder, T. (1993a). *Trans-disciplinary play-based assessment.* Baltimore: Brookes.

Linder, T. (1993b). *Trans-disciplinary play-based intervention.* Baltimore: Brookes.

McClellan, J. M., & Werry, J. S. (2003). Evidence-based treatments in child and adolescent psychiatry: An inventory. *Journal of the American Academy of Child and Adolescent Psychiatry, 42*(12), 1388–1400.

McDonough, S. C. (2004). Interaction guidance: Promoting and nurturing the caregiving relationship. In A. Sameroff, S. McDonough, & K. L. Rosenblum (Eds.), *Treating parent–infant relationship problems: Strategies for intervention* (pp. 79–96). New York: Guilford Press.

Muns, E. (2003). Thera play: Attachment-enhancing play therapy. In C. E. Schaefer (Ed.). *Foundations of play therapy* (pp. 156–174). Hoboken, NJ: Wiley.

Muratori, F., Picchi, L., Bruni, G., Patarnello, M., & Romagnoli, R. (2003). A two-year follow-up of psychodynamic psychotherapy for internalizing disorders in children. *Journal of the American Academy of Child and Adolescent Psychiatry, 42*(3), 331–348.

Ormland, E. K. (1993). Abreaction. In C. E. Schaefer (Ed.) *The therapeutic powers of play* (pp. 143–165). Northvale, NJ/London: Jason Aronson.

Perry, B. D., Pollard, R. A., Blakley, T. L., Baker, W. L., & Vigilante, D. (1995). Childhood trauma, the neurobiology of adaptation, and "use-dependent" development of the brain: How "states" become "traits." *Infant Mental Health Journal, 16,* 271–291.

Piaget, J. (1962). *Play, dreams and imitation in childhood.* New York: Norton.

Ray, D., Bratton, S., Rhine, T., & Jones, L. (2001). The effectiveness of play therapy: Responding to the critics. *International Journal of Play Therapy, 10*(1), 85–98.

Reid, M. J., Webster-Stratton, C., & Baydar, N. (2004). Halting the development of conduct problems in Head Start children: The effects of parent training. *Journal of Clinical Child and Adolescent Psychology, 33*(2), 279–291.

Rogers, S. (2005). Play interventions for young children with autism spectrum disorders. In L. Reddy, T. Files-Hall, & C. Schaefer (Eds.), *Empirically based play interventions for children* (pp. 215–239). Washington, DC: American Psychological Association.

Russ, S. W. (2004). *Play in child development and psychotherapy: Toward empirically supported practice.* Mahwah, NJ: Erlbaum.

Sameroff, A. J. (2004). Ports of entry and the dynamics of mother–infant interventions. In A. Sameroff, S. McDonough, & K. L. Rosenblum (Eds.), *Treating parent–infant relationship problems: Strategies for intervention* (pp. 3–28). New York: Guilford Press.

Sameroff, A. J., & Chandler, M. J. (1975). Reproductive risk and the continuum of caretaking casualty. In F. D. Horowitz, M. Hetherington, S. Scarr-Salapatek, & G. Siegal (Eds.), *Review of child development research* (Vol. 4, pp. 187–244). Chicago: University of Chicago Press.

Scarlett, W. G. (1994). Play, cure and development: A developmental perspective on the psychoanalytic treatment of young children. In A. Slade & D. P. Wolf (Eds.), *Children at play: Clinical and developmental approaches to meaning and representation* (pp. 48–61). New York/Oxford, UK: Oxford University Press.

Schaefer, C. E. (2003). Prescriptive play therapy. In C. E. Schaefer (Ed.), *Foundations of play therapy* (pp. 306–320). Hoboken, NJ: Wiley.

Slade, A. (1994). Making meaning and making believe: Their role in the clinical process. In A. Slade & D. P. Wolf (Eds.), *Children at play: Clinical and developmental approaches to meaning and representation* (pp. 81–107). New York/Oxford, UK: Oxford University Press.

Stern, D. N. (1995). *The motherhood constellation: A unified view of parent–infant psychotherapy.* New York: Basic Books.

Stern-Bruschweiler, N., & Stern, D. N. (1989). A model for conceptualizing the role of the mother's representational world in various mother–infant therapies. *Infant Mental Health Journal, 10*(3), 142–156.

Stifter, C. A., & Wiggins, C. N. (2004). Assessment of disturbances in emotion regulation and temperament. In R. DelCarmen-Wiggins & A. Carter (Eds.), *Handbook of infant, toddler, and preschool mental health assessment* (pp. 79–103). Oxford, UK: Oxford University Press.

Sweeney, D. S., & Landreth, G. L. (2003). Child-centered play therapy. In C. Schaefer (Ed.), *Foundations of play therapy* (pp. 76–98). Hoboken, NJ: Wiley.

Target, M., & Fonagy, P. (1994a). Efficacy of psychoanalysis for children with emotional disorders. *Journal of the American Academy of Child and Adolescent Psychiatry, 33*(3), 361–371.

Target, M., & Fonagy, P. (1994b). The efficacy of psychoanalysis for children: Prediction of outcome in a developmental context. *Journal of the American Academy of Child and Adolescent Psychiatry, 33*(8), 1134–1144.

Terr, L. (1990). *Too scared to cry.* New York: Harper & Row.

Terr, L. (2003). "Wild child": How three principles of healing organized 12 years of psychotherapy. *Journal of the American Academy of Child and Adolescent Psychiatry, 42*(12), 1401–1409.

Thomas, A., Chess, S., & Birch, H. (1968). *Temperament and behavior disorders in children.* New York: New York University Press.

Thomas, J. M., & Guskin, K. A. (2001). Disruptive behavior in young children: What does it mean? *Journal of the American Academy of Child and Adolescent Psychiatry, 40*(1), 44–51.

Trebling, J. A. (2000). Short term solutions oriented play therapy for children of divorced parents. In H. G. Kaduson & C. E. Schaefer (Eds.), *Short-term play therapy for children* (pp. 144–171). New York: Guilford Press.

Vondra, J., & Belsky, J. (1991). Infant play as a window on competence and motivation. In C.

Schaeffer, K. Gitlin, & A. Sandgrund (Eds.), *Play diagnosis and assessment* (pp. 13–38). New York: Wiley.

Vygotsky, L. S. (1967). Play and its role in the mental development of the child. *Soviet Psychology, 5*(3), 6–18.

Vygotsky, L. S. (1978). *Mind in society.* Cambridge, Ma/London: Harvard University Press.

Warren, S. L. (2003). Narratives in risk and clinical populations. In R. N. Emde, D. P. Wolf, & D. Oppenheim (Eds.), *Revealing the inner worlds of young children: The MacArthur Story Stem Battery and Parent–Child Narratives.* Oxford, UK: Oxford University Press.

Warren, S. L., Emde, R. N., & Sroufe, L. A. (2000). Internal representations: Predicting anxiety from children's play narratives. *Journal of the American Academy of Child and Adolescent Psychiatry, 39*(1), 100–107.

Webb, P. (2001). Play therapy with traumatized children. In G. Landreth (Ed.), *Innovations in play therapy: Issues, process, and special populations* (pp. 289–302). Philadelphia: Brunner-Routledge.

Webster-Stratton, C. (1985). The effects of father involvement in parent training for conduct problem children. *Journal of Child Psychology and Psychiatry, 26,* 801–810.

Weiss, B., & Weisz, J. R. (1990). The impact of methodological factors on child psychotherapy outcome research: A meta-analysis for researchers. *Journal of Abnormal Child Psychology, 18,* 639–670.

Weisz, J. R., Weiss, B., Han, S. S., Granger, D. A., & Morton, T. (1995). Effects of psychotherapy with children and adolescents revisited: A meta-analysis of treatment outcome studies. *Psychological Bulletin,117,* 450–468.

Werry. J. S., & Andrews, L. K. (2002). Psychotherapies: A critical overview. In M. Lewis (Ed.), *Child and adolescent psychiatry: A comprehensive textbook* (3rd ed., pp. 1078–1083). Philadelphia: Lippincott, Williams & Wilkins.

Westby, C. (2000). A scale for assessing development of children's play. In K. Gitlin-Weiner, A. Sandgrund, & C. Schaefer (Eds.), *Play diagnosis and assessment* (pp. 15–57). New York: Wiley.

Winnicott, D. W. (1965). *The maturational process and the facilitating environment.* New York: International Universities Press.

Winnicott, D. W. (1968). Playing: Its theoretical status in the clinical situation. *International Journal of Psycho-Analysis, 49,* 591–598.

Winnicott, D. W. (1986). *Playing and reality.* London: Tavistock.

Zeanah, C. H. (Ed.). (2000). *Handbook of infant mental health, second edition.* New York: Guilford Press.

Zero to Three. (1994). *Diagnostic classification of mental health and developmental disorders of infancy and early childhood.* Washington, DC: National Center for Infants, Toddlers, and Families.

16

Using Play in Child–Parent Psychotherapy to Treat Trauma

PATRICIA VAN HORN and ALICIA F. LIEBERMAN

Since Freud (1937) described a toddler playing out his concerns about separation by throwing his top out of sight and then pulling it back by a string, psychologists have understood the special role of play in how children structure their internal worlds. Paraphrasing Freud's conceptualization of dreams as the "royal road to the unconscious," Erikson (1950) referred to play as the "royal road" to understanding the childish ego's attempts at synthesis. He proposed that children use play to set up model situations with which they then experiment, testing different solutions to problems and trying out different roles in the drama. In play, the constraints of physical and social reality are suspended, and children can express their fears and wishes, and master challenges and anxieties (Axline, 1947; Schaefer & O'Connor, 1983). As children use play to cope with their anxieties, they can adopt essentially three different stances: They can directly repeat the anxiety-provoking situation in play; they can repeat it in a way that modifies its outcome; or they can use play to avoid the situation altogether (Watson, 1994).

Play is not, however, merely a vehicle for exploring the child's own subjective experience. Development occurs in a relational matrix, and children use play to explore and express not only their internal wishes and fears but also their feelings about their place in the social world of relationships. Although Freud viewed the play of the toddler described earlier as an expression of the child's anxiety about being left alone and losing the object of his love, the same behavior can be seen equally well as play about the child's expectation that his beloved mother will return. She disappears from his sight, but she invariably comes back, and her return brings him relief and pleasure. The toddler's play also expresses something about his view of himself in relation to his mother: We see that he is not left alone. He sees himself as worth returning to. All of these rich intrapsychic and interpersonal meanings are expressed in the simple game of throwing away, and then retrieving a top.

In this chapter we explore a therapeutic model in which play between the child and a caregiver, facilitated in a therapeutic relationship, becomes the vehicle for healing young children who have experienced traumas. We briefly describe child–parent psychotherapy, discussing the centrality of relationships in creating in children the ability to play and the disorganizing impact of trauma on children's relationships and their ability to symbolize. We then use clinical material to demonstrate how child–parent psychotherapy facilitates the joint construction of a narrative that reveals the child's fears and wishes in relation to the trauma, and allows the child and parent to create new meanings about the trauma, and about their relationship to one another.

CHILD–PARENT PSYCHOTHERAPY AND THE TREATMENT OF TRAUMATIZED CHILDREN

Child–parent psychotherapy, a modification of infant–parent psychotherapy (Fraiberg, Adelson, & Shapiro, 1980; Lieberman & Pawl, 1993; Lieberman, 2004), is for children in the first 6 years of life. Like infant–parent psychotherapy, a treatment model developed by Selma Fraiberg to address mental health problems in children from birth to age 3, child–parent psychotherapy has as its theoretical target the web of mutually constructed meanings in the relationship between the parent and the child (Pawl & St. John, 1998; Lieberman, Silverman, & Pawl, 2000). As she intervened with children in the first 3 years of life, Fraiberg focused her therapeutic attention on uncovering the unconscious conflicts that prevented the parent from seeing the baby as a unique individual and offering care attuned to the baby's needs. When an older child is the target of the intervention, the focus of treatment shifts to away from uncovering the parents' early conflicts and toward the growing child's agency and internal world (Lieberman, 2004).

Young children need their caregivers to help them learn to play. Infants and young children often cannot express their wishes and intentions in words or symbols. They rely upon a range of behaviors, including crying, reaching, facial expressions, tantrums, and running way, to express what they need and the intensity with which they need it. If parents can decipher the meaning of their children's behavior and respond to it in a contingent way, then the children will internalize the experience of being responded to and understood. As these experiences accumulate over time, children gain the capacity to organize their own experience in a coherent way and form internal working models (Bowlby, 1969/1982) of themselves as able to make their feelings and wishes understood and to have an impact on others. These developments are precursors to the ability to tell a story, to use symbols, and to play (Slade, 1994). If, however, parents cannot decipher the meaning of their young children's behavior, then they may fail to respond effectively to their children's needs, and may find themselves trapped with their children in a cycle of miscommunication and mutual alienation, in which neither party understands the intentions of the other. In such cases, an infant–parent or child–parent therapist can guide the parent in observing the child and reflecting on the child's behavior, and help the parent to provide the quality of response that will make it possible for the child to feel understood and to develop the capacity to organize his or her own experience.

Infant–parent or child–parent psychotherapy is a suitable intervention for any infant or young child whose development is impeded by conflicts in the parent–child relationship. When trauma is added to the picture, there are additional considerations. In these cases, the trauma itself places the child's development at risk. First, it subjects the child to overwhelming negative affect at a time when the child has not completed the developmental task of learning to self-regulate affect, but still relies upon caregivers for help. Children "keep the score" of the trauma in their bodies (van der Kolk, 1994). The trauma may manifest itself in children's difficulties with self-regulation, lack of trust in their own sensations, risk taking, or avoidance of physical intimacy. Second, but inextricably intertwined with problems with self-regulation, trauma disrupts children's view of their attachment figures as safe havens and protectors. Young children rightly expect that their caregivers will protect them from being overwhelmed and terrified, an expectation that fails during the traumatic experience (Pynoos, Steinberg, & Piacentini, 1999). Third, even after the traumatic event ends, its effects continue to reverberate, as children and their caregivers are exposed to traumatic reminders and secondary adversities, and as their expectations of the ways in which people will behave in relationships are changed by the trauma (Pynoos et al., 1999). Child–parent psychotherapy addresses all of these effects of trauma in the lives of young children.

Child–parent psychotherapy has much in common with other trauma treatments and shares many of their basic goals (Marmar, Foy, Kagan, & Pynoos, 1993), including fostering a realistic response to the traumatic event, maintaining regular levels of affective arousal, rebuilding the capacity for trust and reciprocity in intimate relationships, encouraging a differentiation between reliving and reenacting the trauma in the present and remembering it as something that happened in the past, and, ultimately, placing the traumatic event in perspective and encouraging a return to normal development. Although child–parent psychotherapy incorporates a variety of treatment modalities, including assistance with concrete problems of daily living, offering unstructured developmental guidance, modeling appropriate protective behavior, and interpretation (Lieberman & Van Horn, 2004), play is a core modality of the intervention.

THE ROLE OF PLAY IN CHILD–PARENT PSYCHOTHERAPY

The psychoanalytic understanding of play has traditionally assigned the therapist the role of understanding the deeper symbolic meaning of children's play and offering a verbal interpretation of that meaning. The therapist seeks to discover the unconscious wishes and fears that drive children's play and to translate them into words for the purpose of bringing them to consciousness (Klein, 1932; A. Freud, 1965). Some children, whose caregiving environments are so chaotic that they have not learned to represent their feelings symbolically, are able to develop the capacity for symbolization, narrative, and reflection in the therapeutic relationship (Slade, 1984). In models of individual child therapy, the child's play is interpreted or enabled in a trusting relationship with a therapist.

Child–parent psychotherapy takes a different approach (Lieberman & Van Horn, 2004). It brings traumatized child and their caregivers together in the play space. The therapist's role becomes one of facilitating play between the parent and the child. In the containing environment of the therapeutic relationship, the parent and child learn to play together, to create a narrative that is satisfying to them both, and to understand one another's view of the world. The underlying premise of child–parent psychotherapy with children who have suffered traumas is that the trauma has disrupted the child's ability to maintain a working model of the parent as a reliable protector. If the child is to regain an optimal developmental trajectory, the security of his or her relationship with the parent must be restored. Traumatized children need their parents to witness their fears, to understand them, and to help them grapple with their fears and place them in perspective. Child–parent psychotherapy accomplishes this goal by helping the parent and child play together to tell the story of the trauma and explore their feelings about it. Through the play, the parent comes to understand the child's inner world. Play allows children to share their vulnerabilities with their parents, gives parents a vehicle to help children examine the distorted expectations created by the trauma, and enables the child and parent together to experiment with different outcomes and to place the trauma in perspective.

The child–parent psychotherapist serves as a container for the parent and the child as they play together. The therapist does not focus exclusively on the meaning of the play for the child, but helps the parent understand how the child's play explicates his or her experience. If the parent resists the meaning of the child's play, or cannot tolerate it, the therapist creates a space in which the child can tell the story and simultaneously supports the parent in observing and participating in the play in as full a manner as possible given the parent's own emotional demands. Once the parent is able to assume a role in the play, or to take part in building the narrative, the therapist turns that function over to the parent and returns to the role of facilitating play between the parent and the child (Lieberman & Van Horn, 2004). The case that we discuss below illustrates the ways in which child–parent psychotherapy uses play not only to strengthen the parent–child relationship but also to help the child move from a state of mind disorganized by trauma to a state in which symbolization and the construction of a narrative are possible.

WHAT HAPPENED TO OLGA?

Olga was referred for treatment by her adoptive mother when Olga was 5 years old. In an initial telephone conversation, Olga's mother Claire told the therapist that she was at her wits' end. She said, "I have to get help for Olga. She's already destroyed my marriage."

The therapist met several times with Claire to explore her concerns about Olga. Claire explained that she and her former husband Jim had gone to Eastern Europe to adopt a child after many years of trying unsuccessfully to conceive. Given their great need, they expressed a willingness to adopt an older child. Olga was a little over 3 years old when they brought her home. They had been able to learn little about her background. Olga's birth mother, who was believed to have had a severe drinking problem, abandoned Olga at the orphanage a few weeks before the child's first birthday. For the next 2 years Olga lived in an environment with little stimulation and no consistent caregivers. Claire, however, was deeply fearful that Olga had suffered damage beyond the loss of her mother and living for 2 years in a depriving environment. She said, "Something horrible must have happened to her to make her so mean."

Claire said that the problems with Olga began immediately after they brought her home. "We so looked forward to having a child, but Olga didn't even care whether we were alive." Claire reported that Olga would not look her or Jim in the eye. She would bang her head against the wall, and when they tried to stop her, Olga either went limp and lifeless as a rag doll or physically fought them—hitting, scratching, and biting. She had no language. After several months in Jim and Claire's home, Olga began to say a few words, but they could hardly understand her, and even at 5 she used little language. Neither of them could please her, though both tried. She did not pretend or play games; indeed, nothing seemed to bring her any pleasure.

In response to this situation, Claire immersed herself in obtaining early intervention services for Olga. Jim retreated into long hours at work and drinking. Claire was frustrated at Jim's refusal to help her find services for Olga, and both spouses felt like failures as parents. Claire said, "We watched our dream of a life as a family with a child fall apart around us. We hardly spoke to each other any more. We were both furious with Olga, but we desperately wanted her to love us. One day, after Jim found Olga sitting on our dog and holding a blanket over his face, he took the dog and left. He pays child support, but he hardly ever comes to see us. I'm at my wits' end."

Claire was firm in her conviction that something "horrible and traumatic" must have happened to Olga. The therapist gently remarked that

Olga's loss of her mother and her very bleak early environment might have been enough to account for the problems Claire was seeing. Claire remained adamant that there must have been something more, and she was convinced that in therapy Olga would reveal this mysterious trauma through her play. After several conversations with Claire, the therapist scheduled her first meeting with Claire and Olga together.

Choosing Toys

Selecting toys for the first session with Olga was a challenge. When they are given appropriate toys, children who have suffered traumas often relive their experiences in posttraumatic play (Terr, 1981; Drell, Siegel, & Gaensbauer, 1993), reenacting traumatic events in a driven way that does not relieve their anxiety but seems to exacerbate it. Olga had lost her birth mother when she was nearly 12 months old, an event that is bound to be profoundly traumatic and disorganizing for such a young child (Lieberman, Compton, Van Horn, & Ghosh Ippen, 2003). Although Claire firmly believed that Olga must have suffered other traumas, no one was able to provide any further information about Olga's early life. The therapist was also curious about whether Olga would be able to play. She did not pretend at home, and her language was still limited. In the end, the therapist chose toys that Olga could use to enact scenes of daily family life, if she chose to do so: wooden blocks; toy dishes; a doctor kit; several small doll figures representing adults, children, and babies; and a baby doll and blanket. The therapist's intent was to provide toys that Olga could use both to reenact her early loss and to build enclosures around the dolls, or walls to keep them apart, and toys that she could use to enact and master the struggles in her everyday life with Claire.

The First Child–Parent Session

Olga approached the playroom slowly, walking sideways and looking at neither her mother nor the therapist. Even after Claire walked into the room and sat down, Olga hesitated. She did not respond when Claire called to her but stood silently outside the door for several minutes. Finally she came in. She did not approach Claire or look at her. She didn't go near the toys. Claire, on the other hand, began talking immediately. She was filled with details of the trouble that she was having with Olga: Olga was not responding to her speech therapy or her physical therapy. She needed glasses but had broken three pairs. She didn't cry when she was hurt, and she wouldn't let Claire comfort her. Olga stood silently and absorbed the words and her mother's angry tone. The therapist said, "You are trying so hard and having so many problems." Then, hoping to be able to include Olga, the therapist asked what Claire had told Olga about why they had come to the playroom. Claire shrugged and said that she had not told Olga anything. She said, "I just hope that bringing her here will help." The therapist asked if she might offer Olga an explanation. Claire shrugged again and said, "Go ahead, but she won't listen to you. She doesn't listen to anyone."

The therapist turned to Olga, who was standing silently in the middle of the room. She said, "Your mom has been telling me that you and she have lots of troubles. She's told me that you had a very sad, scary life before you came to live with her. My job is to help you with those sad, scary feelings, and to help you and your mom get along better." Olga turned her back. Claire looked triumphant and continued to talk about how hard it was to take care of a child who would not look at her and listen to her. The therapist listened, then said, "I know that you're having so many problems, but I wonder how Olga feels standing here listening to you talking about how hard things are." Claire fell silent for a few minutes. She and the therapist waited quietly to see what Olga would do. The therapist said, "There are toys for you to play with."

After several minutes of silence, Olga approached the sandbox. She dipped one hand in slowly, at first allowing the sand to touch only her fingers. Then she buried her whole hand in the sand and moved it around. Without changing her facial expression and or looking up, Olga continued to move her had through the sand, and after a few minutes she put her other hand in the sand. Claire said, "Be careful! Don't get sand on the floor." Olga jerked her hands out of the sand, then slowly put them back, one at a time. The therapist said, "She's listening to you. She's being very careful." Claire seemed a little surprised by the therapist's comment, but she looked at Olga thoughtfully and nodded her head in agreement. Then the therapist turned to Olga and said, "I wonder if the sand just feels good on your skin." Olga moved her hands more deeply into the sand. The therapist asked Claire, "Would you like to join her?" Claire shook her head, but moved her chair closer to the sandbox and began to sift some of the sand through her fingers. She drizzled a little sand on Olga's wrist, but otherwise did not touch Olga. For the remaining minutes of the session, Claire and Olga played quietly with the sand.

In this session, the therapist needed to balance two agendas. Claire badly needed some relief from the stress of trying to care for a child who resisted her attempts at closeness. Listening to Claire's long litany of complaints, however, would have been damaging to Olga. Olga, on the other hand, seemed frozen and unable to move, until she discovered the sand. Her quiet intensity as she moved her hands through the sand made the therapist think of a young infant exploring the world. The therapist chose to intervene in a way that she hoped would bring Claire and Olga closer together and allow their relationship to evolve. She saw herself at that point as the holder of the potential for good feelings between this mother and daughter. When Claire accepted the invitation to join Olga in the sand, mother and child had some minutes of quiet communication at a level that had meaning for Olga: the level of the senses, without words. Claire had not shared Olga's infancy, and she could not bring that time back. But they could share these moments of sensory exploration.

The therapist chose not to give words to the experience during this session; rather, she simply provided a safe environment for Olga and her mother to reach out to one another in this new way.

Olga Begins to Play

For the next several sessions, Olga played in the sand. Repeating the pattern that she had begun in the first session, during each succeeding session Claire began with a pressured narrative of how impossible Olga had been during the last week. As before, the therapist continued to respond that Claire and Olga seemed to be having a very hard time; then she said, "I wonder what it is like for Olga to hear you talk about her in this way?" Each time, with difficulty, Claire turned her attention away from her complaints and joined Olga in the sand. The therapist asked Claire if she would like a referral for individual therapy, so that she would have a place to herself, where she could explore the difficulties that she was having, but Claire refused. As she and Olga played with the sand, however, there were moments of closeness. During one session, as they took turns burying each other's hands in the sand, Olga giggled. It was the first sound that she had made in the therapy room. The therapist commented that Olga loved being with her mom and playing together in the sand. Claire responded that it was a nice change for her and Olga just to have fun together.

Near the beginning of the third month of treatment, Olga touched the toys for the first time. She picked up a small baby doll figure, put it in the sandbox, and buried it in the sand. She piled the sand deeper and deeper on top of the baby. Claire looked worried and told Olga that the baby should not be in the sand, because it could not breathe under all that sand. The therapist told Olga that her mom wanted the baby to be safe. Olga continued to pile on the sand. When Claire tried to take the doll out of the sand, Olga pushed her hand away and buried the baby doll deeper. The therapist asked her what was happening to the baby, but Olga did not respond. After a period of silence in which Olga pulled the baby doll from the sand and then buried it again, the therapist said, "Poor baby. She's all alone in the dark under that sand. It feels so heavy on her. No one can hear her if she cries." Claire got an adult doll and brought it to the sand box. She said, "This is the mama. She's come to get the baby." Olga threw the adult doll across the room. Claire retreated to her chair, crying. The therapist said, "It's hard for you to see the baby all alone and buried so deeply. I wonder if you're thinking about what Olga's life was like after her mother left her at the orphanage."

For several weeks the sessions had an uncomfortable sameness to them. Olga buried babies in the sand. She would not talk or answer questions about her play. She resisted all of Claire's efforts to intervene to save the buried babies. Claire often had tears in her eyes as she watched Olga's play. Once she tried to put her arm around Olga, but Olga shrugged it away. The therapist spoke about how alone the baby was, and how Olga wanted her mom to understand that the baby was alone. Sometimes the therapist asked whether anyone could help the baby. Olga never responded.

While Olga pursued her agenda of communicating the baby's loneliness, Claire became more and more anxious. She spoke of her wish to help Olga and how much it hurt her when Olga turned her back. She said, "It's like she won't let herself have a mother." In fact, Olga's play had the earmarks of a child whose early relationships had not provided her with either an organized, coherent world or the experience of having a role in creating such a universe. As Olga played in their presence, her mother and the therapist were able to help her begin to frame a coherent story about her experience. Claire and the therapist talked about how lonely the baby was and how frightening it must be to be all covered with sand. Claire tried again and again to help the baby and to comfort Olga, but Olga seemed stuck in her lonely sorrow.

Over time, Olga became more receptive to the elements of narrative that Claire's and the therapist's comments provided for her play. The therapist spoke of the lonely baby, all by herself, and asked Olga, "Who can help her?" Both Claire and the therapist often picked up adult doll figures and went searching for the baby. They called to her and said how much they missed the baby. The therapist said to Claire, "The baby needs a mother to hold her, and you need a baby to hold." During this period, Claire complained less about Olga's behavior outside the session. One day she told the therapist, with evident pleasure, that she and Olga had gone to visit a friend. Olga had shut the door to the bathroom and had been unable to get out. She had called to Claire for help. Claire's spirits were lifted by this clear evidence that her daughter needed her and could turn to her for help. In turn, Claire felt less rejected and was able to make herself more available to Olga.

Claire Joins the Play

Olga's play shifted gradually. Although she still buried the baby in the sand during every treatment session, she began to explore other toys and to bury them in the sand as well. She buried whole families of animal figures. The therapist said that the baby was not all alone any more. When Claire tried to rescue the baby animals, and this time Olga allowed her mother to pull the little animals from the sand.

Over the next few weeks, Olga's play shifted away from the sandbox. She discovered a box among the toys that contained fences. She painstakingly put the fences together, sometimes approaching Claire for help. Together they built several small enclosures with the fences. At the end of the hour, Olga told the therapist, "Keep them like this," and the therapist promised that she would. During the next session, Olga looked for and found the fences. She sorted animal groups into the enclosures, putting all of the baby animals in one enclosure and all of the adult animals in another. Claire said, "These babies need a mother to take care of them," and moved an adult animal into the enclosure with the babies. Olga did not resist her mother's intervention. She left the adult animal with the babies, then turned to the adult animals, sorting them into pairs.

Olga and Claire played with the animals and the fences for several weeks. The therapist always preserved the enclosures that they built from week to week. She quietly narrated their play, noting that sometimes the baby animals had a mommy to take care of them and sometimes they were alone; she commented, "So many babies and no mother." As Olga moved the baby animals around in the enclosures, the therapist would sometimes ask what they were doing. Olga began to give simple responses. Sometimes she said that the babies were playing, other times that they were sleeping. Once she said that the babies were looking for their mothers.

In examining this sequence of sessions, we can see that Olga used play to organize her experience. In the beginning, her play had an isolated, fragmented quality. She could not accept help from her mother, who, in play as in real life, was pained by Olga's rejection of her bids to help. When Claire was able to set aside her own anxiety and sorrow over her rejection and join the therapist in observing Olga's isolation and loneliness, Olga was able, over time, to tolerate intervention. She began to describe, in a rudimentary fashion, what the characters in her play were doing. She could allow Claire to add to the story, bringing in a mother to protect Olga's isolated babies. She began to seek help from her mother in the play, and to ask the therapist to help by keeping her toys together from one week to the next, indicating that she could grasp the concept that the toys, and the story, could be preserved across time. Most importantly, Olga began to seek her mother's help outside the sessions. Through the vehicle of play, Olga and Claire took small steps to strengthen their relationship.

Olga Tells a Story

After several weeks of playing quietly with the fences and the small animals, Olga's play shifted dramatically. She found a large dinosaur among the toys and turned it into a monster that repeatedly attacked the baby animals. At the first attack, Claire tried to bring an adult animal to fight the dinosaur. She said that the mommy animal would protect the babies. Olga promptly made the dinosaur eat the adult animal. She laughed and, speaking for the dinosaur, said, "Now I'll get those babies." The therapist spoke for the babies, giving voice to their fear in the face of such a huge, fierce monster. Olga made one very brave little baby alligator emerge from the group of babies to fight the dinosaur and save the other babies. Claire tried again to have an adult animal help. Once more, Olga refused the help. The therapist noted that the baby wanted to fight the dinosaur all by herself, saying, "That baby doesn't think anyone can help her. She has to do all of the fighting by herself." The therapist asked Olga if the baby was afraid. Olga said, "No. She'll kill that dinosaur." Then Olga made the baby alligator bite the dinosaur on the foot and the dinosaur fell over, dead.

Olga played out this story again and again, laughing with delight when the tiny baby alligator vanquished the big dinosaur monster. Claire was equally persistent in offering help. Olga would not let Claire help her kill the dinosaur, but she could tolerate Claire's putting an adult animal with the babies to keep them from being frightened of the monster. The therapist made one of her first attempts to tie Olga's play to the story of her life. She said, "Sometimes you didn't have anyone to help you. You were all alone and very scared." Olga did not acknowledge this interpretation, but she did not turn away from the therapist; she continued her play, gleefully sending the baby alligator out to kill the dinosaur.

During the sessions in which the dinosaur play predominated, Claire made an important step in her understanding of Olga. She seemed to accept Olga's abandonment by her birth mother and her life in the neglectful atmosphere of the orphanage as important causes of distress in their own right. She stopped looking for something else "horrible" that happened and began to play with Olga about themes of isolation, fear, and helplessness. As Claire joined more wholeheartedly in this play, Olga's stories became more elaborated until, finally, she allowed Claire to bring in an adult animal to help the baby alligator fight the dinosaur. Olga and Claire put all of the adult animals in the enclosure with the babies, then the two of them together went out to fight and kill the monster. The therapist noted that the monster was very scary and the babies needed some grown-ups to protect them, so they would not be so frightened. When Olga and Claire had killed the monster, they came back to the pen of baby animals and their protectors. Olga said, "The monster is dead. They will have a party, and everyone will eat him." She and Claire took all of the animals over to where the dinosaur lay, then pretended, with quite a lot of enthusiasm, to chew him up.

After the session in which Olga and Claire used animals to kill the dinosaur together, Olga's play shifted again. She reenacted the theme of babies fighting monsters, but this time she used the small doll figures in place of the dinosaurs. With Claire's help, she used the blocks to build a house for the babies. Claire said, "Those babies can't live all alone in the house. They need someone to care for them." Olga chose several adult figures to live in the house with the babies. When the dinosaur came to threaten the house full of babies, Olga took a baby from the house and fought the dinosaur with it. She again resisted having an adult help in the battle against the monster. After telling the story of the baby killing the monster several times, Olga was willing to have Claire join the battle with an adult doll, and the two planned a cooperative strategy to attack and capture the monster and send him away.

Throughout this play, the therapist described the story that was played out. She commented on Olga's glee as her baby doll killed the monster. She gave voice to the feelings of the babies, saying that the ones left behind in the house were afraid of the monster but glad to have some grown-ups to help them. She did not tie this story to Olga's own life. She wondered if the shift from animal to human characters as the focus of the play meant that Olga was moving closer to her personal reality on her own; she believed that if this were the case, an interpretation tying the play to Olga's own life might bring the play too close and prove overwhelming. For the sessions that involved doll play, the therapist chose simply to narrate and ask questions about the play, and not to step outside the play with interpretation (Birch, 1997).

The Roller Coaster

After nearly a year of treatment, Olga and Claire took a 2-week break from treatment to entertain friends visiting from out of town. When they returned, Olga told the therapist, with a great deal of excitement, that they had gone to the park and that they rode the roller coaster. Her face was more animated than the therapist had ever seen it. For the next several weeks, Olga played at recreating the roller coaster in the playroom. She placed the chairs in a row and told Claire and the therapist to sit in them. She said, "You're on the roller coaster! Scream now! There's a ghost!" Claire explained that the roller coaster they rode at the park had gone through dark tunnels, with ghosts and monsters that popped out to startle the riders. She had been afraid that Olga would get too frightened and would cry, but Olga wanted to ride the roller coaster over and over again. In the end, she was only allowed to ride it three times, and was disappointed when the group went on to other activities.

In the playroom, Olga directed her mother and the therapist. "You're going down now. Scream, because you're scared. Here comes a ghost. Here comes a monster. You have to scream." The therapist had never seen Olga so animated or so willing to speak. She and Claire participated enthusiastically in the game, following Olga's directions. After several "rides," the therapist asked Olga if she wanted to have a turn riding. She smiled and nodded. Claire said, "I'll ride with you, so you won't be too frightened." Olga took the therapist's chair, and the therapist asked her in a stage whisper, "What should I say?" Olga said, "Tells us we're going down. Tell us to scream!" For the rest of the session, Olga, her eyes shining with excitement, directed the therapist, then followed the therapist's directions. Sometimes when the therapist told them to be frightened, Olga snuggled closer to Claire's chair. Claire responded by putting her arm around Olga and comforting her. She said, "It's scary, but fun. We'll be okay. I'll take care of you."

The next week, Olga ran into the playroom, put the chairs in a row, and sat down. She said, "Ride with me, Mommy." Claire sat down, and the therapist directed the ride. For several minutes, the therapist asked for directions from Olga. Finally Olga, in response to a question from the therapist, said, "You say." The therapist said, "You trust me not to make the ride too scary for you. You know that your mom will take care of you and you'll be okay and have fun." This speech was too long. Olga said, "Play!"

During the third week of roller coaster play, Olga said spontaneously, "I miss my mommy." Claire said, "But I'm right here." Olga said, "Not you. My other mommy." Claire started to cry. She said that she had talked to Olga about having a birth mother who was too sick to take care of her. She said that she thought Olga had not listened and taken it in. The therapist said, "It seems like Olga listens to you a lot, even when you're not sure that she's hearing you." Claire took Olga on her lap, and Olga sat there without protest. Claire told Olga that she had been born in another country far away. She said, "Your mommy loved you, but she was too sick, and she couldn't take care of you. Some people told me about you and I came to get you, because I wanted a little girl to love and take care of." Olga looked hard at Claire. She said, "Daddy, too?" Claire began to cry again and looked at the therapist helplessly. The therapist said, "Your daddy has been gone a long time." Olga said, "He's all gone." The therapist said, "You worry. Your first mommy is gone. Your daddy is gone." Claire said, "I won't go away, baby. I'll always be here to take care of you."

In the next session, the therapist brought storybooks about adoption and about a little girl who is sad because her father does not come to see her. Olga listened while Claire read the books to her, but she turned the focus back to her own story. "My mommy's gone," she said. "My daddy's gone." It was clear to both Claire and the therapist that Olga found her own story more compelling than the stories in the books.

Claire and Olga brought a small globe to the next session. Claire showed Olga the country where she was born, and the country where they now lived together. She told about the long airplane ride that she took when she went to get Olga, and about the long ride that they took home together. She brought in the court order of adoption to show Olga that she had promised to take care of her forever. The therapist asked whether they talked about these things at home. Claire said that they did not. She said, "I do okay by myself, but then I'm afraid that she'll ask a question that I don't know how to answer." Claire said that she wanted to start a scrapbook for Olga that would tell the story of her life. They agreed that they would use the next therapy sessions to work on the book.

The Story of Olga's Life

For several months, Claire and Olga came to each session with the scrapbook and pictures. They talked with each other and with the therapist about the pictures, some of which were from the orphanage. There were no pictures of Olga's birth mother, so Olga and Claire drew a picture of what Olga thought she would look like. The work on the scrapbook was not constant. Sometimes Olga and Claire returned to play. They played mainly with the animal families, but a new play theme emerged during this time. Olga, who had ignored the baby doll for over a year of treatment, finally picked it up and held it. Often during the next months, Olga and Claire would play with the baby doll together. They rocked it and sang a lullaby. Claire had learned a lullaby in the language of Olga's birth country, and she taught it to Olga.

As Claire and Olga alternately played with the baby and worked on the scrapbook, they gradually became more able to talk about the issue that was most troubling to Olga: why her birth mother and her daddy had left her. Claire offered explanations but was taken aback when Olga's true fear emerged. "I'm too bad," she said one day. This led to several sessions in which the baby doll was bad and was punished. She cried too loudly and had to be spanked. She spit up her food. She wet her diaper. For all of these "sins," Olga decreed that the baby had to be exiled to the corner of the room and left alone. The therapist said, "She's just a baby. That's what babies do. They cry; they wet. They can't help it because they're little." Over time Olga was able to adjust her sense of right and wrong; she became less punitive with the baby and less negative about herself.

Claire and Olga brought the scrapbook up to date in the therapy sessions. It told the story of a child who had lived with her mother when she was very tiny, but then had been left. She missed her mother and cried, but there was no one to take care of her until Claire came.

After slightly less than 2 years of treatment, Claire told the therapist that she finally thought she understood Olga. She said, "Everything that she has played about is about being left and being alone, and not sure who will take care of her and keep her safe." Claire decided that it was time to end treatment, because she was confident that she would be able to comfort Olga.

Predictably, termination was a difficult time for Olga. She began again to punish the baby doll. The therapist said, "I'm not saying good-bye because you're bad. You're a wonderful little girl. I'm saying good-bye because you and your mom understand each other now, and you don't have so many problems." During the last session, Claire took a picture of Olga with the therapist to put in Olga's scrapbook. They wrote three cards together and agreed that the therapist would keep them and mail them to Olga, one a month for the next 3 months. The therapist said, "They will remind you that I'm thinking about you even if we aren't together. We can both think about the time we spent playing together. You will be in my heart even though you don't come to play here any more."

Summary

Olga used play to move from a disorganized psychological state, in which she could not use words and symbols to express her thoughts and feelings about her self, to a more organized, related state, in which she could organize a narrative, ask questions about things that were important to her, and express a variety of emotions. Because her mother was involved in this metamorphosis, Olga's relationship with Claire deepened, becoming more reliable and more flexible at the same time.

Claire, as we have seen, was an essential partner in Olga's treatment. Her active involvement at each step was essential to Olga's development. Claire was there to meet Olga in her first tentative steps toward sensory–motor play. By participating in that play with her daughter, Claire shared and mirrored

Olga's experience. The intimacy that the two of them developed as they moved their hands through the sand made it possible for Claire to join Olga in battling the monsters. Olga's ability to rely on Claire for help in slaying the monsters was a necessary first step to her growing reliance on her mother to be protective in the face of real-life dangers, fears, and losses. As the therapy progressed, both Claire and Olga grew, and they grew closer together.

In the last analysis, although Claire came to the therapist wanting help for Olga, the treatment was for both of them. Both Claire and Olga needed to grow and change, and to develop more open and reality-based views of one another. Olga's history of deprived caregiving experiences made it difficult for her to trust Claire and to anticipate loving care from her. Claire's concerns about the abuses that Olga might have suffered in the past kept her from appreciating the deep impact that deprivation and loneliness had in shaping Olga's view of the world. The therapist's task in facilitating the changes that both Claire and Olga needed to make was to provide a safe environment in which both of them could explore, to give each of them psychological support at times when their different needs led to conflict, to hold the promise that they would be able to attain warmth and understanding in their relationship, and to help them notice the evidence that their relationship was changing for the better at times when the signs were too subtle for them to see on their own.

Claire's successful adaptation to the demands of the therapy is emblematic of her growing understanding of Olga's needs. We see that early in the treatment, words seemed impossibly intrusive for Olga, and "simply playing" (Slade, 1984) was all that was needed to help Olga organize her thoughts and feelings. This extended period of "simply playing" presented a great challenge for Claire, who had much to say, but whose words seemed to leave Olga frozen. It is the magic of child–parent psychotherapy that once Claire began to understand Olga's need to play quietly, she was able to suspend her own agenda and to join her daughter in activities that ultimately promoted change in them both. Together, in the therapy room, they experienced growth in their understanding for one another. Together, they were able to start afresh and tell the story of their lives together.

REFERENCES

Axline, V. M. (1947). *Play therapy.* Boston: Houghton Mifflin.
Birch, M. (1997). In the land of counterpane: Travels in the realm of play. *Psychoanalytic Study of the Child, 52,* 57–75.
Bowlby, J. (1969/1982). *Attachment and loss: Vol. 1. Attachment.* New York: Basic Books. (Original work published 1969)
Drell, M. J., Siegel, C. H., & Gaensbauer, T. J. (1993). Posttraumatic stress disorders. In C. Zeanah (Ed.), *Handbook of infant mental health* (pp. 291–304). New York: Guilford Press.
Erikson, E. H. (1950). *Childhood and society.* New York: Norton.

Fraiberg, S., Adelson, E., & Shapiro, V. (1980). Ghosts in the nursery: A psychoanalytic approach to the problem of impaired infant–mother relationships. *Journal of the American Academy of Child Psychiatry, 14,* 387–342.

Freud, A. (1965). *Normality and pathology in childhood.* New York: International Universities Press.

Freud, S. (1937). *A general selection* (J. Rickman, Ed.). London: Hogarth Press.

Klein, M. (1932). *The psychoanalysis of children.* London: Hogarth Press.

Lieberman, A. F. (2004). Child–parent psychotherapy: A relationship-based approach to the treatment of mental health disorders in infancy and early childhood. In A. J. Sameroff, S. C. McDonough, & K. L. Rosenblum (Eds.), *Treating parent–infant relationship problems* (pp. 97–122). New York: Guilford Press.

Lieberman, A. F., Compton, N., Van Horn, P., & Ghosh Ippen, C. (2003). *Losing a parent to death in the early years: Guidelines for the treatment of traumatic bereavement in infancy and early childhood.* Washington, DC: Zero to Three: National Center for Infants, Toddlers and Families.

Lieberman, A. F., & Pawl, J. H. (1993). Infant–parent psychotherapy. In C. H. Zeanah (Ed.), *Handbook of infant mental health* (pp. 427–442). New York: Guilford Press.

Lieberman, A. F., Silverman, R., & Pawl, J. H. (2000). Infant–parent psychotherapy: Core concepts and current approaches. In C. H. Zeanah (Ed.), *Handbook of infant mental health* (2nd ed., pp. 472–484). New York: Guilford Press.

Lieberman, A. F., & Van Horn, P. (2004). *"Don't hit my mommy!": A manual for child–parent psychotherapy with young witnesses of family violence.* Washington, DC: Zero to Three: National Center for Infants, Toddlers and Families.

Marmar, C., Foy, D., Kagan, B., & Pynoos, R. S. (1993). An integrated approach for treating posttraumatic stress. In J. M. Oldman & A. Talman (Eds.), *American Psychiatric Association review of psychiatry* (Vol. 12, pp. 238–272). Washington, DC: American Psychiatric Press.

Pawl, J. H., & St. John, M. (1998). *How you are is as important as what you do.* Washington, DC: Zero-to-Three: National Center for Infants, Toddlers and Families.

Pynoos, R. S., Steinberg, A. M., & Piacentini, J. C. (1999). A developmental psychopathology model of childhood traumatic stress and intersection with anxiety disorders. *Biological Psychiatry, 46,* 1542–1554.

Schaefer, C. E., & O'Connor, K. J. (Eds.). (1983). *Handbook of play therapy.* New York: Wiley.

Slade, A. (1984). Making meaning and making believe: Their role in the clinical process. In A. Slade & D. P. Wolf (Eds.), *Children at play: Clinical and developmental approaches to meaning and representation* (pp. 81–107). New York: Oxford University Press.

Terr, L. C. (1981). Forbidden games: Post-traumatic child's play. *Journal of the American Academy of Child and Adolescent Psychiatry, 20,* 740–759.

van der Kolk, B. A. (1994). The body keeps the score: Memory and the evolving psychobiology of posttraumatic stress. *Harvard Review of Psychiatry, 1,* 253–265.

Watson, M. W. (1994). The relation between anxiety and pretend play. In A. Slade & D. P. Wolf (Eds.), *Children at play: Clinical and developmental approaches to meaning and representation* (pp. 33–47). New York: Oxford University Press.

17

Early Intervention for Autism

SUSAN FAJA and GERALDINE DAWSON

Autism is a neurodevelopmental disorder involving qualitative impairments in social interaction and communication, and the presence of a restricted range of interests and/or repetitive behaviors. Since Leo Kanner (1943) first characterized autism, much work has explored the etiology and treatment of autism. Although progress has been made, there is no cure for autism, and its etiology remains largely unknown. Currently, 11.1 in 10,000 individuals are estimated to have autism, while the prevalence rate of all pervasive developmental disorders, including autism, is conservatively estimated to be 27.5 in 10,000 individuals (Fombonne, 2003). Thus, autism is no longer considered a rare disorder. As such, the development of effective treatments for autism and related spectrum disorders represents an important educational and public health challenge and priority, because professionals in a wide variety of settings are likely to encounter children with autism spectrum disorders. More importantly, the economic and emotional strain on families of children with such pervasive disorders is profound, underscoring the need for careful scientific evaluation of intervention studies.

Children with a variety of impairments and risk factors, including those with autism, benefit from early, intensive intervention with trained providers using comprehensive, individualized, and ecologically relevant intervention approaches (Ramey & Ramey, 1998). Evidence suggests that early intervention with autism is more effective than later treatment; specifically, children entering intervention programs as younger preschoolers tend to have better outcomes than those entering programs as school-age children (Fenske, Zalenski, Krantz, & McClanahan, 1985; Harris & Handleman, 2000). With recent advances in early detection of autism (e.g., Osterling & Dawson, 1994; Robins, Fein, Barton, & Green, 2001, see review by Bishop & Lord, Chapter 12, this volume), early autism intervention will eventually be available to infants. Indeed, a variety of intervention approaches targeting toddlers with autism have emerged in recent years (Chandler, Christie, Newson, & Prevezer, 2002; Drew et al., 2002; Green, Brennan, & Fein, 2002; Mahoney & Perales, 2003; McGee, Morrier, & Daly, 1999). Such efforts can potentially answer questions about optimal timing of early intervention. Very early interventions hold promise for improving long-term outcomes for individuals with autism, because such interventions are administered at a time of maximal opportunity to affect learning and development in both the child and the family (Mesibov, 1997a). In addition, younger children may benefit more from treatment than older children because of greater neural plasticity and fewer downstream impairments resulting from core deficits (Dawson, Osterling, Meltzoff, & Kuhl, 2000; Dawson & Zanolli, 2003; Rogers & DiLalla, 1991). However, treatment is likely to have significant benefit to all individuals regardless of age or ability level (Bristol et al., 1996).

EVALUATING EARLY INTERVENTION: A NEED FOR INCREASED SCIENTIFIC RIGOR

In a 1996 report to the National Institutes of Health (NIH), Bristol and colleagues set forth guidelines for evaluating treatment of autism. Importantly, assignment to treatment group (experimental and comparison) should be determined randomly, so as not to introduce bias. Evaluation of treatments must be conducted by independent evaluators who are not invested in the study outcome and should include a variety of standardized measures of a range of behaviors—both in a controlled, laboratory setting and in more natural settings. To ensure that the treatment is replicable by others, measures of the integrity of implementation should be used. Finally, in addition to immediate outcomes, Bristol et al. (1996) advised longitudinal designs to allow for evaluation of treatment effects and their stability over time. The report also suggested direct comparison of treatment approaches and development of new measurement approaches to better address the ethical dilemmas faced by comparison of treatment versus placebo. The 1996 guidelines parallel the more general practices for evaluating clinical research in the field of psychology, which are needed to draw solid logical conclusions about the efficacy of a given treatment (Chambless & Hollon, 1998; Lonigan, Elbert, & Johnson, 1998; Task Force on Promotion and Dissemination of Psychological Procedures, 1995). When evaluating potential interventions, *efficacy*, or demonstrable effects with groups of patients in carefully controlled settings, must first be established, then *effectiveness*, or generalized treatment effects beyond the constraints of the research setting.

In addition to the more elaborate and labor-intensive group designs, single-subject designs are often used for testing novel interventions, because they allow for pseudocontrolled conditions and are often more feasible—clinically, ethically, and financially. While careful single-subject designs (e.g., multiple baselines) can allow for some inferences about causality (Kazdin, 2002), they cannot resolve important questions about which types of children respond best to particular treatments, how two differing treatments compare to one another, or which variables predict treatment outcomes; therefore, promising smaller-scale studies of novel treatments should be followed up with large-scale, empirically sound trials. Because it is ultimately important to answer such questions to provide the most scientifically sound interventions, interventions that have been tested using controlled group designs are emphasized in this chapter. The interested reader is referred to reviews of single-subject or small-sample approaches (e.g., Koegel & Koegel, 1995; Odom et al., 2003).

This chapter primarily focuses on comprehensive psychosocial interventions for preschoolers, for which some data on outcome have been collected (see Table 17.1, p. 392). Brief comments on "focal" treatments and medical/biologically oriented approaches are offered. These are followed by conclusions and recommendations for future work.

COMPREHENSIVE EARLY INTERVENTION MODELS

Applied Behavior Analytic Approaches

Ferster and DeMyer (1961) were among the first to demonstrate the potential of behavioral intervention with operant discrimination learning techniques in treating children with autism, giving rise to the development of comprehensive applied behavioral analysis (ABA) interventions. The use of ABA approaches remains popular. Techniques are constantly evolving, with a variety of refinements and applications to target specific behavioral objectives. ABA intervention approaches involve a strong focus on ongoing data collection with systematic measurement and analysis of treatment strategies and child behavior, as well as examination of the environmental factors that influence behavior. A variety of techniques based on operant conditioning (Skinner, 1938) are used, such as shaping, prompting, chaining, and fading. Due in part to the data-driven nature of behavioral treatment, such interventions enjoy relatively strong scientific support.

Discrete Trials: The Lovaas Method

One of the first comprehensive early intervention programs based on ABA approaches, developed by O. Ivar Lovaas (1987; Lovaas et al., 1981), was delivered to a group of preschoolers participating in the UCLA Young Autism Project (YAP). This approach employed operant conditioning (mostly positive reinforcement, with some use of aversive contingencies) and focused on discrete trial training (DTT), which isolates component skills comprising a child's behavioral deficiencies to be taught one-on-one and then chained together. Each discrete trial consists of a concise instruction followed by a prompt, the child's response, and immediate reinforcement (see Smith, 2001, for discussion of this technique). Lovaas also made use of ignoring, time outs,

TABLE 17.1. Review of Early Interventions for Young Children with Autism

Model	Ages	Sample	Intensity	Diagnosis	Evidence
Autism Preschool Program Jocelyn et al. (1998)	24–72 mo w/no prior treatment; $M = 44$ mo	16 in treatment and 19 community standard controls; all in ~ 20 hr day care	15 hr class over 12 week + 3 hr/wk consultation for 10 wk	Autism and PDD NOS (DSM-III-R)	*Promising—a RCT*: language gains; increased maternal and child care worker knowledge of autism, perceived parental control, and satisfaction; no differences in autism severity, or perceptual–motor, cognitive, socioemotional, adaptive, or gross motor development (both groups improved).
Child's Talk Aldred et al. (2004)	$M = 48$ (29–60) mo	14 in treatment; 14 controls	3.5 hr/wk + psychoeducation and 9 consultation sessions	Autism (ADI autism; ADOS within 1 point) No profound MR.	*Promising—a RCT*: decreased symptom severity (particularly in reciprocal social interaction), expressive language, and increased synchrony of communication. No significant difference in adaptive functioning or parental stress.
Denver Model— Colorado Health Sciences Rogers et al. (1991)	$M = 45.77$ mo ($SD = 10.02$)	49 in autism group; 27 in non-ASD group	22 hr over an average of 18 mo	Autism/other PDDs versus group w/other disorders	Improvement in growth rate for all children in language and cognition. Normal growth rate in language. Limitations include lack of control subjects.
Division TEACCH Ozonoff & Cathcart (1998)	24–72 mo	11 in treatment	1 hr consultation + 3.5 hr over 10 wk	Autism	Improved significantly in psychoeducational skills (at double the normative rate); children with higher baselines improved the most. Assignment was nonrandom.
Douglass Developmental Disabilities Center–Rutgers Harris et al. (1990 & 1991)	Segregated class: $M = 58$ (49–66) mo. Integrated class: $M = 55.8$ (52–60) mo.	5 in each group + 4 typicals in integrated class	15–27.5 hr of intervention over 1–2 yr	Infantile autism (American Psychiatric Association, 1980) and relatively high functioning	Increased language growth rate in typical children and ones with autism relative to normative rate; 18 point IQ gain and 8 point language gain for children with autism. No differences between segregated or integrated children. Growth rate in children with autism seemed to accelerate. Nonrandom assignment; both groups with autism had similar treatment other than presence or absence of peers.
Floor Time (DIR) Greenspan & Wieder (1997)	22–48 mo	200 received FT; 53 community controls	At least 2 yr; hours per week not reported	Autism or PDD NOS (DSM-III-R or DSM-IV)	Chart review with clinical descriptive design (nonexperimental, with no statistics reported). Of the 200, 58% had "good-to-outstanding" outcomes (2% in the community group) with spontaneous symbolic abilities, intent and affect, and CARS ratings below the autism cutoff.

(continued)

TABLE 17.1. (*continued*)

Model	Ages	Sample	Intensity	Diagnosis	Evidence
Multisite Young Autism Project Smith, Groen, et al. (2000)	18–42 mo; $M = 36$ mo	15 in intensive group; 13 in parent training	30 hr versus 20–25 hr/wk for 2–3 years	Autism and PDD NOS	*Probably efficacious:* Significant IQ gains; also better on visual–spatial ability and academic achievement, but no difference on language, adaptive, or maladaptive functioning.
Pivitol Response Training–UCSB Koegel et al. (1992, 1998, 1999)	37–65 mo	Ranged from 3 to 6 children	NA	Autism (DSM-III and DSM-IV)	*Empirically promising:* Multiple baseline, repeated reversal, retrospective analysis and uncontrolled group designs. Findings include increased target language responses, fewer disruptive behaviors, more spontaneous initiation across settings, and more favorable long-term outcomes.
Princeton Child Development Institute Fenske et al. (1985)	Enrolled pre-60 mo ($M = 48.9$) and after 60 mo ($M = 101.2$)	$N = 18$; 9 in each age group	27.5 hr/wk for at least 2 yr. Some residential services	Autism (National Society for Autistic Children 1978 criteria)	67% versus 11% positive outcomes in the early versus later enrollment groups (based on educational placement and living situation). Enrollment age groups self-selected, no comparison group receiving different treatment, small sample size, few outcome measures, which were largely unstandardized.
Scottish Centre for Autism Salt et al. (2002)	$M = 42.4$ ($SD = 7.16$) mo for treatment group	12 in treatment; 5 waitlisted	8+ hr/wk for 10 mo in addition to community treatment	Autism (ICD-10)	Significant improvements in joint attention, social interaction, imitation, daily living skills, motor skills, and adaptive behavior.
UCLA Young Autism Project Lovaas (1987); McEachin et al. (1993)	< 40 mo if mute and < 46 mo if echolalic	19 intensive behavioral treatment, 19 nonintensive, 21 community	40+ hr versus 10 hr/wk for at least 2 yr	Autism (DSM-III) No MR	IQ gains 31.1 points higher than the minimal behavioral group and 25.8 higher than the community group at 6–7 yr and relatively better educational placements. Significantly better IQ, educational placement, and adaptive function at follow-up.
Walden Model McGee et al. (1992, 1994)	$M = 44$ mo (30–66)	Single-subject, noncontrolled designs	All day, all year	Autism (DSM-III-R)	With preschoolers, reports in non-peer-reviewed publications (uncontrolled pre–post studies) or single-subject designs of particular aspects of the intervention. Results include language gains and increased peer interaction.

Note. ADI, Autism Diagnostic Interview; ADOS, Autism Diagnostic Observation Schedule; CARS, Children Autism Rating Scale; FT, floor time; MR, mental retardation; RCT, randomized controlled trial.

and shaping of more socially appropriate behaviors to reduce negative behaviors such as aggression and self-harm. A key hypothesis was the importance of time spent in treatment, stemming from the assumption that typically developing children are learning from their environments in most of their waking hours across a variety of settings, and children with autism do not spontaneously learn this way. The resulting UCLA intervention attempted to provide learning opportunities for young children with autism during essentially all of their waking hours (approximately 40 hours per week) and in all of their environments by enlisting a team of therapists and parents to implement an environmental scaffolding engineered to allow children to catch up to typical development. Treatment targeted a progression of aims, beginning with reduction of disruptive and repetitive behaviors, simple receptive language, imitation, and appropriate play. Then, expressive and abstract language and play with peers were targeted, and the treatment setting was expanded to include the preschool classroom. Whenever possible, children were mainstreamed in public preschools for typically developing children, with the development of individualized education plans as needed in subsequent years. Finally, academic tasks, emotions, and imitation of other children's learning and appropriate social behaviors were targeted. In short, the YAP diverged from previous treatments in its intense treatment delivery, empirically derived teaching strategies, focus on young children, and "normal" peer models (Lovaas, Smith, & McEachin, 1989).

Initial outcome was evaluated on the basis of school placement and intelligence testing when children were ages 6–7 years (Lovaas, 1987). The intensively treated group exhibited a markedly higher IQ than the groups receiving less treatment or community care (83 vs. 52 and 57 in the respective control groups) and attained higher educational placements. Long-term outcome data were presented several years later, though the mean age at follow-up varied by treatment group and some data points were missing (McEachin, Smith, & Lovaas, 1993). The educational placement of the intensive-treatment group was relatively stable and statistically superior to either control group. The intelligence scores of the treated group also remained statistically superior to the control group at follow-up. Finally, parent report of adaptive functioning in communication, socialization, and daily living indicated better adaptive functioning in the treatment group and significantly more maladaptive behaviors in the control group. The YAP was notable in its large effect sizes and the long-term academic gains made by some children in the intensive-treatment group.

The work of Lovaas and colleagues with the UCLA YAP was groundbreaking in its comprehensive exploration of intervention with autism. The original and follow-up work of the UCLA group (Lovaas, 1987; McEachin et al., 1993) has been provocative and has stimulated interest both for its potentially promising treatment and its limitations in methodology. Its strengths included direct comparison of treatment with two control groups, use of treatment manuals, careful supervision of intervention, long-term evaluation of treatment stability, relatively large sample size, and some use of independent evaluators. However, evaluation at baseline and of outcome used a relatively narrow range of measures, did not follow a specific protocol, and was not always conducted in comparable settings. The number of treatment hours was not carefully documented, and duration of intervention varied depending on outcome and parent demand for continuation, though all children were treated for at least 2 years. Children with extreme mental retardation were excluded, though McEachin et al. argued that the sample of children included was representative of children with autism. Finally, the most significantly and constantly held criticism of the original Lovaas study was its nonrandom method of assignment to treatment groups.

Randomized Evaluation of UCLA Intervention Program in a Carefully Controlled Setting

Smith, Groen, and Wynn (2000) conducted a replication study of Lovaas's early intensive behavioral intervention (EBI) using a fully randomized design addressing many limitations of previous investigations of the YAP. The methodology (discrete trials followed by more generalized approaches in the second year), treatment goals, and theoretical rationale were similar to Lovaas's, and the same manual was used (Lovaas et al., 1981). However, treatment was less intensive (30 hours per week instead of 40 hours), parents were not required to give up working for a year as they had been by Lovaas, and aversive contingencies were used less frequently. EBI with student therapists supplemented by parents was compared to a parent training intervention based on the same treatment manual. The comparison group received intervention for 10 hours a week that was similar to the treatment group in the use of Lovaas's theoretical framework and 10–15 hours per week of special education programming.

Methodological improvements included random assignment to treatment groups after matching diagnostic severity and intelligence, independent assessment of diagnosis by the same agency, and good characterization of children on a broad range of domains at baseline and follow-up using a protocol of standardized measures. Participating families varied widely in their ethnic and socioeconomic characteristics, yet no families withdrew from either treatment group after being enrolled. Treatment fidelity was addressed by tracking the amount of time each child spent in treatment, following a manualized intervention, requiring extensive training of student therapists, and documenting credentials of therapists and their supervisors. Thus, the study satisfies four of the criteria laid out by Bristol and colleagues in the 1996 Research Council and echoed by the 2001 National Research Council: random assignment, standardized and wide-ranging outcome measures, independent evaluation of treatment, and integrity of treatment implementation. Both Councils also suggested collecting data throughout intervention, which Smith and colleagues (2000) did, and collecting longitudinal data.

Smith, Groen, et al. (2000) found significantly higher IQ scores at initial outcome in the group receiving therapist-implemented, intensive treatment, though the average gain in intelligence was half that observed by Lovaas (1987). And, as Rogers (in press) points out, the children in Smith's treated group were still, on average, classified as mentally retarded, and only 13% of treated children attained "best outcome" status compared with 47% in the original study. The group receiving intensive intervention also made significant gains on measures of visual–spatial ability and academic achievement but did not differ on language (Smith, Groen, & Wynn, 2001), adaptive or maladaptive functioning. Smith attempted to examine differences in response between diagnostic group (autism vs. pervasive developmental disorder, not otherwise specified [PDD NOS]), but small sample sizes and variable performance between both groups limited the ability to detect differences and none were found, despite a trend for higher scores in the group with PDD NOS. Based on these results, Smith, Groen, et al. (2000) concluded that children with PDD NOS might benefit from early behavioral intervention at least as much as, if not more than, children with autism. Finally, both groups of parents felt positively about the quality of intervention, its impact on the family, and their relationships with the treatment team.

While more methodologically sophisticated, the work of Smith, Groen, et al. (2000) is not without limitations, such as sample size. In addition, the selection of treatment in the control group (parent- rather than center-directed intervention with the same manual for fewer hours) leads to difficulty interpreting the differences between treatment groups. The 1996 guidelines (Bristol et al.) specify comparison with either no treatment or with an existing efficacious treatment in order for clear interpretations to be made. Modest benefits in the group with therapist-implemented behavioral intervention suggest that children may benefit from the expertise of an outside provider; however, both groups received treatment following the same theoretical orientation, so the necessity of particular aspects of the YAP remain uncertain. Limitations of this replication study were acknowledged, and Smith has stated that recent work by a multi-site intervention project addresses some of these concerns.

Other Evaluations of Lovaas-Style Intervention Programs: Investigations of Effectiveness

Other groups (Birnbrauer & Leach, 1993; Sheinkopf & Siegel, 1998) have independently implemented and investigated behavioral analytic interventions using group comparison designs, though none did so with methods as rigorous as those used by Lovaas (1987) or by Smith, Groen, et al. (2000). Nonetheless, these partial replications offer important preliminary information about the Lovaas model in other settings. The group at the University of California–San Francisco (Sheinkopf & Siegel, 1998) investigated the efficacy of the Lovaas method when implemented by community providers. Significant gains were reported in IQ in a sample of children with PDD NOS and autism, suggesting that the Lovaas model may have effects even when implemented out-side a university setting. Similarly, the Murdoch University Early Intervention Program (Birnbrauer & Leach, 1993) implemented the Lovaas model using community volunteers, who generally had less experience with behavioral analysis. Higher-functioning children (borderline or above IQ) were excluded. Gains in intelligence were not documented after the first 2 years of treatment, though nonstatistically tested observations of improvement in visual–spatial skills and behavior were reported. Two additional studies (Smith, Buch, & Gamby, 2000; Bibby, Eikeseth, Martin, Mudford, & Reeves, 2001) examined the effects of parent-managed interventions in which the UCLA method was presented in a workshop format, with professionals serving only as consul-tants to parents and the paraprofessional therapists they enlisted (a common method of service delivery). These studies found much smaller effects and fewer "best" outcomes, possibly due to decreased consistency in implement-ing treatment by these therapists.

In summary, the UCLA YAP model (Lovaas, 1987; Smith, Groen, et al., 2000) may now be considered a *probably efficacious* treatment of young chil-dren with autism (Rogers, in press). With investigations of its *effectiveness* being reported, it is awaiting independent replication, as well as investigation of its critical components and its efficacy with different subgroups of children with autism spectrum disorders.

Other Early Intervention Programs Based on ABA Principles

Douglass Developmental Disabilities Center

The Douglass Developmental Disabilities Center (DDDC) intervention devel-oped at Rutgers University targeted language, cognition, socialization, and motor and self-help skills using a sequential developmental approach. Cer-tified special education teachers implemented classroom work, often begin-ning with DTT and eventually working in groups of children. The DDDC model also made use of parent training and regular instruction with a speech and language therapist. The language development of children with autism placed in segregated versus integrated preschool classrooms with peer models was compared (Harris, Handleman, Kristoff, Bass, & Gordon, 1990), as were the effects of integrated classrooms on children with autism and typically de-veloping children (Harris, Handleman, Gordon, Kristoff, & Fuentes, 1991). All children, including the typically developing peer models, progressed in their language development. The presence of peer models did not appear to impact outcome in children with autism, though their presence has been shown to impact social development (Odom & Strain, 1986). However, the children with autism were relatively high functioning, classroom assignment was determined based on severity of behavior, and sample sizes were small. When children with autism were compared to typically developing children, Harris and colleagues (1991) reported relatively accelerated growth rates, though there were no data from a control group with autism. Age and intelligence at entry into the DDDC significantly correlated with long-term outcome, with better responses by younger, higher-functioning children and more modest benefits for older, lower-functioning children (Harris & Handleman, 2000).

Princeton Child Development Institute

Fenske and colleagues (1985) used an ABA approach, with teams of therapists implementing an intervention that targeted language, socialization, self-care, and leisure skills. Children rotated between different therapists every 30 minutes over 5 hours, and treatment duration and the types of service were customized to the needs of each child. Consultation with parents occurred monthly. Outcome was measured by living situation (at home vs. institutionalized) and school placement. Fenske et al. (1985) also attempted to investigate the effects of age at treatment and found that children entering the program prior to 60 months of age had more favorable outcomes than older children. However, age of enrollment was self-selecting and outcome measures were very limited.

Naturalistic ABA Approaches

One of the key criticisms of the DTT approach to behavioral intervention has been difficulty facilitating generalization beyond the treatment setting. As a result, more naturalistic behavioral methods have been developed. Such methods have been recognized as a best practice in intervention (National Research Council, 2001) and are considered an important complement to DTT (Smith, 2001) if their administration is systematic and planned.

Incidental Teaching and the Walden Early Childhood Programs

The earliest behavioral method to emphasize more naturalistic teaching approaches, "incidental teaching," was developed in the 1970s at the University of Kansas to increase language in impoverished children (Hart & Risley, 1974, 1975, 1980) and eventually applied to children with autism (McGee, Almeida, Sulzer-Azaroff, & Feldman, 1992), including preliminary work with toddlers (McGee et al., 1999). Incidental teaching seeks to create controlled, natural environments in which learning can take place by expanding the child's spontaneous behaviors at an appropriate developmental level. The environment may be carefully and creatively structured to promote child initiation. Drawing on ABA principles, this method capitalizes on children's activities by prompting an elaboration of the initial behavior for which children gain contingent access to the desired object or activity and receive praise, thereby reinforcing both the desired communicative behavior and the act of initiating it.

The Walden model described by McGee and colleagues (1999; McGee, Daly, & Jacobs, 1994) emphasizes incidental teaching both in the classroom and in the home (through the Walden Family Program), as well as the essential inclusion of the family. Walden emphasizes both the amount and quality of intervention, using specific methods of facilitating social integration with typical peer models and learning via enjoyable activities in a carefully planned environment. Teachers vigilantly track children's behaviors to make use of "teachable" moments and seek to increase the likelihood of initiation by creating opportunities (e.g., "marketing" an attractive toy). The Walden curriculum was created by an interdisciplinary team to develop expressive language, social interaction with peers and adults, appropriate toy play, and adaptive function. Early goals include responding to teachers and interacting appropriately with classroom materials; then expressive language is targeted, and, finally, conversation and peer interaction, to enable participants to learn from their typical peers. Evidence for the Walden Preschool's effects on language and increased peer interaction comes from both non-peer-reviewed publications (e.g., McGee et al., 1994) and single-subject experiments testing particular components of the model (McGee et al., 1992). An exciting new development, the Walden Toddler Model at Emory University (McGee et al., 1999), is designed for very young children with autism. Children entered the toddler program at an average age of 2 years, 5 months, and participated for at least 6 months. Preliminary findings include improvements from baseline in language function, proximity to other children, engagement in toy play, and adaptive function, but results from a comparison group were not reported.

Pivotal Response Training

While acknowledging that applied behavior analysis based on DTT appears to be useful for many children, Koegel and colleagues (1989; Koegel, Koegel, & Brookman, 2003) have suggested that acquisition of individual skills one at a time using a mass trial approach places too great a demand on all involved—the child, family, and therapist. Thus, the main focus of pivotal response training (PRT) is to teach key "pivotal" skills that can facilitate the rapid acquisition of related skills, resulting in more efficient behavioral change (Kazdin, 1982). This emphasis on efficiency and parsimony distinguishes PRT from other ABA models that emphasize intensive intervention targeting a variety of discrete behaviors, although it also employs a stimulus–response–consequence structure. PRT is delivered in a variety of natural settings by a variety of people, including parents. The curriculum is customized to the child and family, though key pivotal areas emphasize communication and include responsiveness to multiple cues, child initiation, self-regulation, and motivation. PRT techniques include use of preferred materials or activities, opportunities for child choice, natural reinforcers, and balance of maintenance and acquisition tasks to increase child motivation and success. PRT assumes that such approaches achieve the following: increase the likelihood

that the child's attention is naturally drawn to the correct cue; maximize opportunities for shared attention with the therapist; reduce frustration; focus
more child energy on learning rather than avoiding activities; and increase
motivation, which may reduce the need for teaching some discrete, collateral
skills such as eye contact (see Koegel, Koegel, Harrower, & Carter, 1999, for
a review of PRT techniques and philosophy). For example, to target question
initiation, Lynn Kern Koegel hid a child's favorite objects in an opaque bag
and taught the child to say "What's that" to access the bag's contents. Novel
items and new questions followed. Four children, who were comparable to a
"poor outcome" group studied retrospectively, in that they had similar low
levels of initiation prior to treatment, received the "What's that" intervention.
Initiation and adaptive function increased, and markedly different long-term
social, community, and diagnostic functioning were observed compared to the
low-initiation group from the retrospective analysis (Koegel, Koegel, Shoshan,
& NcNerney, 1999). Studies of PRT typically target outcomes related to the
pivotal behavior being tested rather than more global outcomes (e.g., IQ),
and most studies with preschoolers have used single-subject designs rather
than comparing PRT as a whole against other comprehensive treatments (e.g.,
Koegel, Camarata, Valdez-Menchaca, & Koegel, 1998; Koegel, Koegel,
Shoshan, & McNerney, 1999; Koegel, Koegel, & Surratt, 1992). Results from
such studies suggest that PRT can increase language responses and spontaneous initiations, and decrease disruptive behaviors.

Developmental Approaches Emphasizing Social Relationships

Denver Model

Based on the assumption that autism is largely a disorder of social relatedness
and communication, the Denver model developed by Rogers, Herbison,
Lewis, Pantone, and Reis (1986) emphasizes shared affect, joint activities, and
social communication, as well as play, language, and cognition. Central to the
model are three principles: First, given that a central impairment in autism is
difficulty in relating to other people, a primary goal of intervention is to facilitate the child's ability to form relationships with other people (i.e., care is
given to developing a positive relationship between the child and a consistent
classroom teacher). The model attends to the relationship-based aspects of the
interpersonal experience of intervention itself, such as mutual positive affect
fostered through enjoyable activities. Second, the model is sensitive to development in terms of both the child's level of development in different domains
and the approaches that are used to promote the acquisition of new skills.
The third principle of the model is the use of a variety of well-validated ABA
methods ranging from techniques such as incidental teaching, to more structured approaches such as DTT.

The theoretical perspective of the Denver model, expressed by Rogers
and Pennington (1991), proposes that missed early social milestones poten-

tially lead to secondary problems, including isolation from social interactions followed by more missed learning opportunities. Therefore, the child's relationships, including those with family and therapists, are a focus of intervention. To meet the needs of all family members, families are integrally involved with determining the direction of therapy. A multidisciplinary team approach, including special education, speech–language pathology, occupational therapy, psychology, and pediatrics, informs the treatment in terms of both the skills targeted and the treatment strategies.

The most recent and comprehensive summary of empirical findings for the Denver model (Rogers & DiLalla, 1991) included all children (including children with autism spectrum disorder [ASD], as well as a group with other behavioral, emotional, or developmental disorders) who attended the center-based Denver model playschool over a 9-year period. Rather than use of a control group, progress was tracked against expected developmental growth predicted from baseline. Participants with ASDs and other behavioral, emotional, or developmental disorders exhibited higher outcome scores than predicted by the initial growth rate. Although members of the group with ASD initially had more severe impairments in all domains, their growth rate for cognition and language matched that of the group with other disorders, and during treatment, children with autism had a normal language growth rate. Urban and rural replication sites similarly documented positive effects of the Denver model (Rogers, Lewis, & Reis, 1987). Conclusions regarding the efficacy of the Denver model are limited by the lack of a control group with ASD, which would remove ambiguity surrounding the effects of maturation versus the effects of intervention. One methodological strength of this work was the use of a variety of repeated measures to track development over time.

The Denver model communication curriculum was recently compared with the PROMPT (Prompts for Restructuring Oral–Muscular Phonetic Targets) method (Rogers et al., in press). The Denver model emphasizes imitation, learning of receptive language and object associations, and attempts increase vocal approximations, whereas PROMPT draws on neuromotor theory of speech production and employs tactile–kinesthetic information to shape language, cognition, and oral–motor function. Language gains made by preschoolers with ASD who used fewer than five words per day at baseline were measured against expected trajectories. Both groups benefited from receiving these naturalistic, developmental approaches to language intervention, gaining an average of 10 months in their receptive language abilities over approximately 3 months, though no language differences were found between the two treatments in this preliminary study. The groups differed on their amount of imitation and functional play during posttesting.

Autism Preschool Program

Jocelyn, Casiro, Beattie, Bow, and Kneisz (1998) developed a relatively short-term, multidisciplinary intervention to train parents and child care workers in Canadian community day care centers, which served primarily typically developing preschoolers. The Autism Preschool model (Child Development Clinic—Children's Hospital, Winnipeg) is developmental and primarily targets social and communication behaviors by training the adults working with each child to employ functional behavioral analysis, as well as approaches to social interaction and play. Intervention consisted of lectures, consultations, psychoeducation, and support work for families, above and beyond the day care program. Compared with many other intervention models presented, the Autism Preschool Program is relatively brief (3 months), less intense (a few hours a week), and targets the caregivers rather than the child directly. The group of children with trained caregivers and the group receiving day care alone were well matched, assignment was random, and evaluation before and after treatment was carried out by professionals blind to treatment assignment. Despite the limited intensity of intervention, significant positive benefits were observed, including language gains and increased knowledge of autism by caregivers, and perceived parental control. The two groups did not significantly differ on autism symptom severity. Long-term effects cannot be measured, because both groups ultimately received intervention.

Scottish Centre for Autism

Salt and colleagues (2001, 2002) designed a comprehensive, developmentally based program focusing on social development, communication, and flexibility. The Scottish Centre uses a naturalistic, child-directed approach specifically to target autism-related deficits such as imitation, joint referencing, language, adaptive function, emotion and attention regulation, social reciprocity, and play. Treatment techniques include imitation of the child, intrusion into nonsocial play, and parent training to refine communication skills. Although treatment delivery was less intense than many behavioral approaches, children in both groups spent a substantial number of additional hours in the preschool classroom and in outside treatments. Compared with a waitlisted group with significantly higher pretreatment IQ, the group receiving intervention showed significant improvement in socialization, daily living skills, motor function, adaptive behaviors, imitation, and joint attention. Language development improved in both groups, but no significant differences were found. Although the types of gains were qualitatively different than the IQ improvements reported in behavior analytic studies, the effect sizes in observational measures of imitation and joint attention are promising, particularly since these skills have been found to be important predictors of later outcome in autism (Dawson & Adams, 1984; Mundy & Crowson, 1997; Mundy, Sigman, & Kasari, 1990; Sigman & Ungerer, 1984; Stone, 1997). However, conclusions are limited by a small sample size and non-random assignment. Long term effects may not be examined because the waitlisted group was enrolled at the conclusion of the study.

Developmental, Individual-Difference, Relationship-Based Model/Floor Time

Greenspan and Wieder (1999; Greenspan, 1999) developed the Developmental, Individual-Difference, Relationship–Based model (DIR), which is highly individualized and focuses on the current developmental level of the child. DIR draws on literature beyond the study of autism (e.g., motor planning) and incorporates knowledge from other disciplines, including speech therapy, sensory integration, neurobiology, and medicine. The DIR approach begins with an extensive functional–developmental evaluation. Three domains are emphasized: functional emotional development, sensory–motor processing and planning, and relationships. The level and developmental appropriateness of parents' engagement with their children is assumed to be related to the child's cognitive development. DIR also assumes that children have unique, biologically driven sensory–motor–affective profiles, and therefore need special, individualized help with social–emotional and cognitive development. Thus, Floor Time emphasizes affective experiences and relationships, the ability to process and self-regulate emotion, and reciprocal communication, as well as the use of gesture, problem solving, logical thinking, and creativity. A distinguishing feature of Floor Time is that the child directs the interaction and the parent or therapist builds intervention around the play of the child, without targeting specific skills. Evidence for this model (Greenspan & Wieder, 1997) is based on a large-scale chart review of children who received DIR model intervention for at least 2 years compared with children receiving community-based interventions. Over half the children participating in Floor Time had "good to outstanding" outcomes regarding spontaneous symbolic abilities, intent, affect, and symptom severity, compared with only 2% in the community group, and did not differ in emotional function from typical children. However, the sample was nonrepresentative of the population with autism, families were self-selecting, and data were descriptive, based on chart review. Thus, conclusions regarding the efficacy of DIR are very limited.

Child's Talk

This approach to intervention capitalizes on core social and communication deficits in autism (Aldred, Green, & Adams, 2004; Aldred, Pollard, Phillips, & Adams, 2001). It assumes that parents have more resources to invest in the long-run than professionals and targets them in treatment. Using video feedback, specific aspects of the parent–child interaction are examined, and strategies are developed to improve specific aspects of the dyadic communication, making it more synchronous. This provides both parents with the opportunity to evaluate their own interactions and refine the interaction to fit the child's developmental level. Shared attention, parental sensitivity and responsiveness, adapted communication, and modeling are emphasized. Child's Talk is particularly designed for use with children with lower language functioning (i.e., not children with Asperger syndrome), though children with no desire to interact or global developmental delays were excluded in this trial. Intervention begins with psychoeducation for parents, then six monthly consultations, followed by 6 months of less frequent maintenance sessions. Parents are asked to spend 30 minutes a day implementing therapy at home during treatment, with the hope that the effects "spill over" into other parent–child interactions. Child's Talk may be used to complement other treatments. Its effects, compared with community standard care alone, are documented with a methodologically sound, randomized trial, with independent evaluation using standardized measures of a broad range of symptoms. There were no significant group differences between types or amounts of community treatments received. Significant improvements were documented in symptom severity, expressive language, initiation of communication, and parent–child interaction, though not in adaptive function or parent stress.

Structured Teaching Approach

The TEACCH model (Treatment and Education of Autistic and Related Communication-Handicapped Children) was developed at the University of North Carolina, Chapel Hill, by Schopler, Brehm, Kinsbourne, and Reichler (1971; Schopler, Reichler, and Lansing, 1980). This program typically takes place in a classroom setting that is deliberately engineered to exploit the strengths and compensate for the weaknesses associated with autism (e.g., taking advantage of a visual processing advantage by using visual cues such as the location of learning materials or picture schedules). Yet TEACCH may be implemented in a variety of settings, including the home, and across a range of ages, preschool to adulthood. At the preschool level, social and communication development are particularly targeted. Predictability and routine rather than therapist direction are used to create a structured, rule-based environment. This promotes self-direction, which is assumed to be an important learning skill. The TEACCH classroom also makes use of the location of students and may begin by placing children in individual carrels, so that their work environment is quiet and free from distraction. Gradually, the child may progress to a table with dividers and eventually to an open table with other students. This allows for appropriate pacing and individualization of each child's tasks to best suit individual needs. Parents are engaged as cotherapists, directed to seminars and psychoeducation, and are believed to be integral to treatment success. The founders of TEACCH were among the first to advocate for this important relationship with families (e.g., Schopler & Reichler, 1971).

A variety of the published investigations of the TEACCH program are suggestive of positive effects; it is widely used and claims long-term benefits (Mesibov, 1997b). However, most have not used a control group, have used pseudoexperimental or nonexperimental designs, and have not targeted preschoolers. One recent study (Ozonoff & Cathcart, 1998) compared matched groups of young children who were nonrandomly assigned to receive either home-based, parent-implemented TEACCH programming or no home-based intervention. Many children in both groups also received Lovaas-based day programming, which was standard practice in the state where the study took place, and all children received day programming of some kind, suggesting that the combination of these treatments is feasible. The intensity of treatment administered was less than that in many other studies (about 4½ hours per week over 10 weeks). Programming was nonmanualized, following the individual needs of each child and his or her family, but included common elements such as structured teaching, use of visual strengths, schedules, and emphasis on preacademic skills. In general, psychoeducational skills improved significantly in the treated group, and children with higher baseline scores improved most.

COST–BENEFIT ANALYSES

Given the great amount of time and money required to implement early, intensive intervention, it is important to address the question of costs versus benefits. Jacobson, Mulick, and Green (1998) conducted a cost–benefit analysis of early, intensive behavioral intervention (based on ABA) with autism and found that the costs of not treating children greatly outweigh those involved with treatment. Assuming that 40–50% of children with autism or PDD who receive treatment go on to achieve normal functioning, the savings compared to ineffective or no treatment are estimated to be approximately $275,000 through age 22, and from $2.4 to $2.8 million through age 55. As Jacobson and Mulick noted (2000), these analyses are limited by their focus on the financial impact of autism and overlook the emotional and human costs associated with positive versus negative outcomes. They assume that change over time will be linear, and that long-term mental health services will be comparable to current ones in benefit and cost. Various treatment delivery methods were not compared by providing projections for alternative behavioral and developmental approaches. Another important limitation is that the 40–50% recovery rate reported in work by Lovaas (1987) is a relatively large effect size for *normal* outcome compared with other treatment studies, including recent replications of Lovaas's method (e.g., Smith, Groen, et al., 2000). The use of more modest rates of positive outcome would reduce the benefit-to-cost ratio. Marcus, Rubin, and Rubin (2000) further caution that current cost–benefit analyses may not fully incorporate current knowledge that even children with autism who make the most significant gains (i.e., regular education placement) are not likely to be completely "recovered" and often require continued support, particularly in the social domain. On the other hand, although it can be argued that the cost–benefit analysis conducted by Jacobson and colleagues (1998) used optimistic outcome estimations, they did not include the secondary cost savings that are likely to exist when early intervention is provided. These include the costs of (1) prevention of severe problem behaviors in children of all functioning levels, which often require inpatient hospitalization and/or a highly restrictive treatment setting (e.g., one-on-one, 24-hour supervision), and (2) prevention or amelioration of medical and psychological problems that accompany high levels of stress in parents and siblings when appropriate services are not provided. Such problems include depression, anxiety, marital difficulties, and other stress-related physical ailments. Because autism is a chronic condition affecting not only the child but also the family, it is important to understand the effects of treatment not only on the particular symptom or symptoms it targets, but also its effects on the entire child and family.

BRIEF COMMENTS ON "FOCAL" TREATMENTS AND NONPSYCHOSOCIAL INTERVENTIONS

A variety of interventions have also been developed to target specific domains of impairment associated with autism, rather than treating the entire syndrome comprehensively. Many of these interventions are used in conjunction with other comprehensive treatments. A recent sampling of targeted skills includes self-directed play (Morrison, Sainato, Benchaaban, & Endo, 2002), theory of mind (Hadwin, Baron-Cohen, Howlin, & Hill, 1997) and joint attention (Whalen & Schreibman, 2003), although this is by no means a comprehensive list. Finally, recent review of behavioral studies targeting problem behaviors such as inappropriate toileting, self-harm, and aggression was conducted by Horner, Carr, Strain, Todd, and Reed (2002).

Treatments directly targeting the biochemistry of individuals with autism have also been described. Although most medical interventions have not been rigorously tested with very young children, and the theoretical knowledge of the mechanism of effectiveness of various drugs is limited by lack of clear understanding of the neurobiology and genetics of autism, a few key findings are worth mentioning. There is growing recognition for the need to integrate neurochemical findings and treatment approaches with existing behavioral knowledge of autism as the neurodevelopmental and genetic underpinnings of autism become increasingly well understood (Tsai, 2000; Volkmar, 2001). As Volkmar notes, psychopharmacology may be of particular utility when used to complement behavioral intervention targeting social and communication development, because the repetitive behaviors, attention and hyperactivity, sleep disturbances, behavioral inflexibility, and self-injury or aggression that often accompany autism may be clearly targeted biochemically. By reducing disruptive behaviors, children may be better prepared to benefit from psychosocial intervention. A thorough review of psychopharmacological approaches to treatment is provided by Luby, Chapter 14, this volume. Furthermore, it is increasingly recognized that children with autism, like all children, experience a range of medical conditions, such as sleep and gastrointestinal problems, that can interfere with their ability to engage in behavioral interventions. It is important for practitioners to assess and treat such medical conditions, so that the child's ability to benefit from psychosocial intervention can be maximized.

A variety of alternative interventions with a range of proposed theoretical explanations have also emerged. These interventions include auditory or sensory integration techniques, music therapy, communication systems (e.g., facilitated communication), dietary approaches (e.g., gluten- and casein-free diet, vitamins), hormone therapies (e.g., melatonin, secretin), immunological therapies, and work with animals (e.g., swimming with dolphins, therapeutic horseback riding). Although claims have been made about the positive effects of various alternative treatments, there has been scant scientific support of many such methods to date. The heterogeneity of ASDs allows for the possibility that a subset of children may have unique etiological factors that would allow them to respond to some more theoretically based alternative treatments, such as the dietary approaches. However, this possibility and the methods for identifying such children remain to be carefully evaluated scientifically.

A recent evaluation of the prevalence of complementary and alternative medicine usage by Levy, Mandell, Merhar, Ittenbach, and Pinto-Martin (2003) found that almost a third of parents were using some sort of alternative medical intervention, including treatments that involve medical risk (e.g., cod liver oil, anti-infectives, chelation, or withholding of immunizations). It is important for providers to better understand and be sensitive to the reasons that lead parents to select alternative methods of intervention. Such understanding will give providers and developers of psychosocial treatments important information about the process by which parents select treatment, as well as parental factors that may mediate family commitment to treatment, such as perceived positive outcome, intuitively appealing theoretical rationale, social reinforcement, and parental support (Siegel & Zimnitzky, 1998; Smith & Antolovich, 2000). It is also imperative that well-designed clinical studies on the effectiveness of such alternative treatments be conducted. Large placebo effects have been reported in randomized investigations of secretin (Sandler & Bodfish, 2000; Unis et al., 2002), and 75% of parents who participated continued to believe secretin was an effective treatment after being told of the equivocal findings. Although the placebo effect is poorly understood in autism, this phenomenon likely contributes to the perceived efficacy of many treatments, including alternative ones. As Hansen and Ozonoff (2003) point out, the arena of alternative treatments provides practitioners with an opportunity to collaborate with parents by striving for a balance between remaining open-minded and fair toward novel, nonsupported treatments and cautioning against treatments that are potentially harmful or compete for resources with an empirically supported treatment. One way to collaborate positively is to assist parents in repeated online evaluations of treatment effects.

FUTURE RESEARCH DIRECTIONS

A critical question faced by treatment providers and parents is the decision of which treatment is best suited to the individual needs of the child. Despite strong assertions about the need for evidence-based decision making, there is limited evidence addressing this question to date. Importantly, there is no evidence of universal response to even the most promising treatments, underscoring the need to understand individual differences and to investigate the benefits of various treatments with different types of children (Rogers, 1998). Delprato (2001), in a review of mostly multiple-baseline and reversal design studies, compared findings with discrete trial approaches to more naturalistic interventions (e.g., incidental teaching, PRT) in young children, and found support for better language outcomes in children receiving naturalistic interventions, but noted that these approaches may be best used together, because each approach may better facilitate different aspects of language learning. Looking more broadly, there is overlap between treatment types. Eclectically implementing two treatment models has been acknowledged in a variety of studies, and in particular, benefits have been observed when children receiving an ABA approach were treated with a second, more developmental or naturalistic approach (e.g., Smith, 2001; Ozonoff & Cathcart, 1998; Greenspan & Wieder, 1997; Aldred et al., 2004). Finally, a variety of child factors appear predictive of outcome regardless of treatment selection, including cognitive ability, the presence of language (even abnormal echolalic vocalizations), early imitation skills, dysmorphology, and, importantly, age at intervention (e.g., Fenske et al., 1985; Harris & Handleman, 2000; Lovaas, 1987; Mundy et al., 1990; Stoelb et al., 2004).

Although individual responses to treatment remain poorly understood, parents are beginning to have more treatment options backed by substantial scientific support, such as the UCLA model (Smith, Groen, et al., 2000). Such interventions produced effects in at least some children, who received carefully implemented therapy in controlled settings, such that children improved on average. But no approach has been clearly documented in a head-to-head study, and the specific "active ingredients" of such treatments are unknown and need further investigation. Some elements likely to be involved in producing more positive outcomes were identified by Dawson and Osterling (1997): a carefully designed, comprehensive curriculum targeting attention, imitation, language, play, and social interaction; a deliberately structured and supportive environment for initial learning, accompanied by scaffolding to implement generalization to other contexts; predictability and routine; prevention of problem behaviors and a functional approach to reduce or eliminate existing ones; preparation for advancement to kindergarten by fostering independence in the academic setting; inclusion of the family; and high intensity of intervention. Many of these are echoed in the National Research Council recommendations for practitioners (2001). Factors that currently distinguish existing treatments, such as the presence of typically developing peer models or parental communication skills, may be of particular interest when examining which aspects of treatment are most effective with different types of children. Despite recent work identifying common features of accepted preschool interventions as "best practices," current practitioners face a great deal of complexity in navigating available treatment options. Substantial differences exist in the conceptualization of autism and its etiology, short- and long-term treatment goals, and the outcomes emphasized by various treatment methods. In addition, questions such as "How much is enough?" and "Which approach is best for my child?" are currently impossible to answer based on research. Currently, it is recommended that each child be carefully evaluated prior to beginning treatment, followed by repeated evaluations of progress using single-subject experimental designs (Woods & Wetherby, 2003). Based on available evidence, the National Research Council (2001) task force recommended that preschool-age children with autism received at least 25 hours of structured intervention weekly.

Better understanding of predictors and outcome will be made possible by exploring a broader range of variables, overcoming difficulties in measurement, and improving research design. Recent reviews (Kasari, 2002; Wolery & Garfinkle, 2002) recommend a variety of broad, standardized measures that specifically include symptom reduction and treatment fidelity, as well as other risk and protective factors. Wolery and Garfinkle (2002) noted little measurement of imitation, attention, social engagement, or appropriate play, and suggested that measurement of parental perceptions and functioning, as well as other family factors, may uncover important intervening variables in treatment outcome. Improvements in design are also needed (e.g., growth curve analyses, reporting reliability of measures, and examining intervening effects such as treatment fidelity). To advance current understanding, it is clear that larger sample sizes will be needed to resolve most lingering questions (understanding of individual differences, predictors of outcome, essential treatment factors, etc.) Two specific types of analysis would be of particular utility in evaluating outstanding questions: *factor analysis*, which addresses which aspects of treatment are essential to outcome and therefore potentially lead to more efficient use of resources in intervention; and *meta-analysis*, which addresses which kind of treatment best serves different types of children, and the intensity of intervention necessary to produce effects. Clearly however, existing measurement techniques greatly limit the power of factor- and meta-analytic methods. Here again, collaboration among scientists, practitioners, and parents to test treatments, predictive factors, and individual differences is crucial and will likely benefit all involved.

RECENT ADVANCES IN CURRENT UNDERSTANDING

In recent years, several key advances are likely to inform remaining questions about treatment of preschoolers. For instance, the work by Smith, Groen, et al.

(2000) now serves as probably efficacious treatment to which interventions may now be compared. Head-to-head comparison of two existing treatment approaches may be more palatable ethically and practically than comparison of treatment to placebo or no treatment, and both are acceptable methods for determining efficacious treatments. By removing such ethical and practical barriers, the door is now opened to more rigorous evaluation of the efficacy of other interventions for preschoolers. In addition, current replications by the Multisite Young Autism Project (Smith, Groen, et al., 2000) will be very useful in extending the knowledge of a DTT approach, including effectiveness, efficacy, and understanding interactions between children and essential treatment factors.

Two additional advancements stem from federal funding mechanisms that enable more comprehensive investigation of intervention, as well as advancement in clinical methods. First, collaborations with state education systems funded by the Individuals with Disabilities Education Act may provide a beneficial alternative by which to capture outcome. Arick and colleagues (2003) described such a model for measuring gains made by children in the Oregon public schools, which follows a large cohort of children statewide by repeated collection of meaningful standardized measures. The program, which also educates teachers via training, manuals, and classroom observation in behavioral techniques such as DTT, PRT, and functional routines, was viewed positively by most teachers who welcomed the opportunity to track student progress and receive consultation. Collaborations between psychology and education are a potentially positive complement to existing research, providing an opportunity for large-scale assessment of interventions and, possibly, a way to compare different treatment models.

Second, the NIH is promoting multisite collaborative investigations of treatment for autism that leverage the personnel, funding, and expertise necessary to conduct methodologically rigorous intervention research. Participants in such projects may also be enrolled simultaneously in basic research on the etiology of autism, providing better opportunities to understand individual genetic and other biological differences with respect to treatment outcome and to test competing theories in the treatment literature. Studies of novel, early interventions have been incorporated into the NIMH Studies to Advance Autism Research and Treatment (STAART) program. For example, the University of Washington team is examining the efficacy of downward extension of the Denver model that provides comprehensive, intensive early intervention for toddlers with autism. Development of new strategies that can be used with infants and toddlers will be increasingly important as methods of early detection of infants at risk for autism improve.

In conclusion, solid scientific research on the effectiveness of intervention is essential in making long-range public policy decisions, because cost–benefit analyses are, at best, only as good as the current state of the art of treatment research. Careful scientific evaluation of treatments also enables practitioners, educators, and families to better judge immediately what treatments are effective, allowing parents and educational professionals to work together to optimize limited resources. Use of an inappropriate treatment strategy, at best, delays or prevents delivery of more appropriate intervention, impacting the potential positive development of the child with autism, and, at worst, produces unintended negative consequences for the child, causes considerable stress for the family, and wastes valuable resources of time and money. In spite of these compelling reasons for careful evaluation of treatments, parents and practitioners are presented with a vast array of potential treatment options with varying degrees of scientific support. This array of treatment options challenges clinical scientists to conduct timely research and evaluation of newly developed methods, and practitioners to evaluate the current treatment options and provide appropriate recommendations to families.

A wide variety of interventions have been discussed with respect to their different theoretical underpinnings, similarities, techniques, and empirical support. Such a review uncovers a broad range of options for parents to implement, with varying empirical support. Yet little conclusive evidence to date supports one treatment relative to another, understanding of individual difference in treatment response, or factors that may most efficiently lead to positive outcome. A second wave of research with far more sophisticated methodology and larger-scale multisite collaborations is currently underway and offers hope to service providers, families, and young children with autism. Early detection and a shift in focus to increasingly younger ages offer additional hope. At the intersection of research and practice, the clinician provides a unique perspective to the resolution of the large public health issues presented by ASDs, because exploration of center-based, carefully controlled model intervention programs in community settings is a vital next step for researchers.

ACKNOWLEDGMENTS

The writing of this chapter was funded by a program project grant from the National Institute of Child Health and Human Development and the National Institute on Deafness and Communication Disability (No. U19HD34565), which is part of the NICHD/NIDCD Collaborative Program of Excellence in Autism and by a center grant from the National Institute of Mental Health (No. U54MH066399), which is part of the NIMH STAART Centers Program.

REFERENCES

Aldred, C., Green, J., & Adams, C. (2004). A new social communication intervention for children with autism: Pilot randomized controlled treatment study suggesting effectiveness. *Journal of Child Psychology and Psychiatry, 45,* 1420–1430.

Aldred, C., Pollard, C., Phillips, R., & Adams, C. (2001). Multidisciplinary social communication intervention for children with autism and pervasive developmental disorder: The Child's Talk project. *Educational and Child Psychology, 18,* 76–87.

American Psychiatric Association. (1980). *Diagnostic and statistical manual of mental disorders* (3rd ed.). Washington, DC: Author.

American Psychiatric Association. (1994). *Diagnostic and statistical manual of mental disorders* (4th ed.). Washington, DC: Author.

Arick, J. R., Young, H. E., Falco, R. A., Loos, L. M., Krug, D. A., Gense, M. H., et al. (2003). Designing an outcome study to monitor the progress of students with autism spectrum disorders. *Focus on Autism and Other Developmental Disabilities, 18,* 74–86.

Bibby, P., Eikeseth, S., Martin, N. T., Mudford, O. C., & Reeves, D. (2001). Progress and outcomes for children with autism receiving parent-managed intensive interventions. *Research in Developmental Disabilities, 22,* 425–447.

Birnbrauer, J. S., & Leach, D. J. (1993). The Murdoch Early Intervention Program after 2 years. *Behaviour Change, 10,* 63–74.

Bristol, M. M., Cohen, D. J., Costello, E. J., Denckla, M., Eckberg, T. J., Kallen, R., et al. (1996). State of the science in autism: Report to the National Institutes of Health. *Journal of Autism and Developmental Disorders, 26,* 121–154.

Chambless, D. L., & Hollon, S. D. (1998). Defining empirically supported therapies. *Journal of Counseling and Clinical Psychology, 66,* 7–18.

Chandler, S., Christie, P., Newson, E., & Prevezer, W. (2002). Developing a diagnostic and intervention package for 2– to 3–year-olds with autism. *Autism, 6,* 47–69.

Dawson, G., & Adams, A. (1984). Imitation and social responsiveness in autistic children. *Journal of Abnormal Child Psychology, 12,* 209–225.

Dawson, G., & Osterling, J. (1997). Early intervention in autism: Effectiveness and common elements of current approaches. In M. J. Guralnick (Ed.), *The effectiveness of early intervention: Second generation research* (pp. 307–326). Baltimore: Brookes.

Dawson, G., Osterling, J., Meltzoff, A. N., & Kuhl, P. (2000). Case study of the development of an infant with autism from birth to two years of age. *Journal of Applied Developmental Psychology, 21,* 299–313.

Dawson, G., & Zanolli, K. (2003). Early intervention and brain plasticity in autism. In G. Bock & J. Goode (Eds.), *Autism: Neural bases and treatment possibilities* (Novartis Foundation Symposium 251, pp. 266–280). Chichester, UK: Wiley.

Delprato, D. J. (2001). Comparisons of discrete-trial and normalized behavioral language intervention for young children with autism. *Journal of Autism and Developmental Disorders, 31,* 315–325.

Drew, A., Baird, G., Baron-Cohen, S., Cox, A., Slonims, V., Wheelwright, S., et al. (2002). A pilot randomized control trial of a parent training intervention for pre-school children with autism: Preliminary findings and methodological challenges. *European Child and Adolescent Psychiatry, 11,* 266–272.

Fenske, E. C., Zalenski, S., Krantz, P. J., & McClanahan, L. E. (1985). Age at intervention and treatment outcome for autistic children in a comprehensive intervention program. *Analysis and Intervention in Developmental Disabilities, 5,* 49–58.

Ferster, C. B., & DeMeyer, M. K. (1961). The development of performances in autistic children in an automatically controlled environment. *Journal of Chronic Diseases, 13,* 312–345.

Fombonne, E. (2003). Epidemiological surveys of autism and other pervasive developmental disorders: An update. *Journal of Autism and Developmental Disorders, 33,* 365–382.

Green, G., Brennan, L. C., & Fein, D. (2002). Intensive behavioral treatment for a toddler at high risk for autism. *Behavior Modification, 26,* 69–102.

Greenspan, S. I. (1992). *Infancy and early childhood: The practice of clinical assessment and intervention with emotional and developmental challenges.* Madison, CT: International Universities Press.

Greenspan, S. I., & Wieder, S. (1997). Developmental patterns and outcomes in infants and children with disorders in relating and communicating: A chart review of 200 cases of children with autism spectrum diagnoses. *Journal of Developmental and Learning Disorders, 1,* 87–141.

Greenspan, S. I., & Wieder, S. (1999). A functional developmental approach to autism spectrum disorders. *Journal of the Association for Persons with Severe Handicaps, 24*, 147–161.

Hadwin, J., Baron-Cohen, S., Howlin, P., & Hill, K. (1997). Does teaching theory of mind have an effect on the ability to develop conversation in children with autism? *Journal of Autism and Developmental Disorders, 27*, 519–537.

Hansen, R. L., & Ozonoff, S. (2003). Alternative therapies: Assessment and therapy options. In S. Ozonoff, S. J. Rogers, & R. Hendren (Eds.) *Autism spectrum disorders: A research review for practitioners* (pp. 187–207). Washington, DC: American Psychiatric Publishing.

Harris, S. L., & Handleman, J. S. (2000). Age and IQ at intake as predictors of placement for young children with autism: A four- to six-year follow-up. *Journal of Autism and Developmental Disorders, 30*, 137–142.

Harris, S. L., Handleman, J. S., Gordon, R., Kristoff, B., & Fuentes, F. (1991). Changes in cognitive and language functioning of preschool children with autism. *Journal of Autism and Developmental Disorders, 21*, 281–290.

Harris, S. L., Handleman, J. S., Kristoff, B., Bass, L., & Gordon, R. (1990). Changes in language development among autistic and peer children in segregated and integrated preschool settings. *Journal of Autism and Developmental Disorders, 20*, 23–31.

Hart, B., & Risley, T. R. (1974). Using preschool materials to modify the language of disadvantaged children. *Journal of Applied Behavior Analysis, 7*, 243–256.

Hart, B., & Risley, T. R. (1975). Incidental teaching of language in the preschool. *Journal of Applied Behavior Analysis, 8*, 411–420.

Hart, B., & Risley, T. R. (1980). *In vivo* language intervention: Unanticipated general effects. *Journal of Applied Behavior Analysis, 13*, 407–432.

Horner, R. H., Carr, E. G., Strain, P. S., Todd, A. W., & Reed, H. K. (2002). Problem behavior interventions for young children with autism: A research synthesis. *Journal of Autism and Developmental Disorders, 32*, 423–446.

Jacobson, J. W., & Mulick, J. A. (2000). System and cost research issues in treatments for people with autistic disorders. *Journal of Autism and Developmental Disorders, 30*, 585–593.

Jacobson, J. W., Mulick, J. A., & Green, G. (1998). Cost–benefit estimates for early intensive behavioral intervention for young children with autism—General model and single state case. *Behavioral Interventions, 13*, 201–226.

Jocelyn, L. J., Casiro, O. G., Beattie, D., Bow, J., & Kneisz, J. (1998). Treatment of children with autism: A randomized controlled trial to evaluate a caregiver-based intervention program in community day-care centers. *Journal of Developmental and Behavioral Pediatrics, 19*, 326–334.

Kanner, L. (1943). Autistic disturbances of affective contact. *Nervous Child, 2*, 217–250.

Kasari, C. (2002). Assessing change in early intervention programs for children with autism. *Journal of Autism and Developmental Disorders, 32*, 447–461.

Kazdin, A. E. (1982). Symptom substitution, generalization, and response covariation: Implications for psychotherapy outcome. *Psychological Bulletin, 91*, 349–365.

Kazdin, A. E. (2002). *Research design in clinical psychology* (4th ed.). Needham Heights, MA: Allyn & Bacon.

Koegel, L. K., Camarata, S. M., Valdez-Menchaca, M., & Koegel, R. L. (1998). Setting generalization of question-asking by children with autism. *American Journal on Mental Retardation, 102*, 346–357.

Koegel, L. K., & Koegel, R. L. (1995). Motivating communication in children with autism. In E. Schopler & G. B. Mesibov (Eds.), *Learning and cognition in autism: Current issues in autism* (pp. 73–87). New York: Plenum Press.

Koegel, L. K., Koegel, R. L., Harrower, J. K., & Carter, C. M. (1999). Pivotal response intervention I: Overview of approach. *Journal of the Association for Persons with Severe Handicaps, 24*, 174–185.

Koegel, L. K., Koegel, R. L., Shoshan, Y., & McNerney, E. (1999). Pivitol response intervention II: Preliminary long-term outcome data. *Journal of the Association for Persons with Severe Handicaps, 24,* 186–198.

Koegel, R. L., Koegel, L. K., & Brookman, L. I. (2003). Empirically supported pivotal response interventions for children with autism. In A. E. Kazdin (Ed.), *Evidence-based psychotherapies for children and adolescents* (pp. 341–357). New York: Guilford Press.

Koegel, R. L., Koegel, L. K., & Surratt, A. (1992). Language intervention and disruptive behavior in preschool children with autism. *Journal of Autism and Developmental Disorders, 22,* 141–153.

Koegel, R. L., Schreibman, L., Good, A. B., Cerniglia, L., Murphy, C., & Koegel, L. K. (1989). *How to teach pivotal behaviors to autistic children: A training manual.* Santa Barbara: University of California Press.

Levy, S. E., Mandell, D. S., Merhar, S., Ittenbach, R. F., & Pinto-Martin, J. A. (2003). Use of complementary and alternative medicine among children recently diagnosed with autistic spectrum disorder. *Journal of Developmental and Behavioral Pediatrics, 24,* 418–423.

Lonigan, C. J., Elbert, J. C., & Johnson, S. B. (1998). Empirically supported psychosocial interventions for children: An overview. *Journal of Clinical Child Psychology, 27,* 138–145.

Lord, C., Risi, S., Lambrecht, L., Cook, E. H., Leventhal, B. L., DiLavore, P. C., et al. (2000). The autism diagnostic observation schedule—Generic: A standard measure of social and communication deficits associated with the spectrum of autism. *Journal of Autism and Developmental Disorders, 30,* 205–223.

Lord, C., Rutter, M., & Le Couteur, A. (1994). Autistic Diagnostic Interview—Revised: A revised version of a diagnostic interview for caregivers of individuals with possible pervasive developmental disorder. *Journal of Autism and Developmental Disorders, 24,* 659–685.

Lovaas, O. I. (1987). Behavioral treatment and normal educational and intellectual functioning in young autistic children. *Journal of Consulting and Clinical Psychology, 55,* 3–9.

Lovaas, O. I., Ackerman, A. B., Alexander, D., Firestone, P., Perkins, J., & Young, D. (1981). *Teaching developmentally disabled children: The me book.* Austin, TX: PRO-ED.

Lovaas, O. I., Smith, T., & McEachin, J. J. (1989). Clarifying comments on the Young Autism Study: Reply to Schopler, Short, and Mesibov. *Journal of Consulting and Clinical Psychology, 57,* 165–167.

Mahoney, G., & Perales, F. (2003). Using relationship-focused intervention to enhance the social–emotional functioning of young children with autism spectrum disorders. *Topics in Early Childhood Special Education, 23,* 74–86.

Marcus, L. M., Rubin, J. S., & Rubin, M. A. (2000). Benefit–cost analysis and autism services: A response to Jacobson and Mulick. *Journal of Autism and Developmental Disorders, 30,* 595–598.

McEachin, J. J., Smith, T., & Lovaas, O. I. (1993). Long-term outcome for children with autism who received early intensive behavioral treatment. *American Journal on Mental Retardation, 97,* 359–372.

McGee, G. G., Almeida, C., Sulzer-Azaroff, B., & Feldman, R. S. (1992). Promoting reciprocal interactions via peer incidental teaching. *Journal of Applied Behavior Analysis, 25,* 117–126.

McGee, G. G., Daly, T., & Jacobs, H. A. (1994). The Walden Preschool. In S. L. Harris & J. S. Handleman (Eds.), *Preschool education programs for children with autism* (pp. 127–162). Austin, TX: PRO-ED.

McGee, G. G., Morrier, M. J., & Daly, T. (1999). An incidental teaching approach to early intervention for toddlers with autism. *Journal of the Association for Persons with Severe Handicaps, 24,* 133–146.

Mesibov, G. B. (1997a). Preschool issues in autism: Introduction. *Journal of Autism and Developmental Disorders, 27,* 637–640.

Mesibov, G. B. (1997b). Formal and informal measures on the effectiveness of the TEACCH programme. *Autism, 1,* 25–35.

Morrison, R. S., Sainato, D. M., Benchaaban, D., & Endo, S. (2002). Increasing play skills of children with autism using activity schedules and correspondence training. *Journal of Early Intervention, 25,* 58–72.

Mundy, P., & Crowson, M. (1997). Joint attention and early social communication: Implications for research on intervention with autism. *Journal of Autism and Developmental Disorders, 27,* 653–676.

Mundy, P., Sigman, M., & Kasari, C. (1990). A longitudinal study of joint attention and language development in autistic children. *Journal of Autism and Developmental Disorders, 20,* 115–128.

National Research Council, Committee on Educational Interventions for Children with Autism, Division of Behavioral and Social Sciences and Education. (2001). *Educating children with autism* (C. Lord & J. McGee, Eds.). Washington, DC: National Academy Press.

Odom, S. L., Brown, W. H., Frey, T., Karasu, N., Smith-Canter, L. L., & Strain, P. S. (2003). Evidence-based practices for young children with autism: Contributions for single-subject design research. *Focus on Autism and Other Developmental Disabilities, 18,* 166–175.

Odom, S. L., & Strain, P. S. (1986). A comparison of peer-initiation and teacher-antecedent interventions for promoting reciprocal social interaction of autistic preschoolers. *Journal of Applied Behavior Analysis, 19,* 59–71.

Osterling, J., & Dawson, G. (1994). Early recognition of children with autism: A study of first birthday home video tapes. *Journal of Autism and Developmental Disorders, 24,* 247–257.

Ozonoff, S., & Cathcart, K. (1998). Effectiveness of a home program intervention for young children with autism. *Journal of Autism and Developmental Disorders, 28,* 25–32.

Ramey, C. T., & Ramey, S. L. (1998). Early intervention and early experience. *American Psychologist, 53,* 109–120.

Ritvo, E. R., & Freeman, B. J. (1978). National society for autistic children definition for the syndrome of autism. *Journal of Autism and Childhood Schizophrenia, 8,* 162–167.

Robins, D. L., Fein, D., Barton, M. L., & Green, J. A. (2001). The Modified Checklist for Autism in Toddlers: An initial study investigating the early detection of autism and pervasive developmental disorders. *Journal of Autism and Developmental Disorders, 31,* 131–144.

Rogers, S. J. (1998). Empirically supported comprehensive treatments for young children with autism. *Journal of Clinical Child Psychology, 27,* 168–179.

Rogers, S. J. (in press). Empirically supported comprehensive treatments for early autism. *Journal of Child Clinical Psychology.*

Rogers, S. J., & DiLalla, D. L. (1991). A comparative study of the effects of a developmentally based instructional model on young children with autism and young children with other disorders of behavior and development. *Topics in Early Childhood Special Education, 11,* 29–47.

Rogers, S. J., Hayden, D., Hepburn, S., Charlifue-Smith, R., Hall, T., & Hayes, A. (in press). Teaching young nonverbal children with autism useful speech: A pilot study of the Denver Model and PROMPT interventions. *Journal of Autism and Developmental Disorders.*

Rogers, S. J., Herbison, J. M., Lewis, H. C., Pantone, J., & Reis, K. (1986). An approach for enhancing the symbolic, communicative, and interpersonal functioning of young children with autism or severe emotional handicaps. *Journal of the Division for Early Childhood, 10,* 135–148.

Rogers, S. J., Lewis, H. C., & Reis, K. (1987). An effective procedure for training early special education teams to implement a model program. *Journal of the Division for Early Childhood, 11,* 180–188.

Rogers, S. J., & Pennington, B. F. (1991). A theoretical approach to the deficits in infantile autism. *Development and Psychopathology, 3,* 137–162.

Salt, J., Sellars, V., Shemilt, J., Boyd, S., Coulson, T., & McCool, S. (2001). The Scottish Centre for Autism preschool treatment programme: I. A developmental approach to early intervention. *Autism, 5,* 362–373.

Salt, J., Shemilt, J., Sellars, V., Boyd, S., Coulson, T., & McCool, S. (2002). The Scottish Centre for Autism preschool treatment programme: II. The results of a controlled treatment outcome study. *Autism, 6,* 33–46.

Sandler, A. D., & Bodfish, J. W. (2000). Placebo effects in autism: Lessons from secretin. *Journal of Developmental and Behavioral Pediatrics, 21,* 347–350.

Schopler, E., Brehm, S. S., Kinsbourne, M., & Reichler, R. J. (1971). Effect of treatment structure on development in autistic children. *Archives of General Psychiatry, 24,* 415–421.

Schopler, E., & Reichler, R. J. (1971). Parents as cotherapists in the treatment of psychotic children. *Journal of Autism and Child Schizophrenia, 1,* 87–102.

Schopler, E., Reichler, R. J., & Lansing, M. (1980). *Individualized assessment and treatment for autistic and developmentally disabled children: Vol. 2. Teaching strategies for parents and professionals.* Baltimore: University Park Press.

Sheinkopf, S. J., & Siegel, B. (1998). Home-based behavioral treatment of young children with autism. *Journal of Autism and Developmental Disorders, 28,* 15–23.

Siegel, B., & Zimnitzky, B. (1998). Assessing "alternative" therapies for communication disorders in children with autistic spectrum disorders: Facilitated communication and auditory integration training. *Journal of Speech–Language Pathology and Audiology, 22,* 61–70.

Sigman, M., & Ungerer, J. A. (1984). Cognitive and language skills in autistic, mentally retarded, and normal children. *Developmental Psychology, 20,* 293–302.

Skinner, B. F. (1938). *The behavior of organisms: An experimental analysis.* Oxford, UK: Appleton-Century.

Smith, T. (2001). Discrete trial training in the treatment of autism. *Focus on Autism and Other Developmental Disabilities, 16,* 86–92.

Smith, T., & Antolovich, M. (2000). Parental perceptions of supplemental interventions received by young children with autism in intensive behavior analytic treatment. *Behavior Interventions, 15,* 83–97.

Smith, T., Buch, G. A., & Gamby, T. E., (2000). Parent-directed, intensive early intervention for children with pervasive developmental disorder. *Research in Developmental Disabilities, 21,* 297–309.

Smith, T., Groen, A. D., & Wynn, J. W. (2000). Randomized trial of intensive early intervention for children with pervasive developmental disorder. *American Journal on Mental Retardation, 105,* 269–285.

Smith, T., Groen, A. D., & Wynn, J. W. (2001). Randomized trial of intensive early intervention for children with pervasive developmental disorder [Errata]. *American Journal on Mental Retardation, 106,* 208.

Stoelb, M., Yarnal, R., Miles, J., Takahashi, T. N., Farmer, J. E., & McCathren, R. B. (2004). Predicting responsiveness to treatment of children with autism: A retrospective study of the importance of physical dysmorphology. *Focus on Autism and Other Developmental Disabilities, 19,* 66–77.

Stone, W. L. (1997). Autism in infancy and early childhood. In D. J. Cohen & F. R. Volkmar (Eds.), *Handbook of autism and pervasive developmental disorders.* New York: Wiley.

Task Force on Promotion and Dissemination of Psychological Procedures. (1995). Training in and dissemination of empirically validated psychosocial treatments: Report and recommendations. *Clinical Psychologist, 48,* 3–23.

Tsai, L. (2000). Children with autism spectrum disorder: Medicine today and in the new millennium. *Focus on Autism and Other Developmental Disabilities, 15,* 138–145.

Unis, A., Munson, J. A., Rogers, S., Goldson, E., Osterling, J., Gabriels, R., et al. (2002). A randomized, double-blind, placebo-controlled trial of porcine versus synthetic secretin for reducing symptoms of autism. *Journal of the Academy of Child and Adolescent Psychiatry, 41*(11), 1315–1321.

Volkmar, F. R. (2001). Pharmacological interventions in autism: Theoretical and practical issues. *Journal of Clinical Child Psychology, 30,* 80–87.

Western Psychology Services. (1988). *Childhood Autism Rating Scale (CARS)*. Los Angeles: Author.

Whalen, C., & Schreibman, L. (2003). Joint attention training for children with autism using behavior modification procedures. *Journal of Child Psychology and Psychiatry, 44,* 456–468.

Wolery, M., & Garfinkle, A. N. (2002). Measures in intervention research with young children who have autism. *Journal of Autism and Developmental Disorders, 32,* 463–478.

Woods, J. J., & Wetherby, A. M. (2003). Early identification of and intervention for infants and toddlers who are at risk for autism spectrum disorder. *Language, Speech, and Hearing Services in Schools, 34,* 180–193.

World Health Organization. (1992). *International Classification of Diseases* (10th ed.). Geneva: Author.

Index

417